# Midwifery
# by Ten Teachers

# Midwifery by Ten Teachers

**Debbie Holmes** BSc (Hons), RN, RM, PGCE (HE)
Senior Lecturer in Midwifery,
School of Health,
University of Wolverhampton, UK

**Philip N Baker** BMed Sci, BM, BS, DM, FRCOG
Professor of Maternal and Fetal Health,
Director of the Maternal and Fetal Health Research Centre, and
Consultant Obstetrician at St Mary's Hospital,
The University of Manchester, UK

## Hodder Arnold

A MEMBER OF THE HODDER HEADLINE GROUP

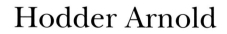

First published in Great Britain in 2006 by
Hodder Arnold, an imprint of Hodder Education and
a member of the Hodder Headline Group,
338 Euston Road, London NW1 3BH

**http://www.hoddereducation.com**

Distributed in the United States of America by
Oxford University Press Inc.,
198 Madison Avenue, New York, NY 10016
Oxford is a registered trademark of Oxford University Press

© 2006 Edward Arnold (Publishers) Ltd

*British Library Cataloguing in Publication Data*
A catalogue record for this book is available from the British Library

*Library of Congress Cataloging-in-Publication Data*
A catalog record for this book is available from the Library of Congress

ISBN-10: 0 340 88879 2
ISBN-13: 978 0 340 88879 7
ISBN-10: 0 340 94159 6   (International Students' Edition, restricted territorial availability)
ISBN-13: 978 0 340 94159 1   (International Students' Edition, restricted territorial availability)

1   2   3   4   5   6   7   8   9   10

Commissioning Editor: Joanna Koster
Project Editor: Clare Patterson
Production Controller: Lindsay Smith
Cover Design: Nichola Smith

Image on chapter openers © Rubberball Productions/Getty Images

Typeset in Minion 9.5/12 pts by Charon Tec Ltd (A Macmillan Company), Chennai, India
www.charontec.com
Printed and bound in India by Replika Press Pvt Ltd

What do you think about this book? Or any other Hodder Arnold title?
Please visit our website: www.hoddereducation.com

# Contents

This book is dedicated to my family, Micheal, Elizabeth, Louise and Robert.

*Debbie Holmes*

# The Ten Teachers

Karen E Bartter MA, RN, RM, ADM, PGCEA
Senior Lecturer in Midwifery, School of Health,
University of Wolverhampton, Walsall

Claire Greig PhD, MSc (Nursing Education), BN, RGN, RM,
ADM, MTD, Neonatal Certificate
Senior Lecturer, Faculty of Health, Life and Social
Sciences, Napier University, Edinburgh

Adela Hamilton MA (Ed), BSc (Hons), Cert Management,
Cert Teaching, RN, RM, E835 Research Design (OU)
Senior Lecturer in Midwifery, Midwifery Department,
City University, London

Debbie Holmes BSc (Hons), RN, RM, PGCE (HE)
Senior Lecturer in Midwifery, School of Health,
University of Wolverhampton, Walsall

Pak Hung RN, RM, ADM, BSc (Hons) Education Studies
(Midwifery), MSc
Senior Lecturer in Midwifery, Supervisor of Midwives,
School of Health, University of Wolverhampton, Walsall

Jayne E Marshall PhD, MA, RN, RM, ADM, PGCEA
Midwife Lecturer/Assistant Director of Midwifery Post
Registration Studies, Faculty of Medicine and
Health Sciences, School of Human Development,
Academic Division of Midwifery,
University of Nottingham, Nottingham

Tracey Mills BSc (Hons), RGN, RM, DPSM, MA
Research Midwife, Maternal and Fetal Health Research
Centre, St Mary's Hospital, Manchester

Sandie Sandbrook RN, RM, ADM, MTD, Cert Ed (FE),
BA (Joint Hons)
Senior Lecturer in Midwifery, School of Health,
University of Wolverhampton, Walsall

Kathy Senessie RGN, RM, BSc (Hons)
Midwife, Maternity Unit, Sandwell and West
Birmingham NHS Hospitals Trust, Birmingham

Gail Williams MSc, BSc, RN, RM, ADM, Cert Ed,
FRSH, ILTM
Director of Midwifery, School of Nursing and
Midwifery Studies, Cardiff University, Cardiff

# Foreword

*Midwifery by Ten Teachers* is a unique collaboration between midwives and their obstetric, nursing and medical colleagues. Within its pages, the reader will find the firm foundations that underpin our art and understanding of normal childbirth set within the context of the complex and competing roles and responsibilities of the midwife of today. Reproductive health with its advances in science and technology is also covered in detail, providing insights into the application and implications of these important developments and consequently the practicalities, problems and provision of both low and high risk maternity care in the twenty-first century.

For many students, practitioners and teachers of midwifery, *Obstetrics by Ten Teachers* will be a familiar textbook, which has over the years provided important insights into obstetric developments and disorders as well as the complication of childbirth and its management. The true value of *Midwifery by Ten Teachers* is to articulate and address such knowledge, insights and understanding and apply it to the work of the midwife in dealing with both normal and abnormal aspects of childbirth within the wider context of the interprofessional team.

An up-to-date and well informed text, *Midwifery by Ten Teachers* provides a broad range of teaching methods and excellent diagrams that make even the most complex of topics accessible. Case histories facilitate engagement with the subject matter and an enquiry based approach helps to contextualize the subject matter in the realities of current midwifery and obstetric practice. Key points enable a ready reference and are important signposts in remembering and recalling the essential elements of the subject matter.

Beginning with the midwife and modern maternity care, the omnipresent social, cultural and political imperatives that make up our global and multicultural society are explored in the context of our history as a profession and some of the more influential reports that have impacted upon our role as midwives.

The early chapters focus on reproductive biology and the physiological changes of pregnancy. Such knowledge is very much a part of current undergraduate education but equally has relevance to the practice of the qualified midwife and will no doubt enhance her ability to better communicate and explain the options and elements of care and assist in the involvement of the woman in decision-making.

The chapters on antenatal care, antenatal imaging and assessment of fetal well-being provide valuable insights into both basic and advanced techniques, including prenatal diagnosis, that seek to facilitate maternal and fetal health; reference to the latest NICE guidelines places such approaches in the context of current recommended practice. This knowledge alongside the chapters on antenatal complications, disorders of placentation, medical complications in pregnancy and perinatal infections are key elements in the continuing role and relevance of the midwife in her care of the mother and family.

Labour and intrapartum care is comprehensively covered in a number of chapters that address the anatomical structures relevant to the process of labour, the management of normal and abnormal labour, induction, comfort in labour as well as instrumental, assisted labour and Caesarean section. The NICE guidelines provide the context of current recommended practice and overall will be a welcome resource for midwives and students alike. Childbirth emergencies are succinctly and well addressed and the continuum of care is covered with chapters on the puerperium, postnatal and neonatal care. The final chapter focuses on the important topic of the law and ethics relating to midwifery practice and rounds off a well structured, relevant, informative and dynamic textbook that will be an asset in the education and development of midwives, and assist them in the enhancement and advancement of their professional knowledge and skills.

*Midwifery by Ten Teachers* is a worthwhile read; it provides knowledge at the graduate level and beyond, and will without doubt make a valuable contribution to the increasingly diverse roles and opportunities that are open to midwives. Its relevance to current midwifery practice and the role of the midwife is one of its many strengths but above all, its engagement with the realities of the midwife's work, in the context of normal and abnormal childbirth, interprofessional working, best practice and evidence based care is likely to make this a well used resource in the pursuit of excellence, understanding and the support of women and their families during pregnancy and childbirth.

*Professor Paul Lewis*
*Academic Head of Midwifery & Child Health*
*Bournemouth University*

# Preface

*Midwifery by Ten Teachers* has evolved from an established and respected text designed for medical students now entitled *Obstetrics by Ten Teachers*, but which when first published in 1917 was known as *Midwifery by Ten Teachers*. The idea for a contemporary midwifery version was suggested by Professor Philip Baker (editor of the 18th edition of *Obstetrics by Ten Teachers*) and supported by myself.

*Obstetrics by Ten Teachers* has been used by many midwives and student midwives to support study and clinical practice. A review of the content indicated that the book was accessed for obstetric information and associated management, but overall the text was rather too medically orientated for the midwifery profession and lacked reference to the role of the midwife.

*Midwifery by Ten Teachers* therefore aims to provide the in-depth knowledge and expertise of *Obstetrics by Ten Teachers* but emphasises the specific role of the midwife in relation to recognition and management of normal and abnormal aspects of childbearing. The reader is taken through the latest best practice guidelines and directed to further reading where appropriate. The contributors have combined their experience and knowledge to provide chapters to support pre- and post-registration midwifery studies. The volume is designed to complement the general midwifery texts available.

The contributors were recruited as enthusiastic experts in midwifery. The original philosophy was based upon individual midwife contributions and has resulted in a unique collection of chapters by teachers of repute. A huge debt is owed to the individuals who make up the team of contributors all of whom are busy clinicians and academics. Many of the midwives were also pursuing their own studies and research during this time.

*Debbie Holmes, June 2006*

# Acknowledgements

*Midwifery by Ten Teachers* is indebted to *Obstetrics by Ten Teachers*. In particular, Debbie Holmes and the publishers would like to thank Philip N Baker, editor of the 18th edition of the obstetrics volume in addition to being co-editor of this midwifery title, and the contributors to the 18th edition who collectively have supported the concept throughout its development and have kindly allowed their material to be reworked for a midwifery audience:

Ian Johnson

Griffith Jones

Lucy Kean

Louise Kenny

Gary Mires

Alec McEwan

Catherine Nelson-Piercy

Janet Rennie

Abdul Sultan

Phillip Hay

In addition, the editors and the publishers would like to extend their thanks to the editors of and contributors to the 17th edition of *Obstetrics by Ten Teachers* who have not been actively involved in the preparation of this adaptation, but whose input in this earlier edition led to the introduction of many of the concepts and features reflected here:

Stuart Campbell, Christoph Lees, James Drife, William Dunlop, Jason Gardosi, Donald Gibb, J.G. Grudzinskas, Kevin Harrington, Des Holden, Richard Johanson, Kypros Nicolaides, Margaret R. Oates, Michael Robson, Neil Sebire, E. Malcolm Symonds, Basky Thilaganathan, J. Guy Thorpe-Beeston.

With thanks to Gillian Wainscott for her help with Chapter 18.

Debbie Holmes would also like to thank the midwifery teachers with whom she works for the support and encouragement that has enabled her to undertake the editing.

# Abbreviations and conventions

Throughout the book, the midwife has been referred to as 'she', and the neonate as 'he'.

Health visitors are now known as 'specialist community public health nurses'. Throughout the book the term 'health visitors' is used. NICE is now known as 'National Institute for Health and Clinical Excellence'. Throughout the book the abbreviation 'NICE' is used.

| | | | |
|---|---|---|---|
| AC | abdominal circumference | CVS | chorion villi sampling |
| ACE | angiotensin-converting enzyme | CW | continuous wave (Doppler) |
| ACTH | adrenocorticotrophic hormone | DCDA | dichorionic diamniotic |
| AED | antiepileptic drug | DHEA | dihydroepiandrosterone |
| AF | amniotic fluid | DIC | disseminated intravascular coagulation |
| AFI | amniotic fluid index | DVT | deep vein thrombosis |
| AFP | alpha-fetoprotein | DOH | Department of Health |
| AFV | amniotic fluid volume | ECC | external cephalic version |
| AIDS | acquired immunodeficiency syndrome | ECG | electrocardiogram/electrocardiography |
| ALT | alanine aminotransferease | EDD | expected date of delivery |
| AP | antero–posterior | EEG | electroencephalogram |
| APH | antepartum haemorrhage | EFW | estimate of fetal/birth weight |
| APS | antiphospholipid syndrome | ELISA | enzyme-linked immunosorbent assay |
| APTT | activated partial thromboplastin time | EPDS | Edinburgh Postnatal Depression Scale |
| ARM | artificial rupture of membranes | ERPC | evacuation of retained products of conception |
| AST | aspartate aminotransferase | | |
| AT | antithrombin | FDP | fibrin degradation product |
| BAPM | British Association of Perinatal Medicine | FEV1 | forced expiratory volume in one second |
| BCG | bacille Calmette–Guérin | fFN | fetal fibronectin |
| BMI | body mass index | FFO | failed forceps outside |
| BP | blood pressure | FFP | fresh-frozen plasma |
| BPD | biparietal diameter | FISH | fluorescence *in-situ* hybridization |
| bpm | beats per minute | FL | femur length |
| BV | bacterial vaginosis | FSH | follicle-stimulating hormone |
| CBG | cortisol-binding globulin | GBS | group B streptococcus |
| CEMACH | Confidential Enquiry into Maternal and Child Health | GGT | gamma glutamyl transpeptidase |
| | | GI | gastrointestinal |
| CEMD | Confidential Enquiry into Maternal Deaths | GnRH | gonadotrophin-releasing hormone |
| | | GP | general practitioner |
| CESDI | Confidential Enquiry into Stillbirths and Deaths in Infancy | GPI | general paresis of the insane |
| | | Hb | haemoglobin |
| CHD | congenital heart defect | HbA1c | glycosylated haemoglobin |
| CIN | cervical intraepithelial neoplasia | HbF | fetal haemoglobin |
| CMV | cytomegalovirus | HC | head circumference |
| CNS | central nervous system | hCG | human chorionic gonadotrophin |
| CPD | cephalopelvic disproportion | HELLP | haemolysis, elevated liver enzymes and low platelets (syndrome) |
| CRF | corticotrophin-releasing factor | | |
| CRL | crown–rump length | hGH | human growth hormone |
| CS | Caesarean section | HIE | hypoxic ischaemic encephalopathy |
| CSF | cerebrospinal fluid | HIV | human immunodeficiency virus |
| CT | computerized tomography | HPA | hypothalamic–pituitary–adrenal axis |
| CTG | cardiotocography | hPL | human placental lactogen |
| CVA | cerebrovascular accident | HPV | human papilloma virus |
| CVP | central venous pressure | HSV | herpes simplex virus |

| | | | |
|---|---|---|---|
| ICP | intrahepatic cholestasis of pregnancy | PEFR | peak expiratory flow rate |
| IDDM | insulin-dependent diabetes mellitus | PGD | pre-implantation genetic diagnosis |
| Ig | immunoglobulin | PGE | prostaglandin E |
| IGF | insulin-like growth factor | PI | pulsatility index |
| IL | interleukin | PID | pelvic inflammatory disease |
| IM | intramuscular | PIH | pregnancy-induced hypertension |
| IOL | induction of labour | PND | postnatal depression |
| ISSHP | International Society for the Study of Hypertension in Pregnancy | PPH | postpartum haemorrhage |
| ITP | autoimmune thrombocytopenic purpura | PPROM | preterm prelabour rupture of the membranes |
| IUGR | intrauterine growth restriction | PT | prothrombin time |
| IV | intravenous | PTL | preterm labour |
| IVF | *in-vitro* fertilization | PTU | propylthiouracil |
| KCT | kaolin cephalin time | PW | pulsed wave (Doppler) |
| LH | luteinizing hormone | RCOG | Royal College of Obstetricians and Gynaecologists |
| LIF | leukaemia inhibitory factor | RCM | Royal College of Midwives |
| LMP | last menstrual period | RDS | respiratory distress syndrome |
| MCDA | monochorionic diamniotic (twins) | REM | rapid eye movement |
| MCMA | monochorionic monoamniotic (twins) | RI | resistance index |
| MCV | mean corpuscular volume | SANDS | Stillbirth and Neonatal Death Society |
| MMR | measles, mumps, rubella (vaccine) | SDD | surfactant deficiency disease |
| MRI | magnetic resonance imaging | SFH | symphysis–fundal height |
| MSLC | maternity services liaison committee | SGA | small for gestational age |
| MSSU | midstream specimen of urine | SIGN | Scottish Intercollegiate Guidelines Network |
| NAS | neonatal abstinence syndrome | | |
| NCT | National Childbirth Trust | SLE | systemic lupus erythematosus |
| NHS | National Health Service | SPD | symphysis pubis dysfunction |
| NICE | National Institute for Health and Clinical Excellence | SROM | spontaneous rupture of the membranes |
| | | SSRIs | selective serotonin reuptake inhibitors |
| NIDDM | non-insulin dependent diabetes mellitus | TB | tuberculosis |
| NMC | Nursing and Midwifery Council | TED | thromboembolic (stockings) |
| NNU | neonatal unit | TPN | total parenteral nutrition |
| NSAIDs | non-steroidal anti-inflammatory drugs | TRH | thyrotrophin-releasing hormone |
| NSF | National Service Framework | TSH | thyroid-stimulating hormone |
| NT | nuchal translucency | TTTS | twin-to-twin transfusion syndrome |
| NTD | neural tube defect | uE3 | unconjugated oestriol |
| OA | occipitoanterior | UKCC | United Kingdom Central Council for Nursing, Midwifery and Health Visiting (superseded by NMC) |
| OP | occipitoposterior | | |
| OT | occipitotransverse | | |
| PAPP-A | pregnancy-associated plasma protein | USS | ultrasound scan |
| PCA | patient-controlled subcutaneous anaesthesia | VKDB | vitamin K deficiency bleeding |
| | | VMA | vanillylmandelic acid |
| PCR | polymerase chain reaction | VZIG | varicella zoster immune globulin |
| PDA | patent ductus arteriosus | WHO | World Health Organisation |
| PE | pulmonary embolus/embolism | WMPI | West Midlands Perinatal Institute |

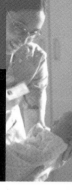

Chapter 1

# The midwife and modern maternity care

## OVERVIEW

The midwife is the expert in normal midwifery care and, as such, should be the lead professional for women identified as low risk for pregnancy and childbirth. However, midwives do not work in isolation, and not all women experience normal pregnancy and childbirth. The midwife works collaboratively with other health professionals, including obstetricians, to provide high-quality, safe, effective care to women who present with obstetric or medical complications. Whatever her role, the midwife also works within a statutory framework, more often than not employed by a National Health Service (NHS) Trust; thus she works with an institution's policies, which include local and national guidelines. The work of the midwife is also subject to social context, the culture of the populations with which she works, and the Government and social norms of the time. This chapter aims to outline some of the political changes that have affected the role of the midwife in maternity care and concludes with issues influencing current practice.

## A 'snapshot' in the history of midwifery

Born in AD23 and author of *Historia naturalis*, Plinius Secundus described the midwife as 'obstetrix' and the role and responsibilities as 'obstetrica' (Hoblyn 1835). In Greek and Roman times, midwives were autonomous practitioners providing care to women during their reproductive cycles. In ancient Egypt, midwives taught the art of obstetrics to physicians (Ghalioungui 1963) at a time when medicine was the business of physicians, and childbearing and gynaecology the business of women and midwives. In ancient Greece, midwives attended normal labour,

and abnormal labour was for the attention of *both* the midwife and physician – collaborative working in ancient times, with both professionals working together for the safety of mother and baby. Most maternity care until the beginning of the twentieth century continued to be provided by midwives.

## Political changes affecting the role of the midwife

In the mid-1870s, the majority of births took place in the home and were attended by midwives, who were very much a part of the community (Donnison 1988).

In 1902, the first Midwives Act was passed and midwifery was recognized as a profession. Although this was a positive change for the professional status of midwives, the ensuing years saw challenges for them as maternal and child health became political issues. In 1929, one of the first Government documents concerning maternal and child health stated a minimum standard for antenatal care that was very prescriptive in its recommendations. Until recently, this was still practised in many regions, despite the lack of research to show that this was effective.

Many Acts have been passed to legislate and control practice. The introduction of the National Health Service Act of 1946 provided for maternity services to be available to all without cost. As part of these arrangements, a specified fee was paid to the general practitioner (GP) depending on whether he or she was on the obstetric list.

Antenatal care became perceived as beneficial, acceptable and available for all. This was reinforced by the finding that the perinatal death rate seemed to be inversely proportional to the number of antenatal visits. In 1963, the first perinatal mortality study showed that the perinatal mortality rate was lowest for those women attending between 10 and 24 times in pregnancy, but failed to take into account poor health and poor education as reasons for decreased visits and increased mortality. However, antenatal care became established, and with increased professional contact came the drive to continue to improve outcomes with an emphasis on mortality (maternal and perinatal), without always establishing the need for or safety of all procedures or interventions for all women.

Even at this time, the apportioning of antenatal care to different professionals was causing problems with little communication between hospital, midwives and GPs. It was not until the late 1950s that the idea of the cooperation card was devised. This allowed a continuous record to be held by the mother and improved communication between professionals, similar to the more complex hand-held records of today.

The ability to see into the pregnant uterus in 1958 with ultrasound brought with it a revolution in antenatal care. This new intervention became quickly established and is now so much part of current antenatal care that the fact that its use in improving the outcome for women at low risk for pregnancy and childbirth was never proven has been little questioned.

The move towards hospital confinement began in the early 1950s. At this time, there simply were not the facilities to allow hospital confinement for all women, and one in three were planned home deliveries. The Cranbrook Report in 1959 recommended sufficient hospital maternity beds for 70 per cent of all confinements to take place in hospital and the subsequent Peel Report (Maternity Advisory Committee 1970) recommended a bed available for every woman to deliver in hospital if she so wished. Midwives continued to care for women and, as the settings for care moved from community to institutions, the midwives followed the women. Midwives were now under the direction of obstetricians, who were perceived to be the experts, and only those midwives who practised independently were able to retain true autonomy.

The trend toward hospital confinement was not only led by obstetricians. Women themselves were pushing at least to be allowed the choice to deliver in hospital. By 1972, only one in ten deliveries were planned for home, and the publication of the Short Report (House of Commons 1980) led to further centralization of hospital confinement. It made a number of recommendations amongst which were the following.

- An increasing number of patients should be delivered in large units; selection of patients should be improved for smaller consultant units and isolated GP units; home deliveries should be phased out further.
- It should be mandatory that all pregnant women should be seen at least twice by a consultant obstetrician – preferably as soon as possible after the first visit to the GP in early pregnancy and again in late pregnancy.

This report led to a policy of increasing centralization of units for delivery and consequently care. Thus, home deliveries became infrequent events with most regions currently reporting less that 2 per cent, the majority of these being unplanned.

The gradual decline in maternal and perinatal mortality was thought to be due in greater part to the medicalization of childbirth and hospital births, although proof for this was lacking. Indeed, the decline in perinatal mortality was least in those years when hospitalization increased the most. As other new technologies became available, such as continuous fetal monitoring and the ability to induce labour, a change in practice began to establish these as the norm for most women. In England and Wales between 1966 and 1974, the induction rate rose from 12.7 to 38.9 per cent. The fact that these new technologies had not undergone thorough trials of benefit prior to their introduction meant that benefit to the whole population of women was never established.

During the 1980s, with increasing consumer awareness, the unquestioning acceptance of unproven technologies was challenged. Midwives and women, supported by groups such as the National Childbirth Trust (NCT), began to question not only the need for any intervention but also even the need to come to the hospital at all. The professional bodies also began to question the effectiveness of antenatal care. The need to attend hospital as often as was occurring was debated and conclusions drawn that the frequency, timing and effectiveness of antenatal visits was a form of care with an unknown effect, which therefore required further evaluation.

In the early 1990s, the whole question of maternity care entered the political arena once again. The Expert Maternity Committee (House of Commons 1992) identified that 72 per cent of women would have liked an alternative to obstetric-led care in hospital and 44 per cent of these women would have preferred a home birth. This survey informed the *Changing childbirth* report (Department of Health 1993).

The Winterton Committee heard evidence from those involved in maternity care on all sides:

> *The Committee was stimulated into conducting the enquiry by its awareness of the fact that it was over a decade since the last major enquiry into maternity services by the then Social Services Committee, and by hearing many voices saying that all was not well with the maternity services and that women had needs that were not being met (House of Commons Select Committee 1992)*

The report culminated in a list of 98 conclusions and recommendations, the most important of which were as follows:

- Given the absence of conclusive evidence, it is no longer acceptable that the pattern of maternity care provision should be driven by presumptions about the applicability of a medical model of care based on unproven assertions.
- We conclude that there is a strong desire among women for the provision of continuity of care and carer throughout pregnancy and childbirth, and that the majority of them regard midwives as the group best placed and equipped to provide this.
- We are persuaded that the present imposition of a rigid pattern of frequent antenatal visits is not

grounded in any good scientific base and that there is no evidence that such a pattern is medically necessary.… There is widespread agreement that this requires a more flexible system, which is based in the community, not in the hospital. The present system of shared care between the hospital and the community should, by and large, be abandoned. Hospitals are not the appropriate place to care for healthy women.

## Changing childbirth

The Government set up an expert committee to review policy on maternity care and to make recommendations. This committee produced the document *Changing childbirth* (Department of Health 1993). This document essentially provided purchasers and providers with a number of action points aiming to improve choice, information and continuity for all women. It outlined a number of indicators of success to be achieved within 5 years:

- the carriage of hand-held notes by women;
- midwifery-led care in 30 per cent of pregnancies;
- a known midwife at delivery in 75 per cent of cases;
- a reduction in the number of antenatal visits for low-risk mothers.

Sadly, those targets that required significant financial input, such as the provision of a known midwife at 75 per cent of deliveries, have never been met. Nevertheless, this landmark report did provide a new impetus to examine the provision of maternity care in the UK and enshrine choice as a concept in maternity care. Since the publication of *Changing childbirth*, a number of new initiatives and research have occurred.

## First class delivery

In 1997, the Audit Commission for Local Health Authorities and the National Health Service in England and Wales published the document *First class delivery: improving maternity services in England and Wales*. This reviewed the provision of maternity care in England and Wales and, very importantly, sent questionnaires to 3570 mothers. The recommendations of this document are as follows.

- Trusts should: (a) ensure clinicians have access to good-quality research, and encourage development of guidelines and protocols; and (b) improve the quality of written information, especially for antenatal screening and testing.

- Commissioners should: (a) actively involve women in maternity services planning; and (b) take local users' views into account as well as cost.

Midwives and women have subsequently worked towards focusing upon normality for women considered 'low risk'. Midwifery-led units and more recently birth centres have been developed to assist in the provision of care. This has gone someway to addressing some aspects of medicalization and has offered women more choice.

## National Institute for Clinical Excellence

More recently, attention has been paid to differences in standards of health care across the UK. The National Institute for Clinical Excellence (NICE) has begun to look at maternity care and has published three important guidelines. The first on fetal monitoring in labour was published in May 2001 and the second on induction of labour soon afterwards in June 2001. The third guideline on antenatal care was launched in October 2003, producing guidelines for antenatal care based on current bodies of research and best practice.

This was the first time antenatal care had been examined in detail since the original recommendations of the 1929 committee. This document should standardize the provision of care across the UK. Postnatal care guidelines are also in the process of development and will be published in 2006, hopefully addressing an area of maternity care that has received little attention as the 'Cinderella of the service'. There is a legal requirement for Trusts to implement the recommendations in these guidelines. These guidelines can be seen on the NICE web site (www.NICE.org.uk).

## National Service Framework

The *National Service Framework* (NSF) *for children, young people and maternity services* establishes clear standards for promoting the health and well-being of children, young people and mothers, and for providing high-quality services that meet their needs (Department for Education and Skills, Department of Health

2004: 5). To enable the delivery of the standards set out in the framework, new roles are emerging within maternity services. Maternity support workers are being appointed to provide clinical and administrative support for midwives. These roles may well provide a pathway for some individuals wishing to pursue a career in midwifery. New advocate and link workers will be required to provide support and care for vunerable or disadvantaged women and their families. Consultant and specialist midwives posts will continue to be developed to address issues such as mental health, domestic violence, sexual health, teenage pregnancy services and substance misuse.

## Confidential enquiries and audit

The Royal College of Obstetricians and Gynaecologists (RCOG) coordinates a national audit in conjunction with other bodies such as the Royal Colleges of Midwives, Paediatricians and Anaesthetists, and the NCT. The most recent audit, published by the RCOG Clinical Effectiveness Support Unit (2001), entitled *The national sentinel Caesarean section audit report*, examined Caesarean sections across the UK. The audit came about as a result of increasing concern regarding the increasing Caesarean section rate. This has provided interesting data for the trends in Caesarean section across the UK.

*The Confidential Enquiry into Maternal and Child Health* (CEMACH; Lewis and Drife 2004) is referenced by the individual contributors in their specific chapters within this text. When a woman dies during or within a year following pregnancy, the Director of Public Health Medicine sends an enquiry form to the midwives, health visitors, obstetricians, general practitioners and any other staff involved in her care. The form requests full information about the case. The completed form is then sent to regional assessors in obstetrics, midwifery, anaesthesia (if appropriate) and pathology. They add their comments and the form is sent to the Chief Medical Officer. It is made anonymous then passed to central assessors of the same disciplines to assess the causes of death and decide whether any aspects of the care were substandard. Every 3 years a national report is published, which collates all the cases, draws attention to areas of 'substandard care' and makes recommendations. The report excludes any details that might allow identification of individual cases.

Summaries from the latest triennial report have identified issues specifically pertinent to midwifery practice, areas where midwives could have influence on care and outcomes. Many risk factors for maternal death are related to the lifestyles of the populations for whom the midwife cares.

- Social exclusion remains a problem for vulnerable groups of women, as does poverty.
- Ethnicity was an important factor and women from other ethnic groups were, on average, three times more likely to die than White women.
- Poor attendance and late booking were features for 20 per cent of the women who died; midwives must find rigorous procedures for following up women who miss appointments.
- A total of 35 per cent of all the women who died were obese, a twenty-first century health issue for the population in general.
- Domestic violence was disclosed by 14 per cent of all the women who died. As this is under-reported in general, this issue could have been influential in more cases.
- A total of 8 per cent of all women who died were substance misusers.
- A continual problem with interprofessional and interagency communication was evident.

A summary of the recommendations in relation to midwifery practice are as follows:

- antenatal guideline recommendations should be incorporated into practice;
- missed appointments/accessible services should be followed up actively;
- women with complex pregnancies should receive collaborative care with the advocacy of a known midwife;
- flexible programmes of care, including early identification of obstetric, medical, psychological or social needs and involvement of specialist care should be adopted;
- professional interpereters should be used to communicate with non-English-speaking mothers.

Perinatal death is about one hundred times more common than maternal death. Perinatal mortality rates, therefore, often seem more relevant to day-to-day practice and, because of the larger numbers of cases, they perhaps give a clearer picture of the problems that may be encountered. However, analysis of individual cases at a national level is more difficult because of the large numbers. As with maternal mortality data, the diagnosis of death is unequivocal. Comparison between countries is often difficult as definitions of the dividing line between miscarriage and stillbirth vary. Until 2003, the reports were written and published by the Confidential Enquiry into Stillbirths and Deaths in Infancy (CESDI). CEMACH has now taken over this role.

## Clinical Negligence Scheme for Trusts

Obstetrics is the highest litigation risk area in the NHS. It is estimated that the outstanding potential obstetric litigation bill is of the order of £200 million. As individual Trusts cannot hope to meet the cost of huge settlements, sometimes running into millions of pounds, an insurance scheme was established. The Clinical Negligence Scheme for Trusts (CNST) was established by the NHS Executive in 1994 'to provide a means for Trusts to fund the costs of clinical negligence litigation and to encourage and support effective management of claims and risk'. The insurance premium is discounted by 10 per cent for a level 1 Trust, 20 per cent for level 2 and 30 per cent for level 3. In 2003, it was decided to assess obstetrics separately, as many Trusts were failing on the obstetric standards only. The standards set by CNST are stringent. They cover the following:

- organization;
- learning from experience;
- communication;
- clinical care;
- documentation and note keeping;
- clinical governance strategy;
- staffing levels.

Trusts are assessed at least every 2 years, but they can bring forward an assessment if they believe improvements have been made, as the financial implications of higher levels of grading are great. This is the first time that improvements in maternity care have been linked to financial incentive, and measurable improvements in many units have been brought about as managers realize the importance of improving standards of care.

## Consumer groups

As well as providing support and advice for women, often at times of great need, they also allow women to have a louder voice in the planning and provision of maternity care. National consumer groups such as the NCT have representatives on many influential panels, such as the National Screening Committee and RCOG working groups. At a local level, each Trust should have a maternity services liaison committee (MSLC). When these committees work well, they can provide essential consumer input into service delivery at a local level. Consumers should make up at least one-third of the membership of the MSLCs. The influence of consumer groups can be huge. The recommendation that all women should have the right to deliver in hospital was essentially consumer led. Interestingly, it was this drive that led to the demise of many local units, centralization of obstetric services and a huge reduction in the numbers of home deliveries, something that consumer groups are now trying to reverse.

Choice is now being sought by consumers in a way never experienced before. *The national sentinel Caesarean section audit* showed that maternal choice, as a reason for Caesarean section, is becoming increasingly common, a move driven at least in part by high-profile women choosing not to labour with their first baby. Consumer groups will need to lead the way in deciding how far choice should be balanced against the financial constraints of a health service that is free at the point of care.

## Midwifery education

Student midwives in the UK are educated to at least diploma level and in many institutions to graduate level, with an equal importance given to theory and practice. Theory is delivered within higher education institutions and practice experience gained within NHS Trusts. Postregistration study is also delivered at these academic levels, and increasingly midwives are undertaking masters/doctorate programmes and are actively involved in undertaking research. Midwifery education, quite rightly continues to promote normality and enthuse the preregistration student about the ability of women to birth their own babies. Students increasingly find difficulty with this philosophy, when in practice there often remains a dependence upon technology and intervention. Students need to be prepared for working within a dichotomous environment where women

may require obstetric intervention for complications in pregnancy and childbirth, and where women may opt for the support of technology or intervention by choice.

Training must remain focused on normality and upon the promotion of good health, both physical and psychological. The skills to detect and refer complex cases are paramount to ensure that the correct plan of care is provided for the individual woman. Training must include the skills to assess and plan care, to cope with emergencies and to care for women who require high-dependency care.

Whether student midwives are qualified nurses or direct entry, they must be educated to recognize subtle signs and symptoms that may be suggestive of changes in women's health that could lead to morbidity or mortality. The triennial report (Lewis and Drife 2004) identified issues surrounding the skills for providing routine postoperative care that may have led to delayed treatment, and it is essential that this is addressed within education.

## Conclusion

The aim of this text is not to highlight and argue the differences between models of care, but to provide an appreciation of the roles and expertise of individual practitioners and promote safe, effective, quality care for women and their families. Midwives must work closely with other professionals in the field of maternity care and women must be provided with the most appropriate care from the most appropriate professional. The latest triennial report identified that some women who died were assigned wrongly to midwifery-led care; assessment must be accurate and appropriate. Conversely, women are also exposed to technology and intervention when there is no clear clinical need and this is just as inappropriate, as it can lead to unnecessary intervention. The development of care pathways (NSF 2004), and the design of maternity services to meet the needs of individual women with an emphasis on maternity-led care can only serve to improve the health of women and their babies. The context of midwifery care is fluid, and midwifery education and professional development must address the issues arising from political, cultural and social change. Midwives must strive to be culturally competent in their professional role.

## 🔑 Key Points

- Midwives are the experts in providing care for 'low-risk' women.
- Maternity care will continue to be on the political agenda.
- Midwives need to be part of service design to ensure women's changing needs are met.
- Midwives should adopt a lifelong learning approach in order to challenge existing practices (see Chapter 20).
- There is increasing public interest in the results of national audits, such as CEMACH and the national sentinel Caesarean section audit.

- The need for Trusts to reduce insurance costs is leading to increased standards of care across the UK.
- National guidelines now cover almost all aspects of maternity care and should lead to standardization of care across the UK.
- Preregistration and postregistration training must address recommendations from CEMACH.
- Midwives have an individual responsibility to ensure they have the knowledge and skills to perform their role.

## References

Audit Commission for Local Health Authorities and the National Health Service in England and Wales. *First class delivery: improving maternity services in England and Wales.* London: HMSO, 1997.

Department for Education and Skills, Department of Health. *National Service Framework for children, young people, and maternity services.* London: HMSO, 2004.

Department of Health. *Changing childbirth.* Report of the Expert Maternity Group. London: HMSO, 1993.

Donnison J. *Midwives and medical men: a history of the struggle for the control of childbirth.* London: Historical Publications, 1988.

Ghalioungui P. *Magic and medical science in ancient Eygpt.* London: Hodder & Stoughton, 1963.

House of Commons. *Perinatal and neonatal mortality.* Second report from the Social Services Committee (Chairwoman R. Short). London: HMSO, 1980.

House of Commons. *Maternity services.* Second report from the Health Committee (Chairman N. Winterton). London: HMSO, 1992.

Lewis G, Drife J (eds). *Confidential Enquiry into Maternal and Child Health; why mothers die 2000–2002.* Sixth report of the confidential enquiries into maternal deaths in the UK. London: RCOG Press, 2004.

Maternity Advisory Committee. *Domiciliary and maternity bed needs* (Chairman: Sir John Peel). HMSO: London, 1970.

Royal College of Obstetricians and Gynaecologists Clinical Effectiveness Support Unit. *The national sentinel Caesarean section audit report.* London: RCOG Press, 2001.

## Key additional reading

CNST Standards for Maternity Services: available online at www.nhsla.com

Cochrane Library (available online at www.nelh.nhs.uk).

Raynor M, Marshall J, Sullivan A (eds). *Decision making in midwifery practice.* London: Churchill Livingstone, 2005.

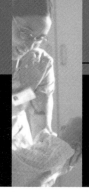

# Conception, implantation and embryology

## OVERVIEW

Many people do not think about whether they are fertile or not. They expect that they will be able to have children at some stage in their lives, if they so wish this to happen. In reality, conception is not always an easy or straightforward process. Knowledge of the fundamental processes involved in human conception, implantation and embryology are vital components in understanding the basic physiology and pathology that surround fertility, infertility, miscarriage, genetic disorders, abnormalities of fetal growth and placental function and, indeed, even other conditions and diseases that may occur in later life.

## Somatic and germ cells

The human body has two types of cells, somatic cells and highly specialized germ cells. The somatic cells of the human body are all diploid cells. This means that each cell contains two copies of each of the chromosomes, one set from the mother and the other from the father. The cells thus contain 22 pairs of chromosomes and two sex chromosomes – X and X for a female, and X and Y for a male. The two copies of each chromosome are described as being homologous.

When somatic cells need to be produced, to replace worn out cells, for example, they duplicate their DNA and then divide to form two exact copies or sister cells, in a process called mitosis. Each sister cell contains exactly the same full amount of chromosomes as all the other somatic, i.e. diploid, cells.

Unlike somatic cells, the mature germ cells, or gametes, are haploid: they have only one copy of each chromosome, and either an X or a Y chromosome. The 23 chromosomes in the germ cell form a pronucleus. Following fertilization, fusion of the pronuclei from the sperm and the ovum re-establish diploidy, and thus result in a somatic cell with a full complement of 46 chromosomes.

## Mitosis and meiosis

Gametogenesis is the process of the formation and development of the gametes or germ cells, through the processes of mitosis and meiosis. It concludes with a reduction of the chromosome number and a change in the shape of the cell.

Mitosis is DNA replication and cell division to provide two exact copies, or daughter cells, of the parent cell, and these copies are complete in every way with the same chromosome complement as the parent cell. Meiosis, on the other hand, is cell division with a reduction of the genetic material in the resulting daughter cells.

Both mitosis and meiosis begin with diploid cells. However, whilst the product of mitosis is two diploid daughter cells, a meiotic division leads to haploid daughter cells. (A diagram comparing mitotic and meiotic divisions is shown in Figure 2.1).

Unlike mitosis, cell division occurs twice in meiosis. At the end of division 1, two daughter cells are produced. During the second division, no DNA replication occurs. Thus, 23 double-stranded chromosomes lined up in metaphase will separate as single-stranded chromosomes to form the nucleus of each haploid daughter cell.

Mitotic cell divisions are important for the exact replication of cells and their genetic material. Meiosis, on the other hand, provides for consistency of the chromosome number from generation to generation, but also provides a random assortment of maternal and paternal chromosomes amongst the gametes, thus ensuring new combinations of genetic material in all the offspring.

## Clinical importance

During the formation of haploid cells by meiotic division, maldistribution of chromosomes may occur. One of each pair of chromosomes should go to each gamete produced. Fertilization then leads to a restored complement of 46 (or 23 pairs) of chromosomes. If an error occurs and both chromosomes in a pair pass to the same daughter cell, two abnormal cells are produced, one with a chromosome complement of 24 and the other 22. Fertilization with a normal haploid cell (with its 23 chromosomes) will then lead to cells with chromosome complements of either 47 or 45.

This error can occur with any chromosome pair. In the majority of such cases, the pregnancy will fail at an early stage (and may even not have been recognized to have occurred). In recognized cases of spontaneous abortion (miscarriage), around 50 per cent can be demonstrated to have had a chromosomal abnormality. Any continuing pregnancy where there is one too many of any chromosome is known as a trisomy. Continuing pregnancy with a trisomy is estimated to occur in one in 200 cases, although many of these will not reach viability (legal viability is the 24th week of pregnancy).

An extra chromosome 21 produces Down's syndrome, the commonest recorded survivable trisomy. Approximately 20 per cent of trisomy 21 cases survive to term if no therapeutic termination of pregnancy is performed. Triple sex chromosomes (44XXX – girl, or 44XXY – boy), are also survivable trisomies, but their exact incidence is not known as there are few external characteristics that denote these conditions. With trisomy 18 (Edward's syndrome) only 4 per cent are likely to survive to term and similarly, in trisomy 13 (Patau's syndrome), there are multiple abnormalities and the prognosis is poor. Monosomies – where there is one chromosome missing, such as in Turner's syndrome (44X and no second sex chromosome) – are less common, occurring in approximately 1 in 8000 live births.

More rarely, there is chromosome breakage, with part of a chromosome being lost, or attaching to another chromosome (translocation). If the transfer of material is between a single pair of chromosomes, then both daughter cells will be abnormal; one will have too much material and the other too little. If the transfer is between unpaired chromosomes, then it is possible for the correct complement to end up in the same haploid cell. If both affected chromosomes go to the same daughter cell, the total genetic complement will be present and this is known as a balanced translocation. Around 1 in 500 'normal' people have a balanced translocation. Formation of their own haploid spermatozoa or oocyte may lead to separation of the two balanced chromosomes. Subsequent fertilization leads to a lack or excess of genetic material in the embryo (and thus an unbalanced translocation), and usually results in a spontaneous abortion of the pregnancy.

Single-gene mutations are base alterations at a single point in the DNA molecule and occur during DNA replication. They are common and most will have no obvious effect, although some are known to cause disease, for instance sickle cell disease. These mutations will be inherited once they have occurred, although the phenotypic effect will depend upon dominance and penetrance. If an abnormal gene is dominant, only one copy is required to reveal the

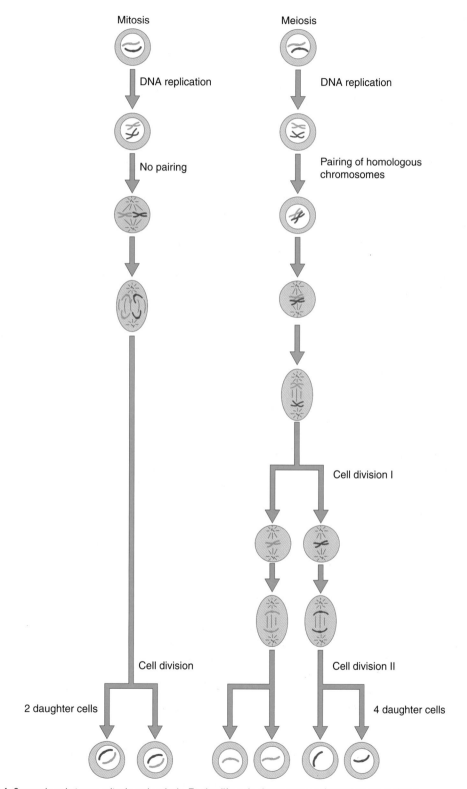

**Figure 2.1** Comparison between mitosis and meiosis. To simplify, only chromosome pair number one is shown.

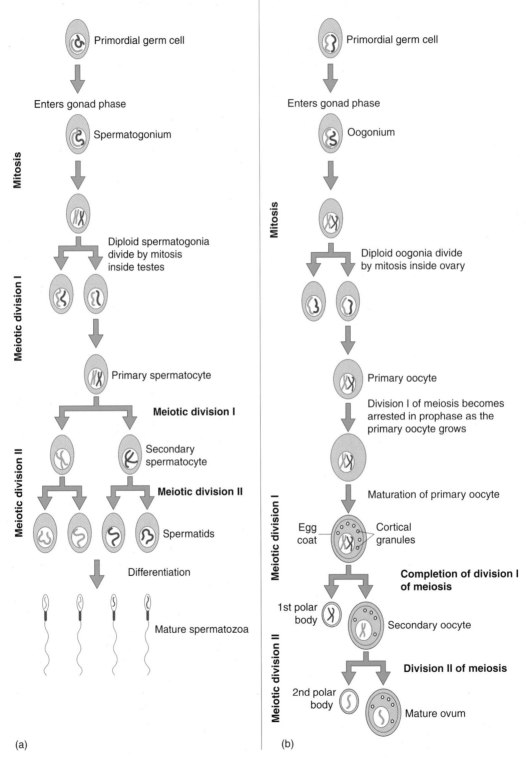

**Figure 2.2** Various stages of spermatogenesis (a) and oogenesis (b). Note that one spermatogonium divides into four haploid mature spermotazoa, whereas one oogonium produces only one haploid mature ovum. The polar bodies eventually degenerate. To simplify, only chromosome pair number one is shown.

disease. If the normal gene is dominant, and so the abnormal one is recessive, both chromosomes need to have the mutation for the gene to be expressed. Achondroplasia is an example of a disease caused by a dominant mutation, and cystic fibrosis is one caused by a recessive mutation. The mutant gene may be on the X chromosome, in which case it will be the only gene available in a male, and thus be dominant and present, but may act as a recessive trait in the female when a second normal X chromosome is present, such as in haemophilia. Other genetic and environmental factors may affect the penetrance of a gene, that is, the actual effect it has on the individual's phenotype, and whether that affected gene acts as recessive or dominant.

## Spermatogenesis

Spermatogenesis is the total process in the production of mature sperm. It occurs in the seminiferous tubules of the testis. The primordial germ cells divide to produce spermatogonia, the precursors of mature sperm. The spermatogonia located at the basal lamina of the tubule begin to divide mitotically at the onset of puberty to produce primary spermatocytes. These undergo a first meiotic division to produce the secondary spermatocytes. The diploid secondary spermatocytes further divide (meiotic division II) to produce the haploid spermatids (Figure 2.2a).

The round spermatids appear like any other somatic cells with a distinct nucleus. During differentiation, a series of changes occur that produce a motile sperm. The most visible change is the reduction in overall size and the formation of a tail, which allows the sperm cell to swim. The chromosomes in the sperm cells are almost crystallized by a special set of sperm-specific proteins called protamines. In fact, this protamine-induced condensation of the sperm chromosomes is so extensive that the size of the sperm nucleus is about one-thirtieth the size of a mature human ovum. This compact structure of the sperm is important for its motility. In humans, it takes approximately 2 months (60–64 days) for the whole process of the completion of mitotic and meiotic divisions and for the spermatogonium to divide and develop into four mature sperm. This process is continuously ongoing in the seminiferous tubules of the testes from puberty well into old age.

## Clinical importance

Production of spermatozoa in the testes requires the presence of germ cells, and their transformation and maturation under the control of hypothalamic and pituitary hormones and testicular androgens. In the survivable trisomy 44XXY or Klinefelter's syndrome, the germ cells are absent and azoospermia results. Deletions of parts of the Y chromosome will have a similar effect. Damage to the germinal epithelium and subsequent azoospermia or severe oligozoospermia may also occur following viral or, less commonly, bacterial infections.

Sperm development may also be affected by impairment of hormonal control, for instance, in the presence of cerebral or testicular tumours. Failure of descent of the testes into the scrotum, cryptorchidism, will also lead to poor sperm quality because of the resulting increase in testicular temperature. Prolongation of this condition is also a serious contributing factor to testicular cancer.

## Sperm transport

Following spermatogenesis, the spermatozoa pass through the seminiferous tubules to the vasa efferentia, to the head of the epididymis where they mature to become fully motile as they progress to the tail of the epididymis and the vas deferens. Figure 2.3 shows a diagram of the male reproductive tract.

The vas deferens from each testis has an ampulla whose function is to collect secretions and act as a secondary sperm store. The ampullae narrow then unite. Excretory ducts from the seminal vesicles join to form the ejaculatory duct, which joins the urethra within the prostate gland. The seminal fluid is made up of secretions from the seminal vesicles, and the prostate and bulbourethral glands. During ejaculation, approximately 2.5 mL of seminal fluid mixes with approximately 250 million sperm. This makes the sperm motile and affords the final chemical changes, so that they will be able to effect fertilization of the oocyte. The sperm now have a complex structure with a head piece (containing the genetic material) and acrosome (for penetrating the oocyte), a midpiece (with mitochondria, which provide the energy source) and a tail section (for propulsion and motility) (Figure 2.4).

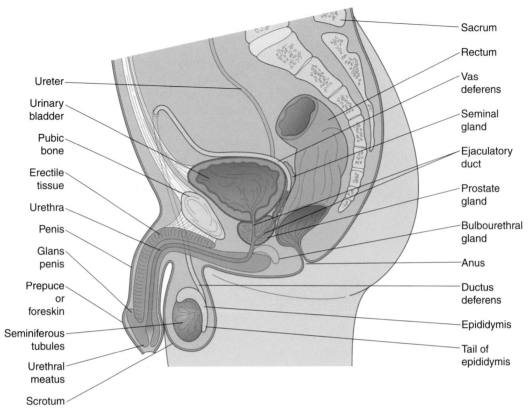

**Figure 2.3** Diagram of the male reproductive system.

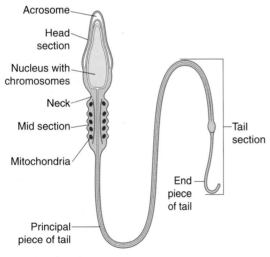

**Figure 2.4** Complete sperm.

The volume of sperm is 60–150 million per mL of ejaculate, with approximately 20–25 per cent of these being abnormal (e.g. double or small heads or tails). The pH of the seminal fluid favours the sperm and assists in offsetting the acidity of the vagina. The sperm must negotiate the acidity of the vagina, the hostile mucus of the cervix and the cavity of the uterus, move through the lumen of the Fallopian tubes to reach the ovum, then release the chemicals in their acrosome to effect penetration of the outer corona radiata and the zona pellucida layer, so that one may gain entry to fertilize the oocyte.

## Clinical importance

Sperm production may be affected by medication and drugs, alcohol and lifestyle activities as well as by infection and disease processes. Obstruction to sperm movement from the testis through the epididymis and vas deferens may result from several causes. Congenital conditions, infections, diseases, blockage following surgery may all prevent the release of sperm. In addition, certain drugs and the impact of psychological conditions may influence effective sexual functions.

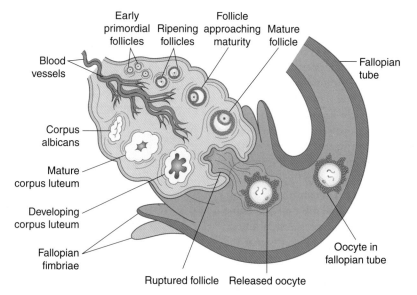

**Figure 2.5** Ovary with ripening follicles.

Movement of spermatozoa from the cervix to the ampulla of the Fallopian tube may be affected by many things:

- condoms, diaphragms and sterilization procedures produce an artificial blockage;
- cervicitis, the presence of pus and organisms in the cervix may reduce sperm mobility;
- pelvic infection, and scarring following infection or the consequences of disease or operations/procedures may prevent passage of sperm through the Fallopian tubes.

## Oogenesis, maturation of follicles and the ovarian cycle

### Oogenesis

In principle, the development of a mature oocyte from a primordial germ cell producing oogonia in the ovary is very similar to that of spermatogenesis in the testis. However, there are some distinct differences. Following the first meiotic division of primary to secondary oocytes, one of the two daughter cells (described as the first polar body) degenerates. Similarly, one of the two daughter cells produced after the second meiotic division (the second polar body) also fails to survive. Therefore, one diploid oogonium after mitotic and meiotic divisions produces one haploid mature ovum (Figure 2.2b). In contrast, one diploid spermatogonium gives rise to four haploid mature spermatozoa.

### Maturation of the follicle and the ovarian cycle

In the cortex of each ovary, approximately two million primordial follicles are present from the third month of fetal development, and they have undergone their first meiotic division by the birth of the female baby. They remain in this stage of arrested development until puberty. Vast numbers of the primordial follicles atrophy in early childhood, and fewer than 400 ever reach maturity and ovulation.

During the first half of the ovarian cycle, a few of the germ cells ripen (Figure 2.5). Each forms a fluid-filled sac or follicle on the ovary surface. One ovum develops faster to mature and is released at about day 14 of the cycle (ovulation). At this time, the fimbriated end of the Fallopian tube comes into close proximity with the ovary. The finger-like processes or fimbriae, waft the released oocyte into the Fallopian tube where the peristaltic contractions of the tube move it into the ampulla, then forward to the uterus. The remaining ripening follicles in the ovary atrophy. The ruptured follicle forms a corpus luteum (yellow body) on the surface of the ovary. This grows and secretes hormones for several days but, in the absence of a pregnancy, atrophies to become a corpus albicans (white body), and a new cycle begins. The secretion of the various hormones in the ovarian cycle influences, to a greater or lesser degree, the whole body. The changes in the endometrium of the uterus are known as the menstrual cycle.

## The menstrual cycle

The beginning of the menstrual cycle is marked by the shedding of the stratum functionale layer of the endometrium down to the stratum baseline; this is known as the mensis or period (Figure 2.6). The pituitary gland releases follicle-stimulating hormone, which initiates follicular growth in, and the release of hormones (specifically oestrogens), from the ovaries. The uterine lining begins to regrow. At the approximate midpoint of the cycle (day 14), the follicle ruptures under the influence of luteinizing hormone from the pituitary gland. Around this time, a variable amount of abdominal pain, known as mittelschmerz, may be felt by some women, and may signal the occurrence of ovulation and Fallopian tube activity. In addition, the basal body temperature may show a slight drop followed by a sustained rise until the end of the cycle. Progesterones are released from the corpus luteum, which further develop the uterine lining. If no pregnancy ensues, the lining is shed from about day 28 of the cycle. Other body changes that occur include changes in the breasts and in the cervical mucus. The cervical mucus is thick and hostile to the sperm (spinnbaskeit mucus) in the first half of the cycle, becoming thinner and more favourable (ferning mucus) after ovulation.

If fertilization of the ovum occurs, the corpus luteum is stimulated by hormones from the developing embryo to release hormones that maintain the uterine lining and the pregnancy, and suppress ovulation until the placenta is sufficiently formed to take over these functions. When this occurs, the corpus luteum becomes a corpus albicans.

## Clinical importance

The formation and release of a mature oocyte is dependent upon the hormones of the ovarian and menstrual cycles, and the efficient working of the hypothalamus and pituitary gland. Interference with the normal pattern of release of any of these hormones is likely to lead to dysfunction in the ovarian or menstrual cycles, which may result in ovulation failure. This frequently occurs naturally in young women shortly after puberty, in women approaching the menopause and, of course, during pregnancy when the cycles are suppressed. During lactation, prolactin production can interfere with the hormonal cycles affecting menstruation and

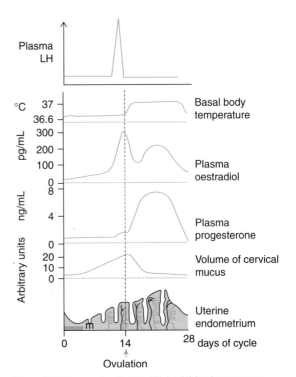

**Figure 2.6** The menstrual cycle. LH, luteinizing hormone; m, mensis. (Reproduced by kind permission of the authors from Jewels C, Tillet A. *One stop doc endocrine and reproductive systems*. London: Hodder Arnold, 2005.)

ovulation, but this cannot be considered as effective contraception. Anovulation can be induced artificially by the hormones used in contraceptive preparations. Endocrinological disease, for instance, polycystic ovarian disease or thyrotoxicosis, may similarly interfere with the hormonal events, causing anovulation and possibly subsequent infertility.

### 🔍 Key Points

- In humans, most cells contain 46 chromosomes; these cells are in a diploid state.
- Meiosis generates mature (haploid) eggs or sperm containing 23 chromosomes.
- A diploid primary spermatocyte undergoes meiosis to produce four haploid mature sperm.
- A diploid primary oocyte undergoes meiosis but produces only one haploid mature ovum (and additional polar bodies).
- During the first meiosis, the primary oocytes remain in meiotic arrest but will resume development once puberty commences.

- All mature oocytes contain 22 chromosomes plus one X (sex) chromosome.
- Mature sperm also contain 22 chromosomes plus either one X or one Y (sex) chromosome.
- The resulting embryo contains 46 chromosomes, of which two will be sex chromosomes; a normal sex combination therefore will be either XX (female) or XY (male).
- The sperm determines the sex of a child.
- Errors in meiotic divisions may lead to trisomies or monosomies or balanced or unbalanced translocation of genetic material.
- Many fetuses in spontaneous abortions (miscarriages) have chromosomal defects.
- New mutations may occur during DNA replication.

## Conception

Conception is the point when the sperm and the ova combine, and it marks the possible beginning of a new life. It occurs as a consequence of several complex events that include the final maturation of the spermatozoa and oocyte, transport of the gametes in the female genital tract and, following the fusion of the male and female gametes, the assembly of a diploid number of chromosomes.

## Fertilization

Fertilization is the process by which the male and female gametes fuse, the process taking approximately 24 hours. Ideally, this occurs in the ampulla region of the Fallopian tube. This is the widest part of the tube, it is close to the ovary and, if fertilization occurs here, there is sufficient time for the cell to attain the correct state for successful implantation in the uterus.

During the first 7–10 hours after coitus, as the sperm ascend the uterus, they become capacitated. Capacitation is the removal of the sperm's glyco-protein coat by proteolytic enzymes from the uterus; this then gives the sperm the capacity to fertilize. In addition, the acrosome becomes reactive and able to release the enzyme hyaluronidase, which acts as a solvent, causing dispersal of the corona cells of the oocyte to allow access to the zona pellucida layer (Figure 2.7). The first sperm that reaches the zona pellucida layer causes a chemical reaction that facilitates penetration of the zona by the sperm head. Further enzymes released at this time alter the zona to prevent penetration by additional sperm. The whole penetration process takes less than 20 minutes and, during this period, the second meiotic division of the oocyte occurs, resulting in the correct chromosome count of 23 in the pronucleus of the oocyte, and one polar body, which is ultimately lost. As the successful sperm completes its passage through the oocyte membrane and towards the oocyte pronucleus, it loses its tail and its nucleus head swells to become the male pronucleus. Then the two pronuclei combine to form a single diploid cell, with its full complement of 46 chromosomes, called a zygote. The coming together of the two haploid sets of chromosomes is called syngamy and is the final phase of fertilization.

## Clinical importance

Fertilization of the oocyte outside of the body is known as *in-vitro* fertilization or IVF (*in vitro* means 'in glass'). IVF has provided the opportunity from many childless couples to become parents.

In IVF techniques the mature ovum is incubated with sperm on day 0. On day 1 the ovum is inspected to ensure that two pronuclei are present, demonstrating that normal fertilization is under way. By day 2 a four-cell pre-embryo, or cleaved pre-embryo, has formed and the eight-cell stage is reached by day 3 (Figure 2.8). In cases where diagnosis of genetic disease is required, it is at this point that two cells can be removed for chromosome and DNA analysis. Only two or three cleaved pre-embryos are returned to the uterus during the 4–8-cell stage. Spare cleaved pre-embryo can be frozen for later use.

GIFT is gamete intra-Fallopian transfer and involves placing retrieved oocytes and many sperm into the ampulla of the Fallopian tube for fertilization to occur within the body.

All practices involving the retrieval, use, storage and disposal of gametes in the UK are strictly controlled under the 1990 Human Fertilization and Embryology Act.

After fertilization the zygote begins mitotic cellular replication and division. Over the next 4 days, cellular division continues, as the zygote travels along the Fallopian tube towards the uterus. Although the DNA increases as the chromosomes replicate and divide, the cytoplasm in the cell does not. The overall size of

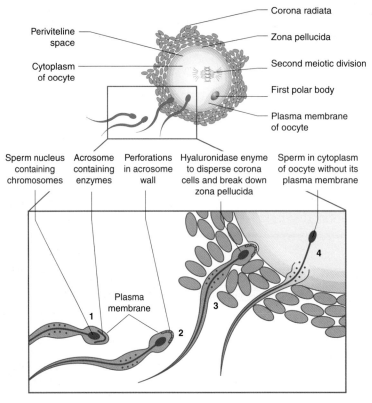

**Figure 2.7** Ovum with sperm entry.

the embryo does in fact slightly reduce as it becomes a dense mass of cells. By day 3, with 12 or more cells, it is known as a morula and, at day 4, as it passes through the isthmus of the Fallopian tubes and into the start of the cavity of the uterus, it is an early blastocyst. With its next divisions, and by day 5, it is a defined blastocyst. At this time, the zona pellucida is shed and the blastocyst consists of a shell of flattened trophoblastic cells (which later form placental tissue) and a central group of about 16 cells, known as the inner cell mass or embryoblast, from which the entire embryo will form. Implantation of the blastocyst into the uterine endometrium commences on about the sixth day after fertilization, at approximately day 20 of the menstrual cycle.

## Implantation and the pre-embryonic period

By day 6, the trophoblastic layer of the blastocyst, comes into contact with the endometrium of the uterus, usually at the upper posterior wall, and begins to implant.

The trophoblastic epithelium closest to the embryoblast becomes cuboidal cytotrophoblastic in structure. These cells undergo many mitotic divisions and form syncytiotrophoblasts. The syncytiotrophoblasts secrete enzymes that erode into the endometrium to assist in the nutrition of the developing embryo and in its anchoring into the endometrium. The syncytiotrophoblasts also produce the hormone human chorionic gonadotrophin (HCG), which stimulates the corpus luteum in the ovary to continue production of oestrogens and progesterones to maintain the pregnancy. HCG can be detected in the blood and the urine about a week after implantation (i.e. around the time of the missed period); this hormone is, therefore, the basis of several pregnancy tests. By the twelfth day after fertilization, the conceptus is completely embedded in the uterine endometrium, with uterine epithelium growing over it. It is at this time that the woman's period is due. During these weeks the uterine endometrium was initially in its proliferation phase. By the time the blastocyst reaches the uterine cavity, the secretary phase of the menstrual cycle is in progress, with the endometrium ready to accept the developing conceptus.

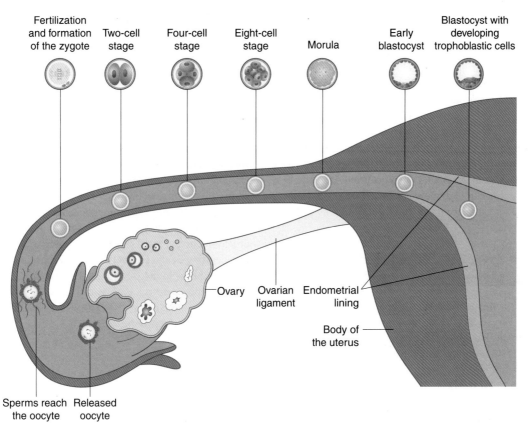

Fertilization and formation of the zygote

Two-cell stage

Four-cell stage

Eight-cell stage

Morula

Early blastocyst

Blastocyst with developing trophoblastic cells

Ovary

Ovarian ligament

Endometrial lining

Body of the uterus

Sperms reach the oocyte

Released oocyte

**Figure 2.8** Fertilized egg showing division to blastocyst.

The 2 weeks from fertilization until the appearance of the primitive steak is known as the pre-embryonic period. The developmental stages within this period include the formation of the morula and the blastocyst, the appearance of the inner cell mass or embryocyst, the embryonic disc becoming visible by day 14, and the visualization of the primitive streak by day 14/15.

The embryonic period runs from day 15 to the end of the eighth week of development or approximately 10 weeks from the first day of the last menstrual period. From this point on, the conceptus is known as a fetus.

## Clinical importance

The pre-embryonic period is crucial in relation to the initiation of the pregnancy. In the embryonic period, all the major organ systems are formed and, by the start of the fetal period, all organs and structures are in place, although complete development, maturity and functioning are not completed until birth at term and beyond. Chromosomal defects, system development abnormalities and interruptions in structural and organ development producing a full range of defects and abnormalities are most likely to manifest in the pre-embryonic and embryonic periods. The highest risk to all the developing systems and organs is at this time, as they are undergoing the most intense and specialized cellular activity. Indeed, up to 45 per cent of all pregnancies may spontaneously abort in the pre-embryonic period, possibly due to abnormality in the developing pre-embryo or in the implantation process.

Delay or obstruction of the passage of the fertilized ovum down the Fallopian tube to the uterus may result in implantation in the Fallopian tube or, more rarely, the ovary or peritoneal cavity. This is known as an ectopic pregnancy and, whilst the pregnancy may continue to develop for some weeks, it will eventually fail. Some cases will cause rupture of the Fallopian tube and will present as an acute emergency.

Within the uterus, implantation failure may be due to deficiencies in the pre-embryo or in the state of readiness of the endometrium, or its ability to accept the blastocyst. Failure or incomplete implantation may be a cause of early pregnancy loss, as may chromosomal abnormalities. It is likely that, in a majority of these cases, this will be unknown to the woman, as she may associate the bleeding as a normal or slightly late menstrual loss and not a lost pregnancy. More subtle deficiencies in implantation are likely to be part of the processes leading to obstetric diseases, such as pre-eclampsia or intrauterine growth restriction later in pregnancy. Inappropriate implantation may also, although more rarely, lead to morbid adherence of the placenta in conditions such as placenta accreta.

## Embryology – week by week

This is the period from the appearance of the primitive streak, day 15 of development, until the end of the eighth week, that is, approximately 10 weeks from the first day of the last menstrual period.

### The third week

Morphogenesis (development of the body form) is the most significant event *initiated* in the third week, and is centred on the primitive streak, which differentiates into three germ layers. These layers are the ectoderm, mesoderm and endoderm, and they are the primitive origins of all tissues and organs.

- Ectoderm – epidermis, hair and nails; central and peripheral nervous systems, and various other structures.
- Mesoderm – skeleton and bone marrow; muscles and connective tissue; reproductory and excretory glands, and blood vessels and blood cells.
- Endoderm – epithelial lining of the respiratory, digestive and urinary tracts; and the glandular cells of various organs such as the liver and pancreas.

The primitive streak also defines the polarity of the embryo, with clear cranial or cephalic and caudal poles (Figure 2.9a). Symmetry and laterality are also defined, which are fundamental at the outset of organogenesis, so that appropriately sited organ-system and limb development occurs. During the third week, two other structures become apparent on the embryonic disk – the neural plate and the somites. The somites develop from mesoderm, and appear as distinct symmetric elevations on either side of the

midline, going on to give rise to most of the axial skeleton and associated musculature. As the somites are visible from the end of the third week and are so prominent during the fourth and fifth weeks, they are used as criteria for determining the embryo's age.

Other structures developing at this time are: the neural fold and neural groove, which go on to form the neural tube; the beginnings of the thyroid gland; the heart tubes which begin to fuse; and the primitive yolk sac. The yolk sac is an important organ for exchanging metabolites between the mother and the embryo at the time when there is no placenta but there are some chorionic villi undergoing vascularization. The life span of the yolk sac is limited; it attains full development by day 32 and its complex wall starts degenerating by the end of the sixth week. The amniotic membrane is also developing and, by day 17, it is closely apposed to the embryonic disk. However, it will be some time before the embryo is suspended in a well-expanded amniotic sac.

### The fourth week

The organ systems develop during the fourth to eighth weeks. This is known as the differentiation phase and it is during this period that exposure to teratogens (drugs or viruses that produce or increase the incidence of congenital abnormality) may cause major defects.

During the fourth week, and continuing through the next two weeks, rapid growth of the embryo takes place. A major landmark of this is embryonic folding. The embryonic disc folds into an embryonic cylinder (Figure 2.9b). The cranial and caudal ends fold to give a curved long axis, which assists in locating organs into their correct body position, and incorporates some of the yolk sac into the body. Some of the yolk sac becomes the foregut, developing into the respiratory and upper digestive tracts, etc., in the upper body, and some of the yolk sac forming the hindgut develops into the lower intestinal and urinary tracts in the lower body. Simultaneously, folding occurs in the horizontal plane. Here part of the yolk sac forms the midgut, developing into the intestines, etc. Closure of the abdominal wall, with initial development of the umbilical cord, and closure of the neural tube begins.

By the end of the fourth week, early eye structure, the beginnings of limb buds, and a rudimentary or

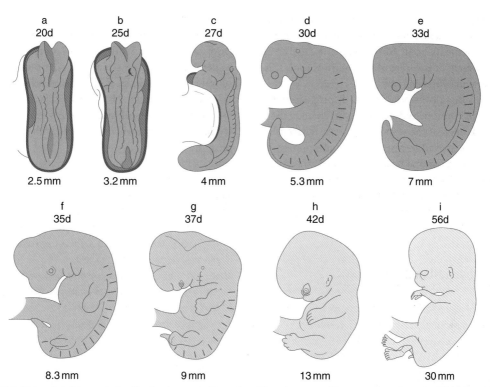

a
20d

b
25d

c
27d

d
30d

e
33d

2.5 mm

3.2 mm

4 mm

5.3 mm

7 mm

f
35d

g
37d

h
42d

i
56d

8.3 mm

9 mm

13 mm

30 mm

**Figure 2.9** Sequential changes during the development of the external form in a normal human embryo from day 20 (a) through to the 56th day (i) postfertilization (add 2 weeks to consider the gestational time from the last menstrual period). The crown-rump length is expressed in millimetres.

attenuated tail are visible. The embryonic heart is beating (Figure 2.9c).

## The fifth week

During the fifth week, changes are minor compared with the fourth week. Growth of the head, however, exceeds that of all the other regions (Figure 2.9d). This is due to the rapid development of the brain. The upper limbs begin to develop differentiation at the elbow and hand plates, and primordial digits begin to develop here from day 33 onwards. Early spontaneous twitching movements of the upper limbs and trunk are possible from the end of the fifth week (Figure 2.9e and f).

## The sixth week

The sixth week shows rapid differentiation in the upper limbs and lower limb-bud development is occurring. By the end of the sixth week, the head and

trunk have begun to straighten, the head is much larger, the eyes are now obvious, grooves are visible on the sides of the head that will develop into the external ear structures, and the oral and nasal cavities and structures are forming (Figure 2.9g).

## The seventh week

In this week, the yolk sac is dramatically reduced, the primitive gut becoming located in the body of the embryo and the abdominal wall begins its closure. During this week, considerable growth and changes occur in the limbs (Figure 2.9h). Over the non-placental area, villi are being lost and a smooth chorion is developing as the placenta differentiates and develops.

## The eighth week

At the beginning of this last week of embryonic life, the digits of the hand are short and webbed, and notches are visible on the feet plates. But by the end of this week, all regions of the limbs are apparent and the digits have lengthened and separated. Purposeful limb movements occur from this point on. The tail is still present at the start of the eighth week but has disappeared by the end of it.

Now, although its head is still disproportionately large, the embryo has clear human characteristics. The eyes, open at the start of the week, have eyelids, which have started to fuse. The ears are present but are still set low on the head. Only a small amount of the intestines are in the proximal portion of the umbilical cord. The external genitalia are gender specific but not distinct enough to permit accurate sex identification (Figure 2.9i).

## Clinical importance

The three essential phases of human development – growth, morphogenesis and differentiation – take place from conception until the end of the eighth week. In the crucial early stages, the woman may not even know she is pregnant. When teratogenic risks are highest, the woman may be still not have had the pregnancy confirmed, or may be suffering from early pregnancy ailments, so that attention to good diet and avoidance of potential teratogens may be far from her mind. Good preconception and early pregnancy health, therefore, are to be promoted at every opportunity by all health care professionals.

Ultrasound examination is commonly used to detect early intrauterine pregnancies. Using transvaginal ultrasound, a gestation sac may be seen in the uterus between the fourth and the fifth week after the last menstrual period (2–3 weeks after fertilization). The rudimentary fetal heart will be seen to be beating from the end of the fifth or beginning of the sixth weeks after the last menstrual period. Abdominal ultrasound examination can be used to identify the gestation sac but it will not be seen by this method until 6–7 weeks. Also, identification of the beating fetal heart is delayed by 1 week when compared with transvaginal ultrasound.

## Key Points

- The pre-embryo must produce cytotrophoblastic and syncytiotrophoblastic tissue in order to successfully infiltrate into the endometrial stroma to implant.
- All major organs and systems of the body form from the three germ layers: ectoderm, mesoderm and endoderm.
- As the structures develop, the appearance of the embryo changes so that, by the end of the eighth week, it is unquestionably human; this is approximately 10 weeks from the start of the woman's last menstrual period.
- The most crucial period of organ and systems development is from the fourth to the eighth week.
- The greatest risk from teratogens is during the fourth to eighth weeks.
- It is now thought that cytokines are involved in initiating a localized immunosuppression, which would allow the developing embryo to avoid a rejection-like response from the uterus.
- Leucocyte infiltration of the implantation site has been observed; most of these leucocytes seem to be T-suppressor cells.

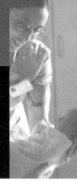

# Normal fetal development and growth

## OVERVIEW

An appreciation of normal fetal development, growth and maturation is important in understanding complications that may occur to the fetus and the neonate. At the end of embryogenesis, organogenesis is complete and the fetus is completely formed. The ensuing 6 months *in utero* will be devoted to maturation and growth.

## Fetal growth and maturation

Determinants of birth weight are multifactorial, and reflect the influence of the natural growth potential of the fetus and the intrauterine environment. The latter is controlled both by maternal and placental factors.

Fetal growth is dependent on adequate transfer of nutrients and oxygen across the placenta. This in itself is dependent on appropriate maternal nutrition and placental perfusion. Factors affecting these are discussed in Chapter 10. Other factors are important in determining fetal growth (e.g. fetal hormones). These affect the metabolic rate, growth of tissues and maturation of individual organs. In particular, insulin-like growth factors (IGFs) coordinate a precise and orderly increase in growth throughout late gestation. Insulin and thyroxin (T4) are required through late gestation to ensure appropriate growth in normal and adverse nutritional circumstances. Fetal hyperinsulinaemia, which occurs when maternal glycaemic control is suboptimal owing to maternal diabetes mellitus, results in fetal macrosomia, causing excessive fat deposition.

Conversely, in growth-restricted fetuses, fetal insulin levels are low, thus further reducing the build up of fetal tissue. Lack of thyroid hormone results in deficiency of skeletal and cerebral maturation, characteristics of cretinism (hypothyroidism) and delayed surfactant production. Cortisol has a limited role in stimulating growth; however, it is essential for the structural and functional development of a wide variety of individual fetal tissues. In the lung, it increases compliance and surfactant release, which ensures that spontaneous breathing can occur at birth. In the fetal liver, cortisol induces beta-receptors and glycogen deposition to maintain a glucose supply to the neonate immediately after birth. In the gut, cortisol is responsible for villi proliferation and induction of digestive enzymes that enable the neonate to switch to enteral feeding at birth.

In developed countries, the average birth weight is about 3.5 kg at the end of a normal pregnancy lasting an average of 40 weeks. About one-third of the eventual birth weight is reached by 28 weeks, half by 31 weeks and two-thirds by 34 weeks. The average fetus gains approximately 25 g/day between 32 weeks gestation and term.

Each baby has its own optimal growth potential, which is, to a degree, predictable from physiological characteristics known at the beginning of pregnancy. The principal known factors are maternal weight and height, parity, race or ethnic group and the baby's sex. Maternal age is also a factor, but the variation is mostly accounted for by parity. These factors are used to produce individualized fetal growth charts within the woman's hand-held antenatal records, on which fundal height is plotted from 24 weeks gestation to standardize the monitoring of fetal growth (National Institute for Clinical Excellence 2003). Of paternal characteristics, height is associated with birth weight but to a lesser extent than any of the maternal variables (see box). The physiological variation in normal birth weight in any heterogeneous maternity population can be considerable (Table 3.1). Such differences become magnified if it is attempted, on the basis of birth weight alone, to determine what is an abnormally small baby. It is important to note that not all

> ## Physiological variables affecting normal fetal growth
>
> - Pre-pregnancy weight and maternal booking weight
> - Maternal height
> - Maternal age and parity
> - Ethnic group
> - Fetal sex
> - Paternal height

small for gestational age (SGA) fetuses are growth restricted; some of these babies are constitutionally small and have reached their full growth potential. In addition, not all growth-restricted fetuses are SGA.

It is important to exclude the known pathological influences on birth weight when calculating the optimal weight that a baby can reach. However, smoking has an all too high prevalence in an average population: about 25 per cent of mothers admit to being smokers at the time of the booking visit, and most of them continue to smoke throughout pregnancy. The effect of smoking on birth weight is significant, consistent and dose dependent (Figure 3.1).

Growth-restricted fetuses that have failed to achieve their growth potential have significantly higher perinatal mortality and morbidity rates than normally grown babies of a similar gestation. They are more

**Table 3.1** – Optimal birth weight. Approximate coefficients used for individually adjusting the predicted birth weight at the end of a normal pregnancy (i.e. pathology-free birth weight). The baseline birth weight for a baby of a non-smoking Anglo-European mother in her first pregnancy, of average height (163 cm) and booking weight (64 kg), is about 3480 g at 40.0 weeks

| | |
|---|---|
| Maternal weight | 9 g/kg |
| Maternal height | 8 g/cm |
| Parity | |
|     Para 1 | +110 g |
|     Para 2+ | +150 g |
| Ethnic group | |
|     South Asian (India, Pakistan) | −185 g |
|     Afro-Caribbean | −130 g |
| Baby's gender (male > female) | ±60 g |

likely to suffer intrauterine hypoxia/asphyxia and, as a consequence, be stillborn or demonstrate signs and symptoms of hypoxic ischaemic encephalopathy, including seizures and multiorgan damage or failure in the neonatal period. Other complications to which these growth-restricted babies are more prone include neonatal hypothermia, hypoglycaemia, infection and

necrotizing enterocolitis. In the medium term, cerebral palsy is more prevalent and, in adulthood, they are at greater risk of cardiovascular complications such as hypertension and ischaemic heart disease, and metabolic disorders such as non-insulin-dependent diabetes.

## Cardiovascular system

The fetal circulation is quite different from that of the adult (Figure 3.2). Its distinctive features are:
- oxygenation occurs in the placenta not the lungs;
- the right and left ventricles work in parallel rather than in series;
- the heart, brain and upper body receive blood from the left ventricle via the umbilical vein, which is richest in oxygen, whilst the placenta and lower body receive mixed blood from both right and left ventricles.

Three temporary structures adapt fetal circulation to take blood away from the quiescent lungs and allow placental oxygenation. This also ensures that

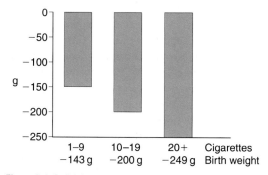

**Figure 3.1** Deficit in birth weight due to smoking as recorded in early pregnancy (adjusted for other variables listed in Table 3.1).

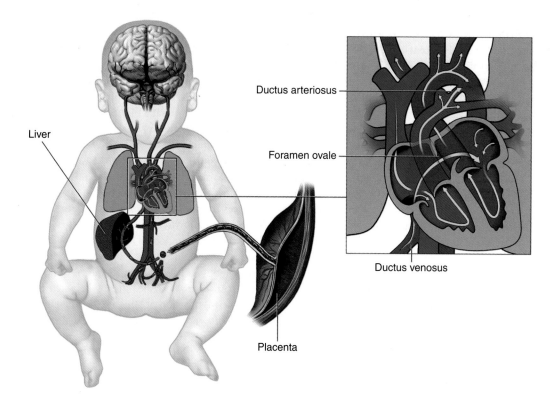

**Figure 3.2** Diagrammatic representation of fetal circulation. (Medical Illustration Copyright © 2006 Nucleus Medical Art, all rights reserved. www.nucleusinc.com).

the best oxygenated blood from the placenta is delivered to the brain. These structures are:

- the ductus venosus, which shunts blood away from the liver;
- the foramen ovale, which shunts blood from the right to the left atrium;
- the ductus arteriosus, which shunts blood from the pulmonary artery to the aorta.

Oxygenated blood from the placenta returns to the fetus through the umbilical vein. This vein divides into two main branches, one that supplies the portal vein in the liver and another narrow vessel, called the ductus venosus, which joins the inferior vena cava as it enters the right atrium. Fifty per cent of the blood will pass to the portal system and 50 per cent to the ductus venosus. The ductus is a narrow vessel and high blood velocities are generated in this vessel. This streaming of the ductus venosus blood, together with a membranous valve in the right atrium (the crista dividens) prevents mixing of the well-oxygenated blood from the ductus venosus with the desaturated blood of the inferior vena cava. The ductus venosus stream passes across the right atrium through a physiological defect in the atrial septum, called the foramen ovale, to the left atrium; from here blood passes through the mitral valve to the left ventricle and hence to the aorta. About 50 per cent of the highly oxygenated blood goes to the head and upper extremities; the remainder passes down the aorta to mix with blood of reduced oxygen saturation from the right ventricle.

Blood from the inferior vena cava and the superior vena cava is directed across the tricuspid valve into the right ventricle. Only a small portion of blood from the right ventricle passes to the lungs, as they are non-functional. Most of the blood is directed through a narrow vessel called the ductus arteriosus into the descending aorta below the origin of the head and neck vessels from the aortic arch. By this means, the desaturated blood from the right ventricle passes down the aorta to enter the umbilical arterial circulation and thence to the placenta.

Prior to birth, the ductus remains patent owing to the production of prostaglandin E2 and prostacyclin, which act as local vasodilators. Premature closure of the ductus has been reported with the administration of cyclo-oxygenase inhibitors.

At birth, the cessation of umbilical blood flow causes cessation of flow in the ductus venosus, a fall in pressure in the right atrium and closure of the foramen ovale. Ventilation of the lungs opens the pulmonary circulation, with a rapid fall in pulmonary vascular resistance. The ductus arteriosus begins to constrict at birth in response to bradykinin, released from the lungs on their initial inflation. The effect of bradykinin is dependent on the $PO_2$ in the blood passing through, once this reaches 50 mmHg, the ductus will close. In the healthy neonate, the ductus normally closes within the first few days of life; however, in premature infants and those with persistent hypoxia, it may remain patent for 2–3 months. In the premature infant, the patent ductus can result in congestion in the pulmonary circulation and a reduction in blood flow to the gastrointestinal tract and brain, and is implicated in the pathogenesis of necrotizing enterocolitis and intraventricular haemorrhage.

Occasionally, this transition from fetal to adult circulation is delayed, usually because the pulmonary vascular resistance fails to fall despite adequate breathing. This delay, termed persistent fetal circulation, results in left to right shunting of blood from the aorta through the ductus arteriosus to the lungs. The baby remains cyanosed and can suffer from life-threatening hypoxia.

## Fetal blood

The first fetal blood cells are formed on the surface of the yolk sac 14–19 days after conception. Haemopoiesis continues from this site until the third postconceptual month. During the fifth week of embryonic life, extramedullary haemopoiesis begins in the liver and to a lesser extent in the spleen. The bone marrow starts to produce red cells at 7–8 weeks and is the predominant source of red cells from 26 weeks' gestation.

Most haemoglobin in the fetus is fetal haemoglobin (HbF), which, having a higher affinity for oxygen, enhances the transfer of oxygen across the placenta. HbF has two gamma-chains (alpha 2, gamma 2) in place of the adult haemoglobins HbA (alpha 2, beta 2) and HbA2 (alpha 2, delta 2). Ninety per cent of fetal haemoglobin is HbF between 10 and 28 weeks' gestation. From 28 to 34 weeks, there is a switch to HbA and, at term, the ratio of HbF to HbA is 80:20; by six months of age, only 1 per cent of haemoglobin is HbF. Owing to the higher haemoglobin concentration of HbF at birth, the neonate's mean capillary haemoglobin is 18 g/dL.

Abnormal haemoglobin production results in thalassaemia. The thalassaemias are a group of genetic haematological disorders characterized by reduced or absent production of one or more of the globin chains of haemoglobin. Beta-thalassaemia results from reduced or absent production of the beta-globin chains. As the switch from HbF to HbA described above occurs, the absent or insufficient beta-globin chains shorten red-cell survival with early destruction of these cells within the bone marrow and spleen. Beta-thalassaemia major results from the inheritance of two abnormal beta-genes; without treatment, this leads to severe anaemia, fetal growth restriction, poor musculoskeletal development and skin pigmentation owing to increased iron absorption. The severest form of alpha-thalassaemia, in which no alpha-globulin chains are produced, results in severe fetal anaemia with cardiac failure, hepatosplenomegaly and generalized oedema. These infants are stillborn or die shortly after birth.

## Respiratory system – lung

Full differentiation of capillary and canalicular elements of the fetal lung is apparent by 20 weeks' gestation. Alveoli develop after 24 weeks. Numerous, but intermittent, fetal breathing movements occur *in utero*, especially during rapid eye movement (REM) sleep and in the presence of adequate amniotic fluid volume. Fetal breathing occurs for 15 per cent of the observation time in the second trimester, rising to 30 per cent in the third trimester. The fetal lung is filled with fluid, the production of which starts in early gestation and ends in the early stages of labour. At birth, the production of this fluid must cease and the fluid present is absorbed. Adrenaline, to which the pulmonary epithelium becomes increasingly sensitive towards term, appears to play a major role in this process.

Lung alveoli are lined by a group of phospholipids, known collectively as surfactant. Surfactant prevents collapse of small alveoli during expiration by lowering surface tension. The surfactant is continually replaced by synthesis from type 2 alveolar cells, with maximal production after 28 weeks. These cells make up 10 per cent of lung parenchyma. The predominant phospholipid (80 per cent of the total) is phosphatidylcholine (lecithin). The production of lecithin is enhanced by cortisol, growth restriction and prolonged rupture of the membranes, and is delayed in diabetes. Other phospholipids may be more potent in reducing surface tension. For example, levels of phosphatidylglycerol in the amniotic fluid are more predictive of respiratory distress syndrome, especially in pregnancies complicated by diabetes.

Normal lung development requires an adequate amniotic fluid volume and fetal breathing movements. Oligohydramnios, decreased intrathoracic space (e.g. diaphragmatic hernia) or chest wall deformities can result in pulmonary hypoplasia, which leads to progressive respiratory failure from birth.

Respiratory distress syndrome (RDS) often occurs in babies born prematurely and is associated with surfactant deficiency. It typically presents within the first few hours of life with signs of respiratory distress including tachypnoea and cyanosis. It occurs in over 80 per cent of infants born between 23 and 27 weeks' gestation, falling to 10 per cent of infants born between 34 and 36 weeks. Acute complications include hypoxia and asphyxia, intraventricular haemorrhage and necrotizing enterocolitis. The incidence and severity of RDS can be reduced by administering steroids antenatally to mothers at risk of preterm delivery.

## Immune system

The fetus requires an effective immune system to resist intrauterine and perinatal infections. Lymphocytes appear from 8 weeks and, by the middle of the second trimester, all phagocytic cells, T and B cells and complement are available to mount a response. Early infection with any of the TORCH organisms (toxoplasmosis, rubella, cytomegalovirus and herpes) will affect a number of systems including the immune defences themselves. Immunoglobulin G (IgG) originates mostly from the maternal circulation and crosses the placenta to provide passive immunity. The fetus normally produces only small amounts of IgM and IgA, which do not cross the placenta. Detection of IgM/IgA in the newborn, without IgG, is indicative of fetal infection. General immunological defences include the amniotic fluid (lysosymes, IgG), the placenta (lymphoid cells, phagocytes, barrier), granulocytes from liver and bone marrow, and interferon from lymphocytes.

## Skin and homeostasis

Fetal skin protects and facilitates homeostasis. The thickness of the skin increases progressively from the first month of gestation until birth. A stratum corneum forms in the fifth month and, after approximately 23 weeks, the appearances of the skin approach that of the adult epidermis. Vernix caseosa appears on the fetal skin from 20 weeks' gestation. It is a thick white substance consisting of desquamated skin cells, cholesterol and glycogen; its function is to protect the skin and act as an insulator. Preterm babies have little vernix and thin skin; this allows a proportionately large amount of insensible water and heat loss.

Thermal control in cool ambient temperatures is limited by a large surface-to-body volume ratio and poor thermal insulation. Heat may be conserved by peripheral vasoconstriction and can be generated by brown fat catabolism, but this is deficient in preterm or growth-restricted babies because of the small amount of subcutaneous fat and immaturity of vascular tone regulation in the former. The response to warm ambient temperatures is also poor, because the poor responses of the sweat glands will preserve heat and can result in overheating of the infant.

## Alimentary system and energy stores

The primitive foregut and hindgut are present by the end of the fourth week and, at this stage, the intestine is almost a straight tube suspended by the mesentery from the dorsal body wall. The abdominal cavity is too small to accommodate the enlarging liver and intestine and, as a consequence, the midgut herniates into the base of the umbilical cord during the sixth week. While herniated, the gut undergoes rotation prior to re-entering the abdominal cavity by 12 weeks. Failure of the gut to re-enter the abdominal cavity results in the development of an omphalocele.

From the time that the gastrointestinal tract is fully formed, the lumen is patent. The swallowing reflex develops and matures gradually. The fetus continually and increasingly swallows amniotic fluid, up to approximately 20 mL per hour at term. A failure in this swallowing mechanism either as a consequence of a neurological abnormality (e.g. anencephaly) or an obstruction in the gut (e.g. atresia of the oesophagus) will result in an increase in fluid within the amniotic cavity (polyhydramnios).

Peristalsis in the intestine occurs from the second trimester. The large bowel is filled with meconium at term. Defecation *in utero*, and hence meconium in the amniotic fluid, is associated with post-term pregnancies and fetal hypoxia. Aspiration of meconium-stained liquor by the fetus at birth can result in meconium aspiration syndrome and respiratory distress.

While body water content gradually diminishes, glycogen and fat stores increase about five-fold in the last trimester. Preterm infants have virtually no fat and a severely reduced ability to withstand starvation. This is aggravated by an incompletely developed alimentary system, and may manifest in a poor sucking, uncoordinated swallowing mechanism, delayed gastric emptying, and poor absorption of carbohydrates, fat and other nutrients. Growth-restricted fetuses also have reduced glycogen stores and are, therefore, more prone to hypoglycaemia within the early neonatal period.

## Liver and gallbladder

The primitive liver appears at about the 18th day of embryonic life as a diverticulum arising from the duodenum. By the 25th day it has developed into a T-shaped outgrowth, which is invaded by blood vessels. The larger portion of this diverticulum gives rise to the parenchymal cells and the hepatic ducts, while the smaller portion gives rise to the gallbladder. *In utero*, the normal metabolic functions of the liver are performed by the placenta. For example, unconjugated bilirubin from haemoglobin breakdown is actively transported from the fetus to the mother with only a small proportion being conjugated in the liver and secreted in the bile (the mechanism after birth). The fetal liver also differs from the adult organ in many processes. For example, the fetal liver has a reduced ability to conjugate bilirubin because of relative deficiencies in the necessary enzymes such as glucuronyl transferase. Following birth, the loss of the placental route for excretion of unconjugated bilirubin results in physiological jaundice of the newborn. This may become severe in the premature infant owing to the continuing deficiencies of necessary enzymes for the conjugation of bilirubin.

The fetal liver plays an important role in haemopoiesis, which starts at 6 weeks, peaks at 12–16 weeks and continues until approximately 36 weeks. Glycogen is stored within the liver in small quantities from the first trimester but storage is maximal in the third trimester with abundant stores being present at term. Growth-restricted and premature infants have deficient glycogen stores; this renders them prone to neonatal hypoglycaemia.

## Kidney and urinary tract

After regression of the mesonephros or Wolffian duct, the metanephros forms the renal collecting system (ureter, pelvis, calyces and collecting ducts) and induces the formation of the renal secretory system (glomeruli, convoluted tubes and loops of Henle) from the mesenchyme of the nephrogenic cord. Nephrogenesis is complete by 36 weeks, but the maturation of excretory and concentrating ability of the fetal kidneys is gradual. It is immature in the preterm infant, and this may lead to abnormal water, glucose and sodium or acid–base homeostasis.

Fetal urine forms much of the amniotic fluid, which is a protein- and sugar-free hypotonic ultrafiltrate of fetal plasma. Fetal urine production rises gradually with fetal maturity, from about 12 mL per hour at 32 weeks to 38 mL per hour at 40 weeks. Renal agenesis will, therefore, result in severe reduction of amniotic fluid (oligohydramnios).

## Fetal behaviour

Fetal movement begins at around 8 weeks' gestation but the mother does not perceive these movements for several weeks. Known as 'quickening' fetal movements, they are felt by the mother at about 16–18 weeks in the multiparous woman and 18–20 weeks in the primigravid woman. Self-monitoring of fetal movements is encouraged: women are asked to become familiar with the daily pattern of fetal movements and to report any decreases. A sensation of diminished fetal activity may be associated with chronic hypoxia and growth failure, and may be a precursor of fetal death. Reduced fetal movements are an important screening tool for further investigation.

With maturation of the central nervous system, the fetus develops more complex patterns and well-defined behavioural states that have been named 1F to 4F. State 1F is similar to quiet (non-REM) sleep, with absence of eye and body movements. In state 2F, periodic eye and body movements are present (REM sleep). State 3F has eye movements but no body movements (i.e. is equivalent to quiet wakefulness), while 4F is an active phase with ongoing eye movements and fetal activity. For most of the time (>80 per cent), the fetus alternates between the sleep cycles 1F and 2F. This is particularly relevant when interpreting tests of fetal well-being, for example, cardiotocography (CTG) and the biophysical profile. An unreactive CTG may reflect the fact that the fetus is in a sleep pattern (1F; 2F) and not compromised. In this situation, providing there are not other indicators of potential compromise, the trace should be repeated after a reasonable time interval when the fetus is in a more active behavioural state (4F).

## Amniotic fluid

By 12 weeks' gestation, the amnion comes into contact with the inner surface of the chorion. The two membranes become adherent, but never intimately fuse. Neither the amnion nor the chorion contains vessels or nerves, but they do contain a significant quantity of phospholipids as well as enzymes involved in phospholipid hydrolysis. Choriodecidual function is thought to play a pivotal role in the initiation of labour through the production of prostaglandins E2 and F2a.

Amniotic fluid (AF) is a clear pale straw-coloured fluid, initially secreted by the amnion but, by the tenth week, it is mainly a transudate of the fetal serum via the skin and umbilical cord. The AF is constantly circulated by the fetus swallowing and inhaling existing fluid and replacing it through urination and exhalation. From 16 weeks' gestation, the fetal skin becomes impermeable to water and the net increase in AF is through a small imbalance between the contributions of fluid through the kidneys and lung fluids, and removal by fetal swallowing. AF volume increases progressively (10 weeks, 30 mL; 20 weeks, 300 mL; 30 weeks, 600 mL; 38 weeks, 1000 mL) but, from term, there is a rapid fall in volume (40 weeks, 800 mL; 42 weeks, 350 mL). The reason for the late reduction in AF volume has not been explained.

The functions of the amniotic fluid are listed below.
- It protects the fetus from mechanical injury.
- It permits movement of the fetus, promoting development of the musculoskeletal system.
- It prevents adhesions between the fetus and the amnion.
- It permits fetal lung development in which there is two-way movement of fluid into the fetal bronchioles. Absence of AF in the second trimester is associated with pulmonary hypoplasia.
- It maintains a constant temperature.

- During labour, it equalizes intrauterine pressure, preventing marked interference with placental circulation.

Major alterations in AF volume occur when there is reduced contribution of fluid into the amniotic sac in conditions such as renal agenesis, cystic kidneys or intrauterine growth restriction; oligohydramnios results. Reduced removal of fluid in conditions such as anencephaly and oesophageal/duodenal atresia is associated with polyhydramnios (see Chapter 8).

## CASE HISTORY 1

A 26-year-old is admitted to the labour ward at 32 weeks' gestation. She gives a history suggestive of preterm rupture of membranes and is experiencing uterine contractions. On vaginal examination, the cervix is found to be 8 cm dilated and she rapidly goes on to deliver a male infant weighing 1650 g. At birth, he is intubated because of poor respiratory effort and transferred to the neonatal intensive care unit.

### As a premature infant, which complications is he particularly at risk of?

- *Fetal growth* – deficient glycogen stores in the liver increase the risk of hypoglycaemia. This is compounded by the increased glucose requirements of premature infants.
- *Cardiovascular system* – patent ductus arteriosus (PDA) may result in pulmonary congestion, worsening lung disease and decreased blood flow to the gastrointestinal tract and brain. The duct can be closed by administering prostaglandin synthetase inhibitors (e.g. indomethacin) or by surgical ligation.
- *Respiratory system* – respiratory distress syndrome and apnoea of prematurity may lead to hypoxia. The administration of antenatal steroids to the mother reduces the risk and severity of RDS. For benefit to be gained, steroids need to be administered at least 24 hours before delivery. In this case, delivery occurred too rapidly for steroids to be administered. The severity of RDS can also be reduced by giving surfactant via the endotracheal tube used to ventilate the baby.
- *Fetal blood* – anaemia of prematurity is common because of low iron stores and red cell mass at birth, reduced erythropoiesis and decreased survival of red blood cells. Treatment is by blood transfusion, iron supplementation or, in some cases, the use of erythropoietin.
- *Immune system* – preterm babies have an increased susceptibility to infection owing to impaired cell-mediated immunity and reduced levels of immunoglobulin. Suspected infection should be treated early with antibiotics because deterioration in these premature small infants can be rapid.

- *Skin and homeostasis* – hypothermia is common in preterm infants secondary to a relatively large body surface area, thin skin, lack of subcutaneous fat and lack of keratinized epidermal layer of skin. High insensible water losses owing to skin immaturity may aggravate dehydration and electrolyte problems secondary to immaturity in renal function (see later). The environment can be controlled by nursing this type of infant in an incubator.
- *Alimentary system* – necrotizing enterocolitis is an inflammatory condition of the bowel leading to necrosis, and is thought to be secondary to alterations in gut blood flow, hypotension, hypoxia, infection and feeding practices. Feeding problems are common in preterm infants because they have immature sucking and swallowing reflexes, and poor gut motility. Parenteral nutrition is usually required in these very premature infants with gradually increasing volumes of milk given by nasogastric tube.
- *Liver and gallbladder* – jaundice (hyperbilirubinaemia) secondary to liver immaturity and a shorter half-life of red blood cells is common in premature infants. Treatment with phototherapy is required because premature infants are at greater risk of bilirubin encephalopathy.
- *Kidney and urinary tract* – immaturity if the kidneys can lead to poor ability to concentrate or dilute urine. This can result in dehydration and electrolyte disturbances: hypernatraemia and hyponatraemia, hyperkalaemia and metabolic acidosis.
- *Neurological* – periventricular and intraventricular haemorrhage result from bleeding from the immature, rich capillary bed of the germinal matrix lining the ventricles. Such haemorrhages are more likely in the presence of hypoxia. Major degrees of haemorrhage can result in hydrocephalus and neurological abnormalities such as cerebral palsy. Periventricular leucomalacia is ischaemic necrosis in the white matter surrounding the lateral ventricles, and commonly leads to cerebral palsy.

## CASE HISTORY 2

A 16-year-old woman is admitted to the labour ward at 38 weeks' gestation. She gives a history suggestive of rupture of membranes and is experiencing uterine contractions. She was seen at 10 weeks gestation for consideration of termination of pregnancy and had a scan at that time which confirmed the gestational age. She opted to continue with the pregnancy but did not attend for antenatal care. She admitted to smoking 20 cigarettes per day. Vaginal examination confirms that the cervix is 8 cm dilated. A cardiotocograph demonstrates a baseline fetal heart rate of 165 beats per minute (bpm) with variable decelerations, and a fetal scalp pH is 7.14 with a base deficit of 12 mmol/L. A Caesarean section is performed and a male infant weighing 1900 g is delivered. Apgar scores are 3 at 1 minute and 8 at 5 minutes.

### Which complications are such severely growth-restricted infants particularly at risk of?

Reduced oxygen supply *in utero* can result in the fetus being *stillborn* or suffering damage from acute *asphyxia*. In the latter case, the neonate may demonstrate features of *hypoxic ischaemic encephalopathy* (HIE), which may lead to death from multiorgan failure. If the infant survives, neurological damage and *cerebral palsy* may result. Chronic hypoxia *in utero* can also result in neurological damage without the acute manifestations of HIE. Other consequences of reduced oxygen supply *in utero* include increased *haematopoiesis* and *cardiac failure*. Increased haemopoiesis can in turn result in coagulopathy, polycythaemia and jaundice in the newborn.

Neonatal *hypothermia* and *hypoglycaemia* are also more common in this type of infant and result from reduced body fat and glycogen stores. Both of these conditions, if untreated, can lead to increased mortality and neurological damage.

Reduced supply of amino acids *in utero* can impair immune function increasing the risk of *infection* in the newborn.

Growth-restricted babies are also at increased risk of *chronic diseases*, such as coronary heart disease, stroke, hypertension and non-insulin-dependent diabetes in adulthood. This is thought to be because the fetal adaptation to undernutrition *in utero* results in the permanent resetting of homeostatic mechanisms and this leads to later disease.

### Key Points

Determinants of birth weight are multifactorial, and reflect the influence of the natural growth potential of the fetus and the intrauterine environment. The following applies to normal fetal development:

- The fetal circulation is quite different from that of the adult. Its distinctive features are:
  - oxygenation occurs in the placenta not the lungs;
  - the right and left ventricles work in parallel rather than in series;
  - the heart, brain and upper body receive highly oxygenated blood from the left ventricle via the umbilical vein while the placenta and lower body receive mixed blood from both right and left ventricles.
- Surfactant prevents collapse of small alveoli in the lung during expiration by lowering surface tension. Its production is maximal after 28 weeks. Respiratory distress syndrome (RDS) usually occurs in babies born prematurely and is associated with surfactant deficiency.
- The fetus requires an effective immune system to resist intrauterine and perinatal infections. Lymphocytes appear from 8 weeks and, by the middle of the second trimester, all phagocytic cells, T and B cells, and complement are available to mount a response.
- Fetal skin protects and facilitates homeostasis.
- *In utero*, the normal metabolic functions of the liver are performed by the placenta. The loss of the placental route of excretion of unconjugated bilirubin, in face of conjugating enzyme deficiencies, particularly in the premature infant' may result in physiological jaundice of the newborn.
- Growth-restricted and premature infants have deficient glycogen stores; this renders them prone to neonatal hypoglycaemia.

## Reference

National Institute for Clinical Excellence. *Antenatal care: routine care for the healthy pregnant woman.* London: RCOG Press, 2003.

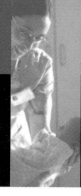

# Physiological changes in pregnancy

## OVERVIEW

This chapter will outline the major maternal physiological adaptations to pregnancy. An in-depth knowledge of the altered physiology in pregnancy is essential for midwives to enhance understanding of the so-called 'minor disorders of pregnancy' and to enable identification of more serious complications that require referral. This chapter begins at a cellular level, examines the individual systems and concludes with some of the more common 'minor' disorders of pregnancy. Some of these conditions arise because the physiological changes of pregnancy exacerbate many irritating symptoms that in the normal non-pregnant state would not require specific treatment. These 'minor' problems of pregnancy are in no way dangerous to the woman but can be troublesome on a day-to-day basis; most are considerably improved by simple treatments or helpful advice.

## Systemic changes

### Volume homeostasis

One of the most fundamental systemic changes of normal pregnancy is fluid retention, which accounts for between 8 and 10 kg of the average maternal weight gain of 11–13 kg. There is some increase in intracellular water but the most marked expansion occurs in extracellular fluid volume, especially circulating plasma volume (Figure 4.1).

This change is pivotal to a series of other physiological adaptations, notably increases in cardiac output and in renal blood flow. It also has important consequences for the interpretation of haematological

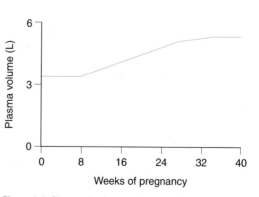

**Figure 4.1** Changes in plasma volume during normal human pregnancy. There is an increase in mean values from 3 L in the non-pregnant state to between 4 and 4.5 L during late pregnancy (between 30 and 50 per cent).

indices in normal pregnancy. Relatively larger increases in plasma volume have been reported in women taking regular exercise during pregnancy and relatively smaller increases occur in the pregnancy complications of intrauterine growth restriction (IUGR) and pre-eclampsia.

The precise mechanisms responsible for this important adaptation remain uncertain. In the non-pregnant situation, sodium is the most important determinant of extracellular fluid volume. There is a net retention of sodium during normal pregnancy, amounting to a total of 900 mmol (or 3–4 mmol per day). In keeping with this finding are the very marked increases in the concentration of the antinatriuretic hormones, aldosterone and deoxycorticosterone observed during pregnancy. However, natriuretic factors, such as atrial natriuretic peptide and progesterone, also increase during pregnancy. Furthermore, a substantial proportion of the retained sodium must be sequestered within fetal tissues (including placenta, membranes and amniotic fluid). Maternal plasma sodium concentration actually decreases slightly during pregnancy and it is, therefore, possible that other factors, such as alterations in intracellular metabolism, may also contribute to the fluid retention.

One noteworthy feature of this change in fluid homeostasis is that plasma osmolality decreases by about 10 mosmol/kg. In the non-pregnant state, such a marked decrease would be associated with a rapid diuresis in order to maintain volume homeostasis. However, the pregnant woman appears to accept this new level of osmolality, as evidenced by infusion experiments where urinary concentration is regulated in order to maintain the new equilibrium. Interestingly, there is also evidence of a decrease in the thirst threshold so that pregnant women feel the urge to drink at a lower level of plasma osmolality than they do in the non-pregnant state.

Not only does plasma osmotic pressure decrease during pregnancy but oncotic pressure (colloid osmotic pressure) is also markedly reduced. Plasma oncotic pressure is predominantly determined by the concentration of albumin, and this decreases by about 20 per cent during normal pregnancy to levels (28–37 g/L), which would be considered pathological in a non-pregnant person. The significance of this change is that plasma oncotic pressure is a major contributor to the Starling equilibrium, which determines the degree to which fluid passes into and out of capillaries (including glomerular capillaries). Thus the decrease in plasma oncotic pressure is one of the factors responsible for the marked increase that occurs in glomerular filtration rate during normal pregnancy. It is also likely to contribute to the development of peripheral oedema, a feature of normal, uncomplicated pregnancy.

The factors contributing to fluid retention are:
- sodium retention;
- resetting of osmostat;
- decrease in thirst threshold;
- decrease in plasma oncotic pressure;
  Consequences of fluid retention are:
- haemoglobin concentration falls;
- haematocrit falls;
- serum albumin concentration falls;
- stroke volume increases;
- renal blood flow increases.

## Blood

The marked increase in plasma volume associated with normal pregnancy causes dilution of many circulating factors. Of particular note is the haemodilution of red blood cells. Although pregnancy is associated with an increase in the production of erythrocytes, this increase is outstripped by the relative increase in plasma volume. Thus haematological indices, which depend upon the proportion of plasma in a measured blood sample, tend to decrease. Such indices include red cell count, haematocrit and haemoglobin concentration.

The mean haemoglobin concentration falls from 13.3 g/dL in the non-pregnant state to 10.9 g/dL at the 36th week of normal pregnancy. This physiological change may be mistaken for the development of pathological anaemia, most commonly owing to iron deficiency. Pregnant women require increased amounts of iron and absorption of dietary iron from the gut is increased. Despite this adaptation, women who do not take supplementary iron during pregnancy show a reduction in stainable iron in the bone marrow as well as a progressive reduction in mean cell volume and serum ferritin. Therefore, pregnant women are often given 'prophylactic' haematinics, notably oral iron. This drug can cause unpleasant side effects, including nausea and constipation. Pregnant women are already predisposed to these symptoms, making compliance with oral iron therapy a well-recognized problem.

The use of supplementary oral iron in pregnancy is controversial. Most would agree that it is indicated if the haemoglobin concentration is less than 10 g/dL, although others have higher cut-off levels. Iron stores are most reliably assessed using serum ferritin measurements. Iron deficiency is endemic in certain parts of the world and there are many women who for personal or cultural reasons take a diet that is relatively deficient in iron. Furthermore, certain pregnant women, such as those with multiple gestations, have a greater than normal dietary iron requirement. Iron supplementation should, therefore, be considered after careful assessment of individual need.

Folic acid supplementation is also widely advocated to prevent macrocytic anaemia. Renal clearance of folic acid increases substantially during normal pregnancy and plasma folate concentrations fall. However, red cell folate concentrations do not decrease to the same extent. Routine folate supplementation for haematinic purposes in women eating an adequate diet and carrying a single fetus is not indicated. However, there is clear evidence that supplementation with folic acid over the time of conception and during the first trimester of pregnancy can reduce the frequency of neural tube defects (see Chapter 7).

Unlike red blood cells, white cell concentrations do not show a dilutional decrease during normal pregnancy. Conversely, the total white cell count increases, and the average value during the third trimester is $9 \times 10^9$/L. This is predominantly because of a substantial increase in the numbers of polymorphonuclear leucocytes. This is especially marked during the immediate puerperium, when values of greater than $20 \times 10^9$/L have been found in healthy women. Alterations in the concentrations of other circulating white cells, including both T and B lymphocytes, are relatively slight in comparison with these changes in neutrophils. There is, however, a slight reduction in the platelet count, with an increased proportion of larger younger platelets.

There are also substantial changes in coagulation during normal human pregnancy, producing a hypercoagulable state. There are significant increases in the production of several procoagulant factors and a reduction in plasma fibrinolytic activity. There is a marked increase in plasma fibrinogen concentration. This is thought to be responsible for the substantial augmentation of erythrocyte sedimentation rate that occurs during pregnancy, since it enhances rouleaux formation. The need for relative hypercoagulability is particularly apparent at the time of placental separation. At term, about 600 mL of blood flows through the placental bed per minute. Without effective and rapid haemostasis, a woman could die from exsanguination within a few minutes. Myometrial contraction is the first line of defence, compressing the blood vessels

supplying the placental bed (see Figure 4.5). Almost immediately fibrin begins to be deposited over the placental site and, ultimately, between 5 and 10 per cent of all of the fibrinogen in the circulation is used up for this purpose. Factors that impede this haemostatic process, such as inadequate uterine contraction or incomplete placental separation, therefore, can rapidly lead to depletion of fibrinogen reserve.

The disadvantage of the potentially life-saving physiological adjustment of hypercoagulation is the substantially increased risks of thromboembolism. Venous thromboembolism remains the largest cause of direct maternal death in the UK (Lewis and Drife 2004). Venous stasis in the lower limbs is a result of reduced venous return caused by the growing uterus and can result in thrombosis.

### 🔑 Key Points

**Haematological changes**
Decreases in:
- red cell count
- haemoglobin concentration
- haematocrit
- plasma folate concentration.
Increases in:
- white cell count
- erythrocyte sedimentation rate
- fibrinogen concentration.

## Cardiovascular system

Early pregnancy is characterized by peripheral vasodilatation. The precise order of events causing this phenomenon is speculative but there is evidence to implicate vasoactive factors derived from the endothelium, such as nitric oxide. Initially, the vasodilatation appears to be perceived centrally as circulatory underfill, similar to that which might occur following haemorrhage. A significant increase in heart rate can be demonstrated as early as the fifth week of pregnancy (3 weeks after conception) and this contributes to an increase in cardiac output detectable at this time.

Cardiac output = Stroke volume × heart rate

However, the increase in stroke volume cannot be detected until several weeks later. This presumably occurs when plasma volume expands, following fluid retention by the mechanisms described above.

Further changes in the factors regulating cardiac output continue as pregnancy advances (Table 4.1 and Figure 4.2). A progressive increase in heart rate continues until the third trimester of pregnancy, when rates are typically 10–15 beats per minute (bpm) greater than those found in the non-pregnant state. There is also a progressive augmentation of stroke volume (10–20 mL) during the first half of pregnancy, probably related to the incremental changes in plasma volume at this time. As a consequence of these changes, cardiac output increases from an average of less than 5 L/min before pregnancy to approximately 7 L/min at the 20th week of pregnancy. Thereafter changes are less dramatic. During the third trimester, the gravid uterus impairs venous return to the heart in the supine position. A proportion of women will in consequence develop significant supine hypotension and loss of consciousness is possible. By rolling over on to her left side, cardiac output is almost instantly restored. This is also of significance when administering cardiac compressions for resuscitative measures and, as such, efforts must be made to displace the uterus by maternal positioning or by manual displacement.

Up to 95 per cent of women will develop a systolic murmur that disappears after delivery due to normal changes in heart sounds during pregnancy.

## Key Points

**Cardiovascular changes in pregnancy**
- Heart rate increases (10–20 per cent)
- Stroke volume increases (10 per cent)
- Cardiac output increases (30–50 per cent)
- Mean arterial pressure decreases (10 per cent)
- Peripheral resistance decreases (35 per cent).

Despite the marked increases in circulating plasma volume and in cardiac output described above, the greater part of normal pregnancy is characterized by a reduction in arterial blood pressure (Figure 4.3). This implies that there must be very substantial decreases in total peripheral vascular resistance during pregnancy and the mechanisms responsible for this dramatic alteration are not fully elucidated. Peripheral arterial tone is the result of a balance of opposing vasoconstrictor and vasodilator influences and, since

**Table 4.1** – Changes in cardiac output with labour

| | Increase in cardiac output (%) |
|---|---|
| Latent phase (cervix <3 cm dilated) | 17 |
| Active labour | 23 |
| Late first stage/second stage | 34 |

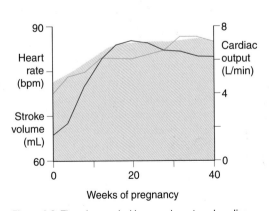

**Figure 4.2** There is a marked increase in maternal cardiac output during pregnancy. Increases in both heart rate and stroke volume contribute but changes in these components are not synchronous.

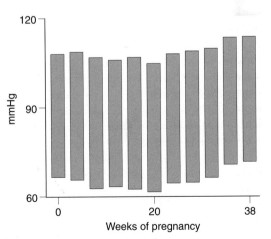

**Figure 4.3** Arterial blood pressure decreases during the first half of pregnancy but gradually increases during the third trimester. This has major implications for the management of hypertensive disorders during pregnancy.

substantial alterations have been reported in the production of both types of agents, it is unlikely that a single simple unifying hypothesis will be sufficient to explain this remarkable physiological phenomenon.

High blood pressure is a major contributor to maternal and perinatal disease and death (Lewis and Drife 2004). The accurate measurement of maternal blood pressure is, therefore, of critical importance in the assessment of pregnancy. The decrease in diastolic blood pressure is more marked during the antenatal period than the decrease in systolic pressure. Thus early pregnancy is associated with a relative increase in pulse pressure. Later, however, diastolic blood pressure increases significantly to levels that are at least equivalent to those found in the non-pregnant state. The precise determination of diastolic pressure is, therefore, critically important. Recent studies have demonstrated that more reproducible and accurate measurements are obtained when the fifth Korotkoff sound (disappearance of sounds) is used rather than the fourth (muffling). This should be standard practice in pregnancy as should be recording of the blood pressure with manual equipment following any detection of a critical reading with an electronic apparatus.

## Reproductive organs

### The uterus

Changes in circulating hormone concentrations markedly affect the tissues of the genital tract. The uterus is formed from fusion of the two Mullerian ducts in the midline, which gives rise to the adult structure of the uterus comprising three layers. These are: a thin inner layer of circular muscle fibres; a thin outer layer consisting predominantly of longitudinal muscle fibres; and a thicker central layer of interlocking fibres. In addition, the ratio of muscle to connective tissue increases from the lower part of the uterus towards the fundus. High levels of maternal oestradiol and progesterone stimulate both hyperplasia and hypertrophy of the myometrial cells, increasing the weight of the uterus from 50–60 g prior to pregnancy to 1000 g by term.

In early pregnancy, uterine growth is independent of the growing fetus and occurs equally rapidly with an ectopic pregnancy. As gestation increases, myometrial cell division is less important and hypertrophy of

individual cells accounts for most of the increase in uterine size. The growing size of the uterine contents is an important stimulus at this stage, with individual muscle fibres increasing in length by up to 15-fold. In the second half of pregnancy, a growth-restricted fetus (see Chapter 10) may be detected on abdominal palpation, by finding a uterine size smaller than expected for gestational age.

The uterine arteries also undergo hypertrophy in the first half of pregnancy, although, in the second half of gestation, the increasing uterine distension is matched by arterial stretching. The spiral arteries are invaded by the trophoblastic tissue and lose their vasoactive response; this occurs around 10–16 weeks and again around 16–20 weeks. If this secondary invasion does not occur, the vessels retain the ability to constrict and reduce the blood flow to the intervillous spaces; this is associated with pre-eclampsia and the growth-restricted fetus (see Chapter 10).

As well as changes in the size and number of myometrial cells, specialized cellular connections also develop with increasing gestation. These intercellular gap junctions allow changes in membrane potential to spread rapidly from one cell to another, facilitating the spread of membrane depolarization, and subsequent myometrial contraction. As these junctions mature, uterine contractions become more frequent. These are apparent initially as Braxton-Hicks painless contractions from 8 weeks of pregnancy that are increasingly apparent to the woman in the second half of pregnancy. Subsequently, these allow the pacemaker activity of the uterine fundus to promote the coordinated fundal-dominant contractions necessary for labour.

Conventionally, the uterus is divided into the lower and upper segments. The lower segment is the part of the uterus and upper cervix that lies between the attachment of the peritoneum of the uterovesical pouch superiorly and the level of the internal cervical os inferiorly. This part of the uterus contains fewer muscle and blood vessels, is thinner and is the site of incision for the majority of Caesarean sections.

Immediately after the placenta has separated from the wall of the uterus, the interlocking muscle fibres of the uterus contract (Figure 4.4). This occludes the blood vessels that were supplying the placenta and reduces blood loss. If the placenta has been attached to the lower uterine segment, the relative lack of oblique muscles in this part of the uterus makes the haemostatic mechanism less efficient, and postpartum haemorrhage can occur.

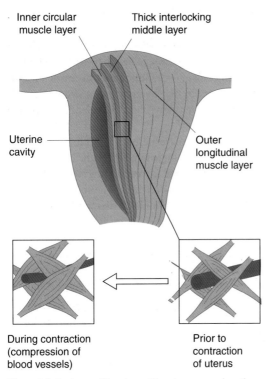

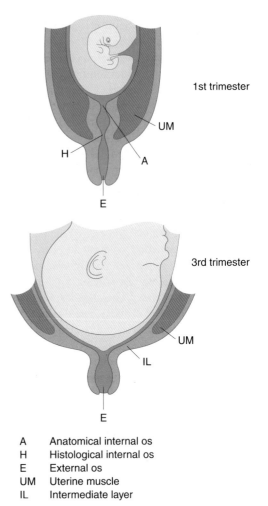

During contraction (compression of blood vessels)

Prior to contraction of uterus

**Figure 4.4** Anatomy of the uterus. The uterus comprises three muscle layers, derived from the layers of the Mullerian ducts. The muscle fibres in the inner layer are arranged in a predominantly circular pattern. The thicker intermediate layer comprises interlocked (oblique) muscle fibres. The outer layer of muscle fibres runs longitudinally, over the fundus.

### The cervix

Under the influence of oestradiol and progesterone, the cervix becomes swollen and softer during pregnancy (Figure 4.5). Oestradiol stimulates growth of the columnar epithelium of the cervical canal that becomes visible on the ectocervix and is called an ectropion. This is of significance as it is a less robust epithelium and is prone to contact bleeding. The cervix is often described as looking 'bluer' during pregnancy. This is a function of increased vascularity. In addition to these changes, the mucus glands of the cervix become distended and increase in complexity. Prostaglandins induce a remodelling of cervical collagen, particularly towards the end of gestation, whilst collagenase released from leucocytes also aids in softening the cervix; during pregnancy, progesterone inhibits this process.

Under the influence of oestrogens, the vaginal epithelium becomes thicker during pregnancy and there is an increased rate of desquamation resulting

| A | Anatomical internal os |
| H | Histological internal os |
| E | External os |
| UM | Uterine muscle |
| IL | Intermediate layer |

**Figure 4.5** Formation of the lower uterine segment. With increasing gestation, uterine stretch occurs. This has the effect of drawing the anatomical internal cervical os (A) further from the histological internal cervical os (H). The retraction of the thick intermediate layer (IL) of muscle with increasing gestation thins the lower segment.

in increased vaginal discharge during pregnancy. This discharge has a more acid pH than non-pregnant vaginal secretions (4.5–5.0) and may protect against ascending infection. Yeast infections, however, thrive in this environment, predisposing to candidiasis (see Chapter 13). The vagina also becomes more vascular with increasing gestation.

### Breasts and lactation

Cyclical changes are seen in breast tissue in response to the menstrual cycle and, during pregnancy, these

Lactation is promoted by early frequent suckling, which stimulates both the anterior and posterior pituitary to release prolactin and oxytocin, respectively. Stress and fear reduce the synthesis and release of prolactin through increased dopamine (prolactin inhibitory factor) synthesis. During the first 2 or 3 days of the puerperium, prolactin promotes breast engorgement, as the alveoli become distended with milk. Oxytocin released from the posterior pituitary causes contraction in myoepithelial cells surrounding the alveoli and small ducts. This squeezes milk into the larger ducts and subareolar reservoirs. In addition, oxytocin may inhibit dopamine release, further promoting successful lactation (Figure 4.6).

## The gastrointestinal tract

Vasodilatation, such as occurs in pregnancy, results from the relaxation of vascular smooth muscle. Other organs that have a significant component of smooth muscle also exhibit a change in function during pregnancy. Thus, in the alimentary tract, there is delay in gastric emptying (important in the management of women requiring general anaesthesia owing to the risk of Mendelson's syndrome) and reduced colonic motility (contributing to constipation). Other gastrointestinal changes are discussed under minor disorders later in the chapter.

## The urinary tract and renal function

Similarly, the urinary tract becomes dilated during pregnancy. By the third trimester, about 97 per cent of women have been shown to have some evidence of stasis or hydronephrosis. This physical change, together with certain alterations in the composition of the urine itself (see later), predispose pregnant women to ascending urinary tract infection, a common and important complication of pregnancy.

One consequence of vasodilatation, reduction in blood pressure, has already been discussed. Another important consequence is increase in blood flow. There is evidence that pregnant women increase blood flow to many organs, notably the uterus, breasts and skin (hence the glow of health with pregnancy). There is also a marked (60–75 per cent) increase in renal blood flow. This leads to a substantial augmentation

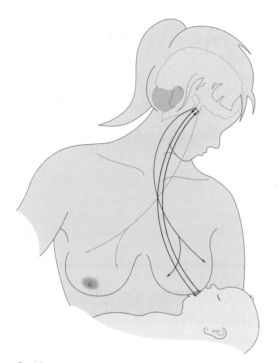

Suckling causes:
Afferent signals to posterior pituitary increasing oxytocin release, inducing myoepithelial cells to contract and express milk.
Afferent signals to anterior pituitary increasing prolactin release, thus increasing milk synthesis.

**Figure 4.6** Schematic representation of lactation. Suckling induces afferent signals to the anterior and posterior pituitary. This results in the release of prolactin and oxytocin. Prolactin induces milk production by the glandular tissue of the breast. Oxytocin causes contraction of the myoepithelial cells surrounding the glandular ducts, squeezing milk towards the nipple.

changes are amplified. There is considerable deposition of fat around the glandular tissue. The number of glandular ducts is increased by oestrogen, whilst progesterone [and human placental lactogen (hPL)] increases the number of gland alveoli. hPL may also stimulate alveolar casein, lactoglobulin and lactalbumin synthesis.

Although the serum prolactin concentration increases throughout pregnancy, it does not result in lactation, as its effect is antagonized at an alveolar receptor level by oestrogen. It is the rapid fall in oestrogen concentration over the first 48 hours after birth that removes this inhibition and allows lactation to begin. Towards the end of pregnancy and in the early puerperium, the breasts produce colostrum, a thick yellow secretion, rich in immunoglobulins.

of glomerular filtration rate, by about 50 per cent (Figure 4.7). Filtration of the plasma is of critical importance in the maintenance of fluid balance, the excretion of waste products and the regulation of essential nutrients.

The increase in glomerular filtration rate is responsible for an increase in the clearance of a number of substances from the bloodstream. Thus the plasma concentrations of urea and creatinine, used as markers for the severity of renal disease, are reduced during normal pregnancy. It is important to use appropriate pregnancy-specific normal ranges when managing both normal pregnancies and those in women with renal diseases. There is also an increase in total protein excretion (particularly microalbuminuria) during pregnancy. The upper limit of urinary protein excretion in pregnancy increases to 0.3 g per day.

Glycosuria, which is rare in the absence of diabetes in the non-pregnant state, is very common during pregnancy. Glycosuria varies during any given pregnancy and does not relate reliably to disorders of carbohydrate metabolism. It is not a reliable screen for gestational diabetes. The increase in glomerular filtration rate may be partially responsible for this glycosuria and a reabsorptive mechanism in the proximal renal tubule may become saturated so that the

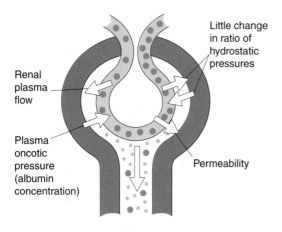

Renal plasma flow

Plasma oncotic pressure (albumin concentration)

Little change in ratio of hydrostatic pressures

Permeability

● Plasma protein     · Other solute

**Figure 4.7** Factors contributing to enhanced glomerular filtration during pregnancy. The marked increase in renal blood flow is the major factor, but there are significant contributions from the decrease in plasma oncotic pressure and enhanced permeability. Although systemic arterial pressure decreases during pregnancy, there is little difference in the relative pressures at either end of the glomerular capillary loop nor in intrarenal pressure.

'renal threshold' is exceeded, explaining the increased amount of this solute in the urine. Glucose reabsorption occurs secondarily to the absorption of sodium and, therefore, other factors contributing to volume homeostasis and sodium retention may be involved in the physiological glycosuria in pregnancy.

### ⚲ Key Points

**Renal changes**
- Blood flow increases (60–75 per cent)
- Glomerular filtration increases (50 per cent)
- Clearance of most substances is enhanced
- Plasma creatinine, urea and urate are reduced
- Glycosuria is normal.

## Respiratory tract

Increases in cardiac output affect both sides of the heart. Therefore, pregnancy is associated with very substantial increases in pulmonary blood flow. There is also a significant increase in tidal volume and the lungs are, therefore, able to function more efficiently, facilitating gas transfer. In consequence, there is a marked decrease (15–20 per cent) in the partial pressure of carbon dioxide, $PCO_2$. Furthermore, there is a slight increase in the partial pressure of oxygen, $PO_2$. These changes facilitate gas transfer to and from the fetus.

During pregnancy, there is an increase in 2,3-diphosphoglycerate (2,3-DPG) concentration within maternal erythrocytes. This anion, which binds preferentially to deoxygenated haemoglobin, promotes the release of oxygen from the red cell at relatively lower levels of haemoglobin saturation; this increases the availability of oxygen within the tissues. Furthermore, the fetus is also adapted to take maximum advantage of this alteration in maternal physiology and oxygen transfer from mother to fetus is facilitated.

There are significant changes in the mechanical aspects of ventilation during pregnancy. These are of particular importance in the management of women with chronic respiratory diseases. Dyspnoea is a common symptom during normal pregnancy. Even in dyspnoeic women, the enhanced ventilation of pregnancy appears to result from increased tidal volume rather than from an increase in respiratory rate. In pregnancy, the ribcage is displaced upwards and increases in transverse diameter; such changes improve airflow along the bronchial tree to compensate for the decrease in the vital capacity of the lungs. Women with respiratory problems tend to deteriorate less during pregnancy than those with other chronic disorders, such as cardiac failure. The physiological changes do not affect the interpretation tests of ventilation, such as forced expiratory volume in one second (FEV1) and peak expiratory flow rate. Therefore, these tests may be used in the management of pregnant asthmatics and women with other obstructive pulmonary disorders.

### Key Points

**Blood gas and acid–base changes**
- $PCO_2$ decreases (15–20 per cent)
- $PO_2$ increases (slight)
- Oxygen availability to placenta and tissues improves
- pH alters little
- bicarbonate excretion increases.

**Ventilatory changes**
- Thoracic anatomy changes
- Tidal volume increases
- Vital capacity decreases
- Functional residual capacity decreases.

### Hormones produced within the pregnant uterus

**Pregnancy-specific**
- Human chorionic gonadotrophin (hCG)
- Human placental lactogen (hPL)

**Hypothalamus-related**
- Gonadotrophin-releasing hormone (GnRH)
- Corticotrophin-releasing factor (CRF)

**Pituitary-related**
- Prolactin
- Human growth hormone (hGH)
- Adrenocorticotrophic hormone (ACTH)

**Other peptides**
- Insulin-like growth factor I and II (IGF)
- 1,25-Dihydroxycholecalciferol
- Parathyroid hormone-related peptide
- Renin
- Angiotensin II

**Steroids**
- Oestradiol
- Progesterone

Note that this list is not exhaustive.

### Endocrinological changes

Complex endocrinological changes occur in pregnancy. Many of the peptide and steroid hormones, produced by the endocrine glands in the non-pregnant state, are produced by intrauterine tissues during pregnancy (see box). The precise contributions of these alternative sources to circulating concentrations of hormones, as well as their possible feedback activities, are not fully understood. Many hormones exert their actions indirectly, by interacting with cytokines and chemokines. The production and activity of many of these substances are also significantly altered during human pregnancy.

Many pregnancy-specific peptides are produced within the uterus but not all have been shown to have definite endocrine roles. Of those that have, the best known is human chorionic gonadotrophin (hCG). This hormone is composed of alpha- and beta-subunits and the beta-subunit is pregnancy specific, being widely used in modern practice as a sensitive pregnancy test. The hormone is produced by trophoblast cells and is detectable within the maternal circulation in small quantities within days of implantation. Production of hCG is influenced both by the cytokine leukaemia inhibitory factor (LIF) and by an isoform of gonadotrophin-releasing hormone (GnRH), which is also produced within the placenta. hCG has a major role during early pregnancy in maintaining the function of the corpus luteum. When the importance of this ovarian source of maternal progesterone diminishes (as placental production of progesterone becomes dominant during the later weeks of the first trimester) concentrations of circulating hCG decrease from peak values around the tenth week of pregnancy to plateau after the 12th week (Figure 4.8).

The alpha-subunit of hCG differs only slightly from the alpha-subunits of luteinizing hormone (LH), follicle-stimulating hormone (FSH) and thyroid-stimulating hormone (TSH) and can interact with receptors for at least some of these hormones. For example, hCG is widely used clinically in assisted reproduction to mimic the physiological LH surge in order to induce ovulation from stimulated ovarian follicles. During normal pregnancy, hCG suppresses secretion of FSH and LH by the gonadotrophs of the anterior pituitary gland, perhaps by similar hormone–receptor interaction at the hypothalamic level.

Human placental lactogen, another peptide produced from the placenta, has partial homology with both prolactin and human growth hormone (hGH). hPL has major effects upon maternal production of these hormones (see later).

Sex steroid hormones are produced in large quantities by the placenta and fetus. Concentrations of oestrogens, including the active hormone oestradiol, and progesterone increase substantially from the earliest weeks of pregnancy, then plateau for the remainder of the pregnancy. These hormones were previously used to assess fetal well-being but this practice has been superseded by more specific biophysical methods. Both oestrogen and progesterone have effects upon the myometrium (oestrogen encourages cellular hypertrophy, whereas progesterone discourages contraction) and, together with prolactin, upon the tissues of the breast (see 'The breast', page 279). It is likely that they exert effects on many other target tissues during pregnancy, such as the smooth muscle of the vascular tree and of the urinary and gastrointestinal tracts.

Concentrations of prolactin reach levels during pregnancy that would be considered pathological in a non-pregnant woman. Oestrogen may have a stimulatory role in this process and hPL may be inhibitory. The endocrinological mechanisms that regulate prolactin production in the non-pregnant state, such as sleep (which increases prolactin concentrations) and dopamine agonists (which reduce them) remain effective during pregnancy. Therefore, prolactin production by the lactotrophs of the anterior pituitary gland probably continues despite intrauterine production especially from cells within the decidua. Receptors for prolactin are present on trophoblast cells and within the amniotic fluid. The increased prolactin production is essential for lactation.

In contrast to prolactin, there is evidence that hGH production by the anterior pituitary gland is suppressed during pregnancy. A reduction has been reported in the number of pituitary somatotrophs and responses to conventional provocation tests are blunted. Circulating concentrations of hGH are also reduced during pregnancy. It is likely that hPL suppresses hGH release by the maternal pituitary: In women who have a pregnancy in which hPL is deficient (e.g. in trophoblastic disease), it appears that pituitary growth hormone production is not suppressed.

## Factors controlling carbohydrate metabolism

During the first half of pregnancy, fasting plasma glucose concentrations are reduced but there is relatively little change in plasma insulin levels. A standard oral glucose tolerance test at this time shows an enhanced response compared to the non-pregnant state, with a normal pattern of insulin release but reduced blood glucose values. This pattern changes during the second half of pregnancy, at least in women who take a Western-style diet. There is a delay in reaching peak glucose values and an increase in these values throughout the test despite significant increases in plasma insulin concentrations, a pattern suggestive of relative insulin resistance. This change may involve hPL or other growth-related hormones, which reduce peripheral insulin sensitivity. Pregnancy is also associated with alterations in the characteristics of insulin binding to its receptor, similar to those described in non-pregnant women who are obese or have non-insulin-dependent diabetes mellitus. If such women become pregnant, they are liable to have babies of higher mean birth weight than normal women. Whether this phenomenon

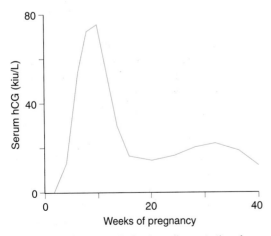

**Figure 4.8** Serial changes in the plasma concentration of human chorionic gonadotrophin (hCG) during pregnancy. Note the marked increment during the first trimester.

results from increased transplacental transfer of glucose or from the growth-promoting characteristics of insulin and somatomedins (see earlier) is unclear.

## Thyroid function

Human chorionic gonadotrophin has thyrotrophic activity (perhaps as a result of alpha-subunit homology with TSH) and maternal TSH production may be suppressed during the first trimester of pregnancy, when hCG levels are maximal. The TSH response to injection of thyrotrophin-releasing hormone (TRH) is blunted during the first trimester but later returns to normal.

Some have suggested a role for hCG or TSH in the nausea and vomiting often experienced by normal pregnant women, which usually improves after the first trimester. Hyperemesis gravidarum, an extreme and pathological form of nausea and vomiting, may be associated with a biochemical hyperthyroidism with high levels of free T4 and a suppressed TSH. In general, however, thyroid function is considered to remain normal throughout the remainder of pregnancy.

Maternal iodine requirements increase because of active transport to the fetoplacental unit and because iodine excretion in the urine is increased. Because the plasma level falls, the thyroid gland increases iodine uptake from the blood. If there is already dietary insufficiency of iodine, the thyroid gland hypertrophies in order to trap sufficient iodine.

## Factors controlling calcium metabolism

In the circulation, about 40 per cent of calcium is bound to albumin. Since plasma albumin concentrations decrease markedly during pregnancy, total plasma calcium concentrations also decrease. There is little change in the circulating concentration of unbound ionized calcium. There is a substantial fetal demand for calcium and transplacental flux rates of about 6.5 mmol per day have been calculated. Such a quantity would represent about 80 per cent of the net amount absorbed from the upper gastrointestinal tract in a non-pregnant woman. However, the pregnant woman increases absorption and slightly decreases excretion, thereby coping with little net change in transfer rates into and out of bone stores. This new equilibrium is finely poised: women who are unable to sustain this level of fetal transfer from dietary sources alone may develop osteopenia during and after pregnancy.

## Placental corticotrophin-releasing factor and the onset of human labour: the placental clock theory

From mid-pregnancy onwards, the trophoblast is able to synthesize corticotrophin-releasing factor (CRF). CRF stimulates the fetal pituitary to increase fetal adrenocorticotrophic hormone (ACTH) and thereby fetal dihydroepiandrosterone (DHEA) production by the fetal adrenal is increased. DHEA is the main precursor for placental oestrogen secretion. The high levels of oestrogens towards the end of pregnancy increase gap junction synthesis between uterine myometrial cells, aiding conduction and, therefore, regular uterine contractions. CRF synthesis is regulated in a positive feedback loop by oestrogens.

The placental regulation of its own metabolism via effects on the fetus, with subsequent effects on maternal uterine physiology and possibly the onset of labour, has been christened the placental clock theory.

## Corticosteroids and the renin–angiotensin system

Trophoblast cells produce both CRF and ACTH. These placental hormones have roles in regulating the activity of the fetal adrenal glands and the myometrium. There is a progressive increase in maternal circulating concentrations of cortisol throughout pregnancy, despite a relative decrease in the concentration of ACTH during the later weeks. Much of the cortisol is bound to cortisol-binding globulin (CBG), which doubles in concentration during pregnancy, but there is also a slight increase in unbound cortisol. The lack of diurnal fluctuation of cortisol and the attenuated response to dexamethasone suppression suggests that placental ACTH may have a role in regulating maternal cortisol levels.

Circulating concentrations of the antinatriuretic hormones aldosterone and deoxycorticosterone increase up to ten-fold in pregnancy. Progesterone has natriuretic properties and other factors that may influence aldosterone production, notably atrial natriuretic peptide and angiotensins, are produced in increased amounts during pregnancy. The increased production of angiotensins, including the vasoactive angiotensin II, is the result of an augmented production of the enzyme renin and its substrate angiotensinogen. Intrauterine tissues, both maternal and fetal in origin, also produce the elements of this system.

---

### 🔑 Key Points

**Endocrine changes**

- Prolactin concentration increases markedly
- Human growth hormone is suppressed
- Insulin resistance develops
- Thyroid function changes little
- Transplacental calcium transport is enhanced
- Corticosteroid concentrations increase.

---

## 'Minor' disorders of pregnancy

### Backache

Backache occurs frequently in pregnancy as progesterone and relaxin cause softening and relaxation of the ligaments of the pelvis. The weight of the pregnant uterus causes an exaggerated lumbar lordosis and increases back strain, leading to pain. Pregnancy can also exacerbate the symptoms of a prolapsed intervertebral disc, occasionally leading to complete immobility.

The midwife's advice to the woman should include maintenance of correct posture, limiting physical activity including lifting heavy objects, wearing low-heeled shoes and taking adequate rest. Supportive pillows beneath the knees and abdomen, and local heat applications may also help to reduce the discomfort. In order to further reduce back strain when getting up from a lying position, the woman should be advised to turn on to her side and sit up as she lowers her legs down from the bed/couch using her arms for support. A physiotherapist may teach the woman back and abdominal muscle exercises to strengthen these muscles or apply a sacroiliac or trochanteric support. Simple analgesia, such as paracetamol or paracetamol–codeine combinations may also be given to help relieve the pain. Other therapies, such as swimming, can be suggested with a cautionary note that prolonged breast stroke can increase lumbar lordosis.

### Oedema

Oedema is common and occurs to some degree in most pregnancies. There is generalized soft tissue swelling and increased capillary permeability, causing intravascular fluid to leak into the extravascular space. In pregnancy, the fingers, toes and ankles are usually worst affected, and the symptoms are aggravated by hot weather. The midwife can advise the woman to take frequent periods of rest with leg elevation in order to reduce the oedema associated the ankles and feet. Occasionally, support stockings or tights may be indicated. It is important for the midwife to recognize that generalized (rather than lower limb) oedema may be a feature of pre-eclampsia, and thus the woman's blood pressure should be assessed along with urinalysis for signs of any protein. More rarely, severe oedema may suggest underlying cardiac impairment or nephrotic syndrome.

### Carpal tunnel syndrome

Compression neuropathies occur in pregnancy owing to increased soft-tissue swelling during the second and third trimesters of pregnancy. The most common of these is carpal tunnel syndrome, where the median nerve in the wrist is susceptible to compression. The symptoms include numbness, tingling and weakness of the thumb and forefinger, with often quite severe pain occurring at night. The midwife should refer the woman to a physiotherapist for application of a light splint to support the wrist, especially at night. In addition, simple analgesia can be advised to ease the discomfort. Surgical decompression is very rarely performed in pregnancy. Although there is no realistic prospect of a cure, the symptoms usually resolve completely after the birth of the baby. However, there is a tendency for carpal tunnel syndrome to recur in subsequent pregnancies and there is also a risk of such women developing the syndrome in later life.

### Nausea and vomiting

Nausea and vomiting are common disorders affecting over 50 per cent of pregnant women, and are often most pronounced in the first trimester. Vomiting occurs when either the emetic centre in the medulla or the chemoreceptor trigger zone situated on the lateral wall of the fourth ventricle is stimulated. However, the aetiology is not proven, but it is thought that high levels of circulating hCG may contribute to the condition, and thus the symptoms are much worse in a molar or multiple pregnancy. For some pregnant women, the symptoms occur mainly upon waking and, consequently, it is often erroneously referred to as morning sickness. However, for others, the nausea and vomiting continue throughout the day. The midwife may suggest having a milky drink at bedtime, and eating a dry biscuit or cracker with a drink before rising in the morning, avoiding spicy or pungent odours, and eating small frequent meals in order to maintain the body's blood sugar levels. In addition, devices that transmit electrical stimulation via the wrist to trigger sensory and neurological impulses that control vomiting, acupuncture, homeopathic and herbal remedies may also help to minimize the discomfort of this condition. For the majority of women, the nausea and vomiting generally improves between the 16th and 22nd week of pregnancy. A small proportion of women (0.3–2 per cent) will develop a more serious condition known as *hyperemesis gravidarum* that requires urgent medical referral (see Chapter 8).

## Heartburn

This is very common in pregnancy. The symptoms are of retrosternal burning in the chest or discomfort, often on lying down. If persistent, it may be a symptom of reflux oesophagitis resulting from the regurgitation of acidic stomach contents. Heartburn is caused by the weight effect of the pregnant uterus affecting stomach emptying and the effects of progesterone relaxing the lower oesophageal (cardiac) sphincter. The woman should be advised to eat small frequent meals, and avoid fatty foods and very cold liquids. Furthermore, smoking, alcohol, coffee, chocolate and eating before bedtime may increase gastrointestinal irritation. An upright position and avoiding lying down after meals may be helpful, and nocturnal heartburn may be alleviated if the woman sleeps propped up with extra pillows. The woman may be advised that certain homeopathic remedies for heartburn may also be effective. However, should these simple measures be ineffective, referral to a doctor may be necessary. Antacids may also relieve symptoms in some women but, in cases where there are severe refractory dyspeptic symptoms, a gastroenterology referral is warranted to determine whether the cause may be a stomach ulcer or hiatus hernia.

## Constipation

In pregnancy, the general slowing down and decreased peristalsis of the colon owing to the relaxation of smooth muscle by progesterone, can give rise to constipation. In addition, the problem may be exacerbated by increased fluid absorption from the colon owing to the increased levels of aldosterone and angiotensin, and as a consequence of the administration of oral iron tablets. A high-fibre diet with extra fruit, vegetables and fluid should be encouraged. Laxatives should only be used as a short-term measure in conjunction with information and education on diet to prevent recurrence of constipation. Lactulose, a hyperosmotic mild non-stimulant laxative, is usually prescribed rather than senna preparations, which are generally badly tolerated by the pregnant woman, causing abdominal pain and discomfort.

## Varicose veins

Varicosities may develop during pregnancy in 40 per cent cases and are usually seen in the veins of the legs. However, they may also develop in the vulva and anal area as haemorrhoids. All are thought to be due to the relaxant effect of progesterone and relaxin on the smooth muscle of the vein walls and the dependent venous stasis caused by the weight of the pregnant uterus on the inferior vena cava. There is a tendency for varicose veins to become worse in later pregnancy; however, if surgical treatment is warranted, this will be reviewed following the birth of the baby.

Varicose veins of the legs may be symptomatically improved with support tights, although constricting or tight clothing should be avoided. The midwife can encourage the woman to keep her legs elevated when at rest, to increase her rest periods and avoid standing for prolonged periods. Furthermore, exercise, such as walking and swimming, and avoiding excessive weight gain should also be encouraged. Although thrombophlebitis may occur in a large varicose vein, it is more common during the postnatal period. Should a large superficial varicose vein be traumatized, it may bleed profusely and the leg must be elevated with direct pressure applied.

Although vulval and vaginal varicosities are uncommon, they can be symptomatically troublesome and the woman may require analgesia to reduce the discomfort. It is also important that trauma to the varicosity, such as lacerations, an episiotomy or the use of instruments, be minimized in order to reduce the risk of excessive bleeding arising during the birth of the baby. The discomfort associated with haemorrhoids may be improved during pregnancy with the use of local anaesthetic/anti-irritant creams and a high-fibre diet.

## Skin pigmentation

Increased pigmentation of the skin is very common in pregnancy, affecting up to 90 per cent of all pregnant women. Although the cause is unclear, it is thought to be attributed to increased oestrogen, progesterone, adrenal hormones, beta-endorphins or an increase in melanocyte-stimulating hormone. Consequently, the face (*chloasma*), nipples, areola, vulva, perineum and perianal areas darken. Freckles, naevi and abdominal scars may also darken. In addition, the tendonous midline of the linea alba that stretches from the umbilicus to the symphysis pubis, increases in pigment and becomes known in pregnancy as the linea nigra. Following childbirth, the pigmentation fades but may never completely disappear. Skin pigmentation may be more noticeable in darker skinned women.

## Striae gravidarum (stretch marks)

Striae gravidarum may appear as red–purple linear streaks on the breasts, abdomen, thighs and buttocks during pregnancy as the tension within the dermal layer of the skin is increased. It is thought that their appearance may be related to increased levels of free cortisol during pregnancy. Following pregnancy, the striae fade to a silver colour. Despite there being a number of topical preparations available, their use remains controversial as none have been proven to reduce/prevent the development of striae.

## Other common 'minor' disorders

These are:
- itching;
- urinary incontinence;
- nose bleeds;
- thrush (vaginal candidiasis);
- headache:
- fainting;
- breast soreness;
- tiredness;
- altered taste sensation;
- insomnia;
- leg cramps.

---

### ⚲ Key Points

**'Minor' disorders of pregnancy**
The following are the most common 'minor' disorders of pregnancy:
- Backache: usually low back, aggravated by movement
- Heartburn: worse on lying down, better when sitting up
- Varicose veins and piles: often coexist, worse if pre-existing
- Carpal tunnel syndrome: worse at night, may require splint
- Oedema: worse in hot weather and when walking, better when resting with the feet up.

---

## Reference

Lewis G, Drife J (eds). *Confidential Enquiry into Maternal and Child Health; why mothers die 2000–2002*. Sixth report of the confidential enquiries into maternal deaths in the UK. London: RCOG Press, 2004.

## Key additional reading

Stables D, Rankin J (eds). *Physiology in childbearing: with anatomy and related biosciences,* 2nd edition. London: Elsevier, 2005.

Wylie L. *Essential anatomy and physiology in maternity care.* Edinburgh: Churchill Livingstone, 2000.

# Antenatal care

## OVERVIEW

The aim of antenatal care is to provide effective and holistic care for the mother, her baby and her family through appropriate screening, preventative and treatment interventions. The midwife has a significant role in the care and support of the mother, her baby and family in respect to their physical, psychological, social and spiritual needs. The provision of antenatal care aims to serve the multifaceted elements of this primary and public health in obtaining the best possible outcome for the mother and baby.

## Aims of antenatal care

The role and responsibilities of the midwife in accordance with the European Union (1980) *Second midwifery directive* 80/155/EEC Article 4 – 'activities of a midwife' (amended by European Union Directive 89/594/EEC) are:

- to diagnose pregnancies and monitor normal pregnancies; to carry out examinations necessary for the monitoring of the development of normal pregnancies;
- to prescribe or advise on the examinations necessary for the earliest possible diagnosis of pregnancies at risk;
- to provide a programme of parenthood preparation and a complete preparation for childbirth including hygiene and nutrition.

## Confirmation of the pregnancy

Many women may experience early signs and symptoms of pregnancy. *Probable signs* of pregnancy are breast changes and tenderness, nausea and vomiting, amenorrhoea, frequency of micturition and increasing abdominal girth. *Positive signs* of pregnancy are confirmed by positive urinary or serum hormonal testing; by ultrasound scan showing a viable fetus, fetal heart sounds via a Pinard stethoscope and ultrasound sonicaid; and palpation of fetal parts and fetal movements in the second and third trimester.

## First appointments

The National Institute for Clinical Excellence (NICE 2003) guidelines recommend that the first booking visit needs to be before 12 weeks' gestation period. An in-depth medical and obstetric history-taking and a large volume of information are required to help assess and establish the risk factors of the woman, as well as a full physical examination and routine assessments (NICE 2003, Appendix F). This may determine the model of care to which the mother may be allocated. The mother will also need to be given relevant and appropriate information at this stage to help her to adjust her lifestyle and consider her options for the antenatal screening options. It is also vital to establish that the fetus is viable and establish the expected date of delivery (EDD).

## The booking examination

A thorough and in-depth assessment of the mother's past medical, surgical, obstetric and gynaecological histories is crucial in establishing the needs of the mother. The standardization of antenatal booking maternity records has been implemented by the West Midlands Perinatal Institute (WMPI) in order to help midwives to gain as much key information from the mother and her family.

Midwives should ensure that adequate time is allowed to conduct this initial booking interview; such interviews can take up to 2 hours. It should be conducted in an environment that is quiet and free from interruptions, as it is important to establish effective communications and foster a positive and trusting relationship. Many Trusts have now employed maternity 'support link workers' who help to translate for women who do not speak English as their first language to overcome communication barriers.

## Past medical history

The past and current medical, surgical and psychiatric history of a woman may play a major part in the success or failure or continuation of the pregnancy. Certain conditions, the pathology or treatments may adversely affect the fetus in a number of ways. The pregnancy may cause an improvement or deterioration in the existing medical condition. Medications taken by the mother may have potential teratogenic effects on the fetus (e.g. anticonvulsive drugs for the treatment of epilepsy). The women must have coordinated and collaborated care with the midwife, specialist medical physicians and the obstetrician.

NICE have advocated that women should be screened for psychiatric illnesses in early pregnancy and be referred for a full psychiatric assessment, as early interventions can reduce perinatal or postnatal depression (PND). Women should not be assessed antenatally using the Edinburgh Postnatal Depression Scale (EPDS), as it is not a reliable indicator for predicting the development of PND (see Chapter 18).

## Past obstetric and gynaecological history

The age ranges at either end of the reproductive ages have been linked with increased risk of pregnancy complications, such as pregnancy-induced hypertension (PIH), as well as an increased risk of chromosomal disorders (e.g. Down's syndrome). Previous obstetric complications, such as the need for a Caesarean section, will require careful discussion with the mother as to the possible mode of delivery for the impending delivery. If the mother has a history of recurrent miscarriages, there will be an increased risk of miscarriage as well as the potential for preterm labours and other associated problems. There are increasing numbers of mothers who have undergone female genital mutilation and early antenatal examination will allow effective planning for intrapartum care and mode of delivery.

## Family and social history

Family history and social factors are also key determinates in how the pregnancy may be affected. Race groups may raise concerns regarding risks such as sickle cell or thalassaemias that may affect the baby. For example, the antenatal sickle cell and thalassaemia screening programme as recommended by Department of Health is offered to all eligible parents in some Trusts, but to selected cases in others.

A family history of PIH experienced by the maternal grandmother and the pregnant woman's female siblings is likely to place the woman in a higher risk category for developing PIH.

Poor socioeconomic status of the mother may be a predisposing factor for a poorer obstetric outcome owing to poor dietary and nutritional health. Moreover, modern-day social factors, such as domestic violence and substance misuse, can cause a whole range of maternal and fetal adverse outcomes. Health care professionals should be aware of the signs of domestic violence, and offer early help and support to women who may disclose their sufferings.

## Physical examination

Historically, a full 'top to toe' physical examination was carried out at the first booking visit by either the midwife and/or the medical practitioner. This involved assessment of the respiratory and cardiovascular system and a full abdominal, pelvic and breast examination. The relevancy of this practice has been questioned and also the practice of the pelvic examination coupled with the collection of a cervical smear sample was strongly criticized, as it was associated with possible spontaneous miscarriages after the event. NICE have recommended minimal interventions for low-risk mothers and that high-risk mothers should have individualized specialist care if the need arises. Nonetheless, the midwife's top to toe examination is a simple and effective means of assessing the physical state of the mother and fetus.

The midwife should be able to ask after the mother, as to her general well-being and how she feels about her progress in the pregnancy. Moreover, the midwife will also be able to ask the mother to assess her baby's well-being.

## Investigations

There are a whole range of investigations that are offered to women antenatally. The role and responsibilities of the midwife are to ensure that she provides information that is accurate, truthful and presented in such a way that it is easily understood. The information must be objective, unbiased and evidence based, so that the mother will be able to make an informed choice about the care, and the treatments and interventions that she may receive.

NICE has recommended the following screening tests.

### Haematological conditions

#### Full blood count for anaemia and thrombocytopenia
Further investigations must be carried out if the haemoglobin levels are below 11 g/dL at first contact

and 10.5 g/dL at 28 weeks and anaemia is indicated. Thrombocytopenia (low platelet count) is a predisposing factor for antepartum haemorrhage (APH) or postpartum haemorrhage (PPH) and problematic for the mother.

#### Blood grouping and red-cell alloantibodies
The mother's blood grouping and rhesus status should be known for potential blood transfusions and routine antenatal anti-D prophylaxis should be offered to all non-sensitized rhesus-negative pregnant women.

## Fetal anomalies

#### Structural anomalies
Pregnant women should be offered an anomalies ultrasound scan between 18 and 20 weeks' gestation to detect any possible fetal defects, and the pregnancy managed according to the outcome of the scan.

#### Screening for Down's syndrome
Women can be offered a range of tests depending on the gestational age of the pregnancy. The tests must be able to have a standard detection rate of 60 per cent and a false-positive rate of less than 5 per cent.

- From 11 to 14 weeks: nuchal translucency (NT); the combined test [NT, human chorionic gonadotrophin (hCG) and pregnancy-associated plasma protein (PAPP-A)].
- From 14 to 20 weeks: the triple test [hCG, alpha-fetoprotein (AFP) and unconjugated oestriol (uE3)]; the quadruple test (hCG, AFP, uE3 and inhibin A).
- From 11 to 14 weeks and 14–20 weeks: the integrated test (NT, PAPP-A + hCG, AFP, uE3, inhibin A); the serum integrated test (PAPP-A + hCG, AFP, uE3, inhibin A).

## Infections (see Chapter 13)

- *Asymptomatic bacteriuria* – routine urinalysis of midstream urine, and early identification and treatment of asymptomatic bacteriuria may prevent preterm labour.
- *Chlamydia trachomatis* – there is a general movement to screen for this disease, as it is asymptomatic in many individuals and can cause

infertility in the woman, and optical nerve damage to the fetus and neonate.

- *Hepatitis B virus* should be routinely screened for, as early postnatal interventions can reduce the risks of mother–child transmission.
- *Human immunodeficiency virus* (HIV) screening should be offered in early pregnancy, as early antenatal interventions can reduce the risks of intrauterine transmission of the disease.
- *Rubella* must be screened for in early pregnancy to identify women at risk of contracting the disease, which can cause severe congenital abnormalities to the fetus; these mothers will require immunization postnatally.
- *Syphilis* must be screened for, as early treatment is beneficial to both mother and fetus.

## For clinical conditions

### Pre-eclampsia

The mother's blood pressure should be monitored routinely on each visit and urinalysis for protein should be undertaken for mapping the overall pattern of the mother's blood pressure status. Other clinical signs and symptoms, such as headaches, visual disturbances, epigastric pain, nausea and vomiting, swelling and gross oedema of the body, should also be monitored by the midwife's top to toe examinations. Mothers and their families should also be alerted to the signs and symptoms so that they are aware of the physical signs and so can call for help quickly.

### Routine urinalysis

This may also be helpful to detect glucose, as an early indicator of gestational diabetes mellitus. The presence of blood and protein are indicators for possible infections and renal dysfuction in the mother. Protein is also associated with pre-eclampsia.

## Fetal growth and well-being

The midwife's role and responsibilities are to assess the development of the fetus clinically. Abdominal palpation for fetal presentation will help the midwife to establish the presentation of the fetus, and may influence the planning and management of the delivery after 36 weeks. The key determinant is whether it is a breech or cephalic presentation.

## Inspection

This should be carried out as follows.
- Assess the shape of the uterus and note any asymmetry.
- Observe for fetal movements. Note any scars (women often forget to mention previous surgical procedures, if they were performed long ago). Striae gravidarum or linea nigra, bruising and skin rashes may also be observed.

## Palpation (measurement of symphysis–fundal distance

There are great controversies and debate regarding the method of uterine fundal height measurement in the antenatal period, concerning its accuracy in detecting small or large for gestational age babies. Nevertheless, regular measurements must be taken and plotted on individualized fetal growth charts to help assessment for fetal growth.

The top of the fundus should be palpated; this is rarely in the midline. Next, the upper border of the symphysis pubis should be located and the tape measure placed here. With the centimetres face down, measure to the previously noted top of the fundus. Turn over the tape measure and read the measurement. Plot this measurement on a symphysis fundal height chart within the hand-held notes (Figure 5.1).

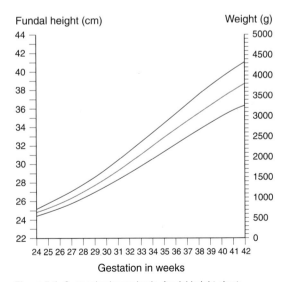

**Figure 5.1** Customized symphysis–fundal height chart. (Courtesy of the West Midlands Perinatal Institute.)

## Fetal lie, presentation and engagement

A large symphysis–fundal height (SFH) raises the possibility of:

- macrosomia;
- multiple pregnancy;
- polyhydramnios.

A small SFH could represent:

- intrauterine growth restriction;
- oligohydramnios.

First, palpate to count the number of fetal poles (Figure 5.2a). A pole is a head or a bottom. If no more than one or two can be felt, it is likely to be a single-ton pregnancy. If you can feel three or four, a twin pregnancy is likely; however, sometimes large fibroids can mimic a fetal pole.

Next, assess the lie by lateral palpation. If there is a pole over the pelvis, the lie is longitudinal regardless of whether the other pole is lying more to the left or right (Figure 5.2b, c, d). If the symphysis fundal height is large and the fetal parts very difficult to feel, there may be polyhydramnios present. If the SFH is small and the fetal parts very easy to feel, oligohydramnios may be the problem.

An oblique lie is where the leading pole does not lie over the pelvis, but just to one side, and a transverse lie is where the fetus lies directly across the abdomen (Figure 5.3). Once it is established that there is a pole over the pelvis, if the gestation is 34 weeks or more, you need to establish what the presentation is. It will be either cephalic (head down) or breech (bottom/feet down). Using a two-handed approach and watching the woman's face, palpate for the presenting part (Figure 5.2b). The head is generally much firmer than the bottom, although, even in experienced hands, it can sometimes be very difficult to tell. If you can feel the whole of the fetal head and it is easily movable, the head is likely to be 'free'. This equates to five-fifths palpable and is recorded as 5/5. As the head descends into the pelvis, less can be felt. When the head is no longer moveable, it has 'engaged' and only one- or two-fifths will be palpable (Figure 5.4). Do not use a one-handed technique (Pawlick's grip), as this is much more uncomfortable.

The fetal position (i.e. whether the fetal head is occipitoposterior, lateral or anterior) is ascertained next prior to auscultation.

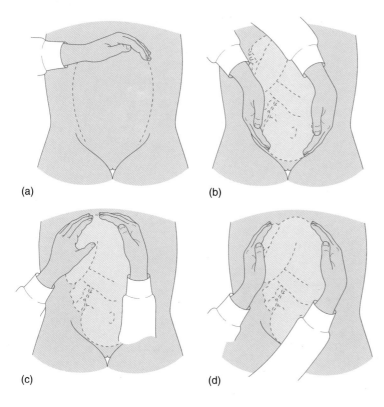

**Figure 5.2** Engagement of the fetal head in the maternal pelvic brim assessed. (a) Palpating the uterine fundus; (b) assessing engagement of the fetal head; (c) and (d) palpating fetal poles.

(a)

(b)

(c)

(d)

## Auscultation of the fetal heart

This helps to confirm that the fetus is alive and fetal circulation is maintained. However, it is not an accurate indication of the potential outcome of the baby. Despite this, many mothers are relieved and reassured to hear the fetal heartbeat.

If you are using a Pinard stethoscope, position it over the fetal shoulder. If you cannot hear the fetal heart, *never* say that you cannot detect a heartbeat. Always explain that a different method is needed and move on to use a hand-held Doppler device. If you have begun the process of listening to the fetal heart, you must proceed until you are confident that you have heard the heart. Hand-held Doppler devices have the advantage that the mother can also hear the fetal heart. With twins, you must be confident that both have been heard.

## Monitoring of fetal movement

Fetal movement charting and counting has been found to be a poor indicator of fetal well-being. The traditional use of the 'Cardiff Count to Ten Kick Chart' has largely been abandoned. However, many mothers still find monitoring their baby's fetal movements comforting and reassuring during the antenatal period, and it promotes alertness to subtle changes that may be significant.

## Cardiotocography

The routine use of cardiotocography in the antenatal period is not advised by NICE, and should only be offered in cases where high risk factors have been shown to exist and there are concerns for the well-being of the fetus.

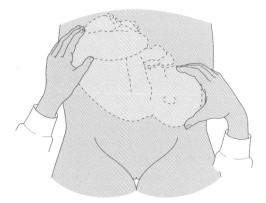

**Figure 5.3** Abdominal palpation of the fetus lying transversely.

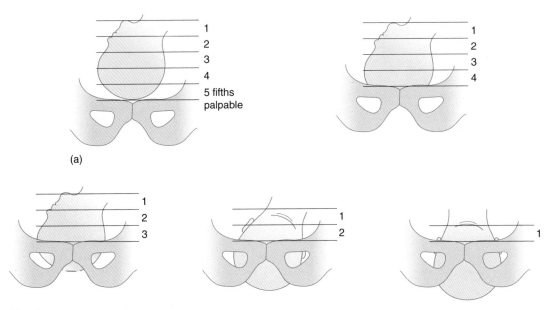

**Figure 5.4** Palpation of the fetal head to assess engagement.

## Ultrasound assessment in the third trimester

NICE guidelines do not recommend the routine use of an ultrasound scan after 24 weeks' gestation for low-risk cases.

## Umbilical and uterine artery Doppler ultrasound

Traditionally, these methods of monitoring maternal placental blood flow and fetal blood flow have been used to predict loss of placental function and ultimate fetal growth restriction as a result of pre-eclampsia or other medical problems. However, NICE has found no real substantive evidence to testify that these procedures are effective in predicting adverse fetal outcome.

## Dating the pregnancy

Many mothers pay great significance to the calculation and setting of the expected day of delivery, as it helps them to focus on their baby. Therefore, the midwife has an important role in ascertaining from the mother the first day of the last menstrual period (LMP), her menstrual pattern and its regularity. Accurate dating of the pregnancy becomes extremely important in cases where the pregnancy is preterm and may influence the timing of the delivery, if there are fetal or maternal problems, or if the pregnancy is prolonged. The gestational age of the fetus is important when specific antenatal screening test are carried out, such as serum screening for alpha-fetoproteins for neural tube defects and Down's syndrome.

There has been great debate concerning the reliability and accuracy of the traditional method of calculating the EDD using Naegele's rule. However, it remains a useful and simplistic means of estimating a likely delivery date. Naegele's rule states that the EDD is calculated by adding 7 days to the first day of the LMP and taking away 3 months, or by adding 280 days (e.g. using 1 January 2005 as the LMP gives 8 October 2006 as the EDD).

Many clinicians use an 'obstetric wheel', which calculates the EDD by 7 days and 9 months. This method assumes the mother has an 28-day menstrual cycle, with ovulation on the 14th day of the cycle and an accurate recollection of the first day of the LMP.

Both methods are considered to be unreliable, as they do not calculate for mothers whose menstrual cycles differ from the 28-day cycle and those who are unable to recall their LMP.

The majority of women will now be offered a dating scan in the first or early second trimester to establish the gestational age of the fetus.

Before 15–16 weeks' gestation there is minimal variation in fetal size between individual pregnancies, so measurements of the crown– rump length, biparietal diameter and femur length can be plotted on standard fetal biometry charts, and the gestation calculated. If the EDD predicted by the dating scan differs by more than 7 days from the menstrual EDD, the scan date is usually chosen as the final EDD.

Beyond 20 weeks' gestation, the effects of genetics and environmental factors will cause significance variability in fetal size. Dating a pregnancy by ultrasound scan becomes less accurate as the pregnancy advances. In the light of this, the WMPI have piloted and implemented the use of individualized fetal growth charts to aid and minimize the misdiagnosis of intrauterine growth restriction or fetal macrosomia.

## Key Points

**Benefits of a dating scan**

- Accurate dating in women with irregular menstrual cycles or poor recollection of LMP.
- Reduced incidence of induction of labour for 'prolonged pregnancy' (see Chapter8).
- Maximizing the potential for serum screening to detect fetal abnormalities (see Chapter 7).
- Early detection of multiple pregnancies.
- Detection of otherwise asymptomatic failed intrauterine pregnancies.

## Individualized antenatal care

Antenatal care forms the basis from which subsequent care and management of the mother and baby and her family can be assessed and reviewed according to their individual needs. The modern-day model of antenatal care, with up to 15 visits to a doctor or midwife in the UK, as set out by Professor John the 1900s, has been greatly criticized by ...ssionals and mothers as ritualistic, not ...ed and inconvenient for many mothers. ...over, studies have found that there are no significant adverse outcomes to both maternal and perinatal mortality and morbidity when the numbers of antenatal visits have been reduced.

Current key recommendations from NICE advocate the following.

- Pregnant women should be offered evidence-based information and support to enable them to make informed decisions regarding their care. Information should include details of where they will be seen and who will undertake their care. Addressing women's choices should be recognized as being integral to the decision-making process.
- A schedule of antenatal appointments should be determined by the function of the appointment. For a woman who is nulliparous with an uncomplicated pregnancy, a schedule of ten appointments should be adequate. For a woman who is parous with an uncomplicated pregnancy, a schedule of seven appointments should be adequate.

The criteria for so-called routine antenatal care have been conceptualized into the current NICE algorithm for healthy pregnant women. There is much debate as to the purpose and function of antenatal care and each visit should have an justifiable purpose (NICE 2003 Appendix F), as well as which particular health professional should be involved or contribute in the delivery of care. In the current climate of clinical risk management and clinical governance, the trend has been to assess and categorize the mothers clinically into low-risk and, in particular, high-risk groups (NICE 2003 Appendix E), in order to assess the level of care that may be required. Risk assessment should be viewed as an ongoing exercise throughout the pregnancy, so that the level and type of care offered to a mother can be changed accordingly, if her level of risk changes. Care must be 'woman centred' and flexible to the individual's needs, as these may alter during the course of the pregnancy.

## Classification of antenatal care

There are many definitions, models and variations in the delivery of antenatal care that are provided for women in both the hospital and community environment, and many have been adapted to the demographic needs of each local National Health Service (NHS) Trust or independent midwifery practitioners.

## Midwifery-led care

Midwifery-led care is care that is led, managed and delivered by the midwife. The midwife may be the sole lead carer and will make the necessary booking appointment, carry out or request routine ultrasound scans and all investigations. This was brought about as a result of the Winterton (House of Commons 1992) and *Changing childbirth* recommendations (Department of Health 1993). In some Trusts, the midwives are responsible both for 'low-risk' and 'high-risk' mothers, and will liaise with and refer mothers to general practitioners (GPs) and hospital consultants. Some Trusts have integrated team midwives who practice in both the community and hospital settings, as they practise case holdings and travel to where ever they are needed by the mother. An example is the Albany Project in London, which is an independent group of midwives who are self-employed and are contracted to a South London NHS Trust to provide care for both high- and low-risk mothers. Independent midwives working privately and who are contracted to individual mothers who employ them can also be said to provide midwifery-led care.

While the midwife may be the lead carer for the mother, the Nursing and Midwifery Council (NMC) Midwives Rules and Standards stipulates that the midwife must always be able 'to recognize the warning signs of abnormality in the mother … which necessitate referral to a doctor' and 'to carry out treatment prescribed by a doctor'. Furthermore, the midwives' responsibilities, and those of other health professionals, are inter-related and complementary. Good team working is in the interest of the woman or baby, and can only be achieved by mutual recognition of the respective roles of midwives and others who participate in their care.

## Shared care

This term is given to antenatal care that is provided jointly by a hospital maternity team, a GP and community midwives. Women booked under this scheme are generally booked under a named hospital consultant and are seen in hospital for either the booking visit or at least one hospital clinical appointment. Some consultants will see mothers at 28–32 weeks and again at 41–42 weeks' gestation, once they have passed their EDD. Many mothers will deliver their baby within the hospital environment, and can also be in a GP unit/GP beds in the consultant unit. Previously mothers who were deemed 'low risk' were allocated this model of care; however, both low- and high-risk mothers may be assigned to this model of care in many Trusts. This enables the high-risk mothers to have extra hospital appointments if their condition requires it.

## Community-based care

This model of care is based on the mother receiving all her care out in the community environment, with minimal or no visits to a hospital unit. Mothers are delivered in either the home or in the hospital. In the past, these have been called the 'domino' schemes. Traditionally, it is low-risk mothers who are allocated to this model of care delivered by the community midwives and the GPs. However, there are innovative models of community-based care that have involved hospital consultants visiting satellite clinics to review high-risk mothers. Examples include the satellite clinics in the St Paul's area in Bristol, and the Scottish Sighthill project in the early 1980s.

## Hospital-based care

Hospital-based care involves mainly care being provided for the mother within a hospital environment. This type of care caters for high-risk mothers who require specialist midwifery or medical management. The mother may have structured care pathways that are based on local and national evidence-based guidelines under which the mother is managed (e.g. insulin-dependent Type 1 diabetic mothers, mothers with antepartum haemorrhages or mothers who develop pregnancy-induced hypertension). Some of these mothers may spend a considerable amount of time either as an in-patient or having repeated visits to a maternity unit during the antenatal period.

Many Trusts have antenatal assessment day units where a mother can be assessed without the full admission into hospital and receive specialist antenatal screening test, such as ultrasound scans, Doppler scans as well as other screening interventions related to their specific antenatal problem or needs. Many

midwives working in the units have specialist skills in sonography, antenatal screening and counselling for mothers. The units help to give a preliminary diagnosis and subsequent care, and assess whether a full admission to hospital or discharge home is the most suitable course of action, thus reducing costs of hospital admissions and disruptions to family life for the mothers.

Whichever form or model of care a pregnant woman is assigned to, she will have a set of patient-held records in which all health care professionals will write each time the mother has contact with them. The WMPI has standardized maternity records for the West Midlands and, hopefully, in the future, nationally standardized maternity records may help to improve records and record keeping, to enhance communication and to allow access for all health care staff to the same information electronically.

## Advice, reassurance and education

The needs of the pregnant mother during the antenatal period are dependent on her physical and psychological health, social and economic status, personal experiences, and previous life and childbirth experiences. They may range from minimal care and support to intensive midwifery care. The midwife must be able to give the necessary supervision, care and advice to women. She has an important task within the family and the wider community in providing antenatal education, preparation for parenthood in all clinical settings and across many other boundaries of health care, such as gynaecology, family planning and childcare.

The midwife has a pivotal role in public health through health promotion in areas such smoking cessation, alcohol and substance misuse (both legal and illegal). In some populations almost a third of women smoke during pregnancy despite the association with fetal growth restriction, preterm labour, abruption and intrauterine death. Smoking-cessation programmes help women to limit these harmful behaviours during pregnancy. Alcohol and substance misuse may require other specialist health professionals (e.g. psychiatric services) and other interprofessional agencies, such as social services, to be involved in the care and management of the mother. Information and advice to mothers regarding the consequences of smoking, alcohol and substance misuse must be provided, so that mothers can make informed choices and decisions about their care. The midwife must work in partnership with the mother and respect the woman's rights to refuse any advice given, or to refuse any treatments or interventions if she so wishes.

The majority of women will require advice, reassurance and education about their changing and developing bodies, including dietary and nutritional advice. Reassurance and explanation on to how to cope with the minor symptoms of pregnancy, such as early morning sickness, heartburn, backache and abdominal discomfort due to the normal physiological changes of pregnancy, may help to relieve unnecessary stress and anxieties (see Chapter 4). Other more serious complications, such as urinary tract infections, headaches and raised blood pressure, must be fully investigated and followed through to determine whether referral to hospital is required or whether mothers can be reassured and managed with simple advice.

Increasingly, the role of the midwife has expanded and extended owing to sociological changes and changes in the relationship between women and midwives. Midwives have been involved with detecting, managing and supporting mothers with domestic violence issues, child protection and criminal legal complications. Midwives must ensure that, whenever possible, they act as advocates for the women and the child or children, and maintain strict confidentiality at all times, as they have a duty of care in ensuring the health and safety of patients and the public in their care.

The establishment of positive and effective relationships between women and midwives is vital. Social, psychological and spiritual support has been valued by women as highly as the physical and practical aspects of care provided by midwives. Antenatal social and psychological support has been found to be effective in the early detection of postnatal depression.

Traditionally parenting skills and the practical elements of childrearing were often learnt through large and extended families. However, with changes in family structures of modern society, many first-time parents are complete novices and look to the midwife for guidance and support. Parent education can be delivered by the midwife via a formal structured programme, within small informal groups or on a one-to-one basis in both the hospital or community environments. The educational programme may discuss a range of topics relating to the pregnancy, labour and care of the newborn. These sessions may help to reduce the anxiety, and increase maternal choice and control for the women and their respective partners. They can also help in socializing with other parents and establishing new support networks and friendships.

## CASE HISTORY

At her first antenatal booking visit with the midwife, Amy, a 28-year-old mother, is 10 weeks pregnant and is wishing to booked to have her second baby at home. She had a previous uneventful first pregnancy, which resulted in a normal vaginal delivery of a live girl weighing 3.4 kg 3 years ago. She sustained a first-degree tear, which was sutured and healed successfully. She is working part-time in her local supermarket at weekends when her husband is able to look after their daughter. She has been well during this pregnancy and has indicated that she wishes to try to breast feed this baby, as she only managed to breast feed for 5 days before giving up owing to sore and cracked nipples.

The type or model of care that should be followed is the 'low-risk' routine antenatal care model as advised in the NICE guidelines. Much of her care will be organized and coordinated by the midwife, with some visits to the hospital for ultrasound scans to confirm dates and for anomaly scanning. The majority of her care will be community based, provided by either the community midwives or an integrated team of midwives. The Supervisor of Midwives and Midwifery Managers will also be involved with the case from a Health and Safety and Clinical Risk Management perspective. In many Trusts, two midwives will attend the home birth. One midwife will focus on caring for the mother, and the other will be responsible for the care of the baby and will have knowledge and experience of neonatal resuscitation, if required. Both midwives will be well trained in dealing with obstetric emergencies in the home environment. Trust policies and guidelines will be discussed with the mother regarding the care and management of a home birth.

The midwife will support and assess the needs of the mother throughout the pregnancy and discuss fully the implications of a home birth, as well as the mother's key wish to breast feed in the postnatal period. Having a baby at home allows the mother to have minimal or no interventions, freedom of movement and to eat and drink fully. She is also able to have her family members to support her, her young daughter and husband. The mother is more able to exercise choice and control over her own labour, and this has been shown to have positive obstetric outcomes for women and their babies. Many women require little or no analgesia, and are aware of a more positive birth experience. Being in her own home environment, the mother is free from the noise and distractions of the busy hospital wards, and may be more relaxed in breast feeding. She will experience less changeover of staff, and have greater continuity of carer and continuity of advice to help support her breast-feeding efforts.

## Conclusion

Effective antenatal care forms the strong foundations from which the midwife will be able to first assess the needs of the mother and her family. It enables the mother and other health professionals to plan and determine her care holistically during the pregnancy. It enables positive relationships to be formed between the mother and the health professionals, so that there is equal contribution to the care and management of the mother and her unborn baby, and that the mother and baby are the central focus of the care and attention, no matter what model of midwife care delivery is being utilized. With proactive health promotional strategies through education and advice, and the wide range of screening programmes available that can be offered and implemented, antenatal care can go some way to reduce the maternal and perinatal mortality and morbidity rates, and improve the health outcome for the mother and her baby.

## New developments in antenatal care

The current NICE antenatal care guidelines are being incorporated into many Trusts' care pathways for antenatal women. Individual units have structured their care management according to the needs of the local demographic population as well as the needs of the individual mother.

Striving for 'normality in childbirth' is the key focus of the midwifery profession, with Trusts and midwives re-examining and reorganizing their practice to ensure that the mother experiences the normal physiological changes of pregnancy with minimal interventions through 'midwifery-led' care.

Technological and medical advances have enabled extensive screening programmes to be made available for mothers and their babies for the detection of abnormalities. The National Screening Committee has set up national screening programmes for all women for a wide variety of diseases and congenital abnormalities.

## Key Points

- Good antenatal care and management sets the foundations for the rest of the pregnancy and childbirth process.
- Thorough and systematic assessment of the mother and fetus is essential in establishing care that is low- or high-risk based.
- There are many models of antenatal care available for women depending on the geographical Trust and demographic needs.
- The midwife has a key role in assessing, planning, implementing and evaluating the care provided for women and their babies by ensuring the care is individualized, effective, coordinated and appropriate to their needs.
- Support, advice and education of women and their families is critical in ensuring the successful bonding relationships between the mother, the baby and the family.
- Care provided is multiprofessional and enhanced by effective communication between the midwife, the different agencies and the mother and her family.
- Antenatal care is multifaceted and multidimensional, ranging from physical, psychological, emotional and spiritual to social support.
- Accurate, unbiased and evidence-based information provision is crucial in ensuring that mothers are able to make informed choices regarding their care.

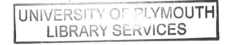

## References

Department of Health. *Changing childbirth*. Report of the Expert Maternity Group. London: HMSO, 1993.

European Union. *Second midwifery directive* (80/155/EEC). Brussels: European Union, 1980.

European Union. Directive (89/594/EEC). Brussels: European Union, 1989.

House of Commons. *Maternity services*. Second report from the Health Committee (Chairman N. Winterton). London: HMSO, 1992.

National Institute for Clinical Excellence. *Antenatal care, routine care for the healthy pregnant woman. Clinical guideline 6*. London: NICE, 2003.

## Key additional reading

Chalmers I, Enkin M, Keirse M. *Effective care in pregnancy and childbirth*. Series. Oxford: Oxford University Press, 1989.

Hall M, MacIntyre S, Porter M. *Antenatal care assessed*. Aberdeen: Aberdeen University Press, 1985.

Villar J, Carroli G, Khan-Neelofur D, Piaggio G, Gulmezoglu M. Patterns of routine antenatal care for low risk pregnancy (Cochrane Review). In: *The Cochrane Library*, Issue 1. Oxford: Update Software, 2002.

# Chapter 6

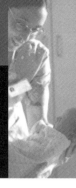

# Antenatal imaging and assessment of fetal well-being

## OVERVIEW

Diagnostic ultrasound has evolved rapidly and is now an integral part of antenatal care in most developed countries. Ultrasound scans are offered routinely to date pregnancy, chart fetal growth and to identify congenital abnormalities. Colour and spectral Doppler ultrasound can identify placental and fetal blood vessels, and provide information on placental function and the fetal circulatory response to hypoxia. The new development of three-dimensional ultrasound can provide further information when a fetal abnormality is suspected. Many antenatal tests of fetal well-being are based on ultrasound techniques and are designed to identify fetuses that are in the early or late stages of hypoxia. Continuous-wave Doppler ultrasound is employed to provide continuous tracings of the fetal heart rate, the patterns of which alter when the fetus is hypoxic. Magnetic resonance imaging is only occasionally used to provide further information when a fetal structural abnormality is suspected.

## Diagnostic ultrasound

### How ultrasound images are formed

Ultrasound images are produced using a transducer, which sends high-frequency (3–7.5 MHz), low-intensity sound waves through the abdomen or pelvis. The transducer contains piezoelectric crystals, usually mounted in a curved array. Small groups of crystals are triggered in sequence and each emits a focused ultrasound beam in a series of pulses, which is reflected when it meets a structure. Reflected signals are detected between the pulses and generate small electric charges that are transformed into visual signals on a screen. The texture and shade of the screen image is determined by the quantity of reflected sound, varying from black (denoting a fluid) to white (denoting a solid structure, e.g. bone). A two-dimensional map of the contents of the uterus is provided in thin slices and, because the complete array is triggered 20 or more times per second, the image is constantly updated in real time, and fetal, cardiac and other movements can be studied.

A small array mounted on a long probe and placed in the vagina is commonly used for first trimester scanning (Figure 6.1a). Transvaginal ultrasound is also useful for examining the cervix later in pregnancy and for identifying the lower edge of the placenta. Generally, after 12 weeks, an abdominal transducer, which is a flat probe with a much wider array, is used (Figure 6.1b).

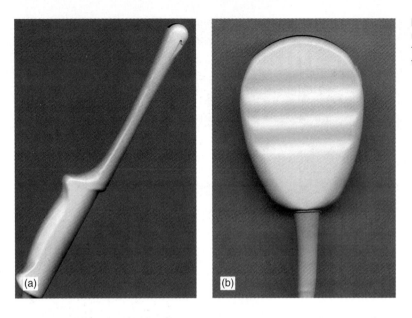

**Figure 6.1** (a) Transvaginal ultrasound transducer; (b) transabdominal ultrasound transducer.

## Ultrasound safety in pregnancy

In common with most medical technologies, ultrasound has the potential to cause harm as well as good and absolute safety should not be assumed. Ultrasound cannot properly be considered a *non-invasive* technique. Sound waves generate energy capable of inducing various effects on body cells, including direct surface heating and cavitation. Cavitation occurs when gas bubbles, which can generate heat through expansion and bursting, are formed in liquids exposed to ultrasound (Ziskin 1990).

The potential for ultrasound to cause direct damage to the developing fetus has been studied *in vitro*, using animal models and in epidemiological studies by analysing the incidence of cancers, dyslexia, speech development and other variables in children exposed to antenatal ultrasound *in utero*. Generally, these studies have been reassuring and there is no conclusive evidence that ultrasound has harmed any woman or baby, but concerns remain regarding certain applications. Transvaginal ultrasound places the source of the ultrasound beam nearer to the target, and colour, pulsed or power Doppler employ higher power outputs than conventional ultrasound and thus have greater potential thermal effects.

Ongoing investigation of ultrasound safety in pregnancy presents particular problems. Extensive worldwide ultrasound use has reduced numbers of unexposed pregnant women, and equipment and techniques are constantly evolving. A randomized controlled trial of 2800 women identified an increased risk of intrauterine growth restriction (IUGR) in fetuses exposed to frequent Doppler (Newnham et al. 1993). This finding was not the primary outcome measure for the study and thus could have occurred by chance. In view of the possible hazards, diagnostic ultrasound should be used only for sound clinical reasons, by properly trained operators. Women should be exposed for the shortest time and to the minimum power output necessary to complete the examination.

## Ultrasound in pregnancy

### Ultrasound in the first trimester

*Early pregnancy problems*
Transvaginal ultrasound enables easier, more detailed visualization of pelvic structures in early pregnancy and has improved the diagnosis of disorders of early pregnancy, such as miscarriage and ectopic pregnancy. Women may perceive transvaginal scanning as potentially uncomfortable or embarrassing; therefore, a clear explanation of the reasons for using this method must be given prior to the scan.

*The early pregnancy scan (11–14 weeks)*
Many centres offer a routine scan at 11–14 weeks' gestation. This is normally performed transabdominally, but in some countries the transvaginal route is preferred.

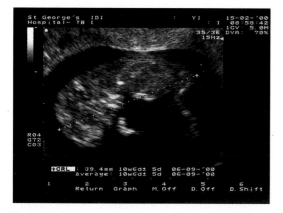

**Figure 6.2** Crown–rump length measurement taken at 12 weeks' gestation. This view is also used for measurement of the nuchal translucency.

The principal aims of this scan are:
- to confirm fetal viability;
- to provide an accurate estimation of gestational age;
- to diagnose multiple gestation and, in particular, to determine chorionicity;
- to identify markers that would indicate an increased risk of fetal chromosome abnormality, such as Down's syndrome;
- to identify fetuses with gross structural abnormalities.

## Estimation of gestational age

Fetal age can be assessed accurately before 12 weeks by measuring the crown–rump length (CRL; Figure 6.2) and from 12–20 weeks by biparietal diameter (BPD), head circumference (HC) or femur length (FL; Figure 6.3a, b and c). At this stage in pregnancy, the range of values around the mean is narrow. In clinical practice, the CRL and BPD are the most often used, because they are the most reproducible measurements. The earlier the measurement is made; the better the prediction and measurements made from an early CRL (accuracy of prediction ±5 days) will be preferred to a BPD at 20 weeks (accuracy of prediction ±7 days). Predictions of gestational age by ultrasound before 20 weeks have been shown to be more accurate than predictions from the last menstrual period, even if the woman is certain of her dates. Conventionally, the ultrasound date is only taken if the discrepancy in the expected day of delivery (EDD) calculated from ultrasound and the date of the last menstrual period is >10 days.

## Multiple pregnancy and chorionicity

Monochorionic twin pregnancies are associated with an increased risk of pregnancy complications and a

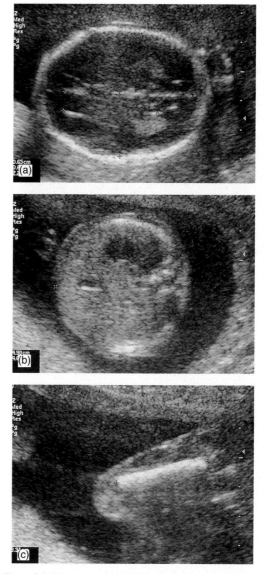

**Figure 6.3** Measurements of (a) biparietal diameter and head circumference; (b) abdominal circumference; (c) femur length at 24 weeks' gestation.

higher perinatal mortality rate than dichorionic twin pregnancies. It is, therefore, helpful to be able to determine chorionicity early in pregnancy (see Chapter 9).

The dividing membrane in monochorionic twins is formed by two layers of amnion and in dichorionic twins by two layers of chorion and two of amnion. Dichorionic twins, therefore, have thicker membranes than monochorionic twins and this can be perceived qualitatively on ultrasound. Dichorionic twin pregnancies ultrasonically in the first trimester of pregnancy have a thick inter-twin separating membrane (septum) flanked on either side by a very thin amnion.

This is in contrast to a monochorionic twin pregnancy, which on two-dimensional ultrasound will have a very thin inter-twin septum.

Another method of determining chorionicity in the first trimester uses the appearance of the septum at its origin from the placenta. On ultrasound, a tongue of placental tissue is seen within the base of dichorionic membranes and has been termed the 'twin peak' or 'lambda' sign. The optimal gestation at which to perform ultrasonic chorionicity determination is 9–10 weeks. Dichorionicity can also be confirmed by the identification of two placental masses and, later in pregnancy, by the presence of different sex fetuses.

### Nuchal thickness measurement and chromosomal abnormalities

In normal pregnancy during the first trimester, a fluid-filled area may be seen on the posterior surface of the fetal neck. This can be measured and an association is now recognized between this nuchal translucency (NT) measurement and chromosomal and cardiac defects. At any given maternal age, the measurement of NT can be used to modify the underlying age-related risk of a fetal trisomy (see Chapter 7).

## Ultrasound in the second trimester

### The mid-pregnancy scan (18–22 weeks)

A routine scan is offered to most pregnant women between 16 and 22 weeks. Many centres now delay this scan to between 20 and 22 weeks, as this improves the diagnosis of cardiac and late developing abnormalities, such as microcephaly.

The aims of this scan are as follows.

- To provide an estimation of gestational age, if an early scan has not been performed, through measurement of the BPD, HC and FL.
- To carry out a detailed fetal anatomical survey to detect any fetal structural abnormalities or markers for chromosome abnormality. This is probably the principal reason for the mid-pregnancy scan. The vast majority of fetal abnormalities will not be anticipated and, therefore, would not be detected without this routine scan.
- To establish the presence of multiple gestation, if an early scan has not been performed, and to determine the chorionicity.
- To locate the placenta and identify the 5 per cent of women who will have a low-lying placenta.

A small percentage of such women will eventually be shown to have a placenta praevia.
- To estimate the amniotic fluid volume.

### Fetal anatomy

Serious fetal structural abnormalities, the most common being central nervous system abnormalities and cardiac defects, occur in around 3 per cent of pregnancies. The most detailed survey of fetal anatomy is carried out at the mid-pregnancy scan at 20–22 weeks' gestation (see box). The detection rate for abnormalities varies between centres and is dependent on the type of anomaly being screened for, the skill of operator, the time allowed for the scan and the quality of equipment. An international systematic review reported detection rates of 45 per cent overall, with a range of 15–85 per cent for different anomalies (Bricker et al. 2000). Fortunately, the false-positive rate is low and termination of a normal fetus because of a mistaken diagnosis is a rare event. Once a serious abnormality is detected, evidence shows that parents will elect to terminate the pregnancy in 80–90 per cent of cases.

---

**Fetal measurements and anatomic features visualized on the routine scan between 18 and 22 weeks' gestation**

**Standard fetal measurements**
- Biparietal diameter
- Head circumference
- Abdominal circumference
- Femoral length

**Fetal anatomic features and measurements**

*Brain*
- Ventricular section: anterior and posterior horns of the cerebral ventricles; measurement: anterior and posterior ventricle-hemisphere ratio
- Posterior fossa section: cerebellum, vermis, cisterna magna, and nuchal skinfold; measurement: transcerebellar diameter and nuchal skinfold thickness

*Skull*
- Shape, e.g. lemon-shaped as in spina bifida

*Face*
- Orbits (and both lenses) measurement: interorbital, external orbital diameters
- Nose, lips, palate, and mandible

*Spine*
- 'Anterior' view of spinous processes down to tip of sacrum; clear view of skin margin throughout length of spine

*Chest*
- Heart: four-chamber view, aortic root and arch, pulmonary artery and ductus
- Lungs

*Abdomen*
- Diaphragm
- Cord insertion
- Liver, stomach and intestines
- Both kidneys for parenchyma and renal pelvis size
- Bladder
- Genitalia

*Limbs*
- Femur, tibia, fibula, foot and toes (both limbs)
- Humerus, radius, ulna, hand, and fingers (both limbs)

*Placenta*
- Morphology and site

*Cord*
- Number of vessels

*Amniotic fluid*
- Volume assessment

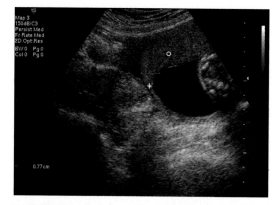

**Figure 6.4** Transvaginal scan showing cervix and placenta covering internal os. o, placenta; +, placenta covering the internal os.

## Placental location

Placenta praevia is a cause of life-threatening haemorrhage in pregnancy. Major antepartum haemorrhage is often preceded by a warning haemorrhage and any woman with a bloodstained vaginal loss should have a scan, at the earliest opportunity, to determine placental location. If the lower edge of the placenta appears to lie close to the cervix, then a gentle transvaginal scan should be performed to determine whether the placenta covers the internal os, indicating a major placenta praevia (Figure 6.4).

In the third trimester, if the lower edge of the placenta lies within 3 cm of the internal os, then the provisional diagnosis would be grade I (minor) placenta praevia. At the mid-pregnancy scan, it is customary to identify women who have a low-lying placenta. At this stage, the lower uterine segment has not yet formed and most low-lying placentas will appear to 'migrate' upwards as the lower segment stretches in the late second and third trimesters. About 5 per cent of women will have a low-lying placenta at 20 weeks and only 5 per cent of this group will eventually be shown to have a placenta praevia. Recent studies have shown that a transvaginal scan performed in women with a low-lying placenta will identify cases of true placenta praevia with more precision.

## Amniotic fluid volume

The fetus has a role in the control of the volume of amniotic fluid. It swallows amniotic fluid, absorbs it in the gut and later excretes urine into the amniotic sac. Congenital abnormalities that impair fetal ability to swallow (e.g. anencephaly or oesophageal atresia) will result in an increase in amniotic fluid. Congenital abnormalities that result in failure of urine production or passage (e.g. renal agenesis and posterior urethral valves) will result in reduced or absent amniotic fluid. Variation from the normal range of amniotic fluid volume calls for a further detailed ultrasound assessment for possible causes.

## Umbilical cord

Some abnormalities of the umbilical cord can be identified by ultrasound during the antenatal period and visualization is improved with the use of colour Doppler. A single umbilical artery is associated with fetal abnormalities and intrauterine growth restriction, and is looked for at the time of the mid-pregnancy scan.

## Ultrasound screening for adverse pregnancy outcome

In some centres, the scope of the mid-pregnancy scan has been extended to include screening for increased risk of adverse pregnancy outcome. Doppler ultrasound examination of maternal uterine arteries is used to predict pre-eclampsia and IUGR; transvaginal measurement of cervical length is used to assess the risk of pre-term delivery.

### Doppler ultrasound and the prediction of adverse pregnancy outcome

The ability to study blood vessels in the uterus, placenta and fetus, and measure aspects of blood velocity has led to major advances in the management of pregnancy. Doppler ultrasound utilizes the principle that ultrasound waves reflected from moving structures (e.g. red blood cells flowing along a vessel) show a variation in frequency corresponding to the speed of movement of the structure. This principle is known as the Doppler frequency shift. If the structures are moving towards the beam, the reflected signal will be at a higher frequency than the transmitted one; if the movement is away from the beam, the reflected signal will be at a lower frequency.

Early obstetric systems used continuous wave (CW) Doppler, where different crystals within the transducer continually send and receive signals. The disadvantage of CW Doppler is that signals are obtained from all vessels in the path of the ultrasound beam. Pulsed wave (PW) Doppler is the preferred mode in modern scanners and has advantages over CW systems in using one crystal to send and receive signals, allowing measurement of depth (or range) at which flow is observed. Additionally, the size of the sample volume (or range gate) can be changed. These features make the isolation of signals from particular vessels easier.

PW ultrasound is used to provide data for Doppler sonograms and colour-flow images, and the Doppler-shifted signals can be displayed in two ways. First, they can be shown as a colour map of blood vessels superimposed on top of the grey scale image. This is called colour Doppler imaging (or just colour Doppler). Blood flowing towards the transducer is shown in shades of red, the brighter shades indicating high velocity. Flow away from the transducer is shown as shades of blue. By this means, nearly all the major blood vessels in the placenta and fetus can be displayed (Figure 6.5). Quantitative information about the velocity or resistance to flow in any of these vessels can be obtained by means of pulsed or spectral Doppler. Signals from a particular vessel can be isolated (gated) and displayed in graphic form, with the velocity plotted against time. Arterial flow is pulsatile; venous flow is usually constant but is pulsatile in veins that are close

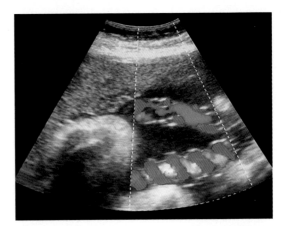

**Figure 6.5** Typical colour Doppler image of fetal vessels.

to the heart (central veins). In general, most studies have been carried out on arterial flow, although recently there has been an increasing interest in central veins.

The pulsatile arterial flow velocity waveform has a systolic and diastolic component. If the angle of the ultrasound beam to the long axis of the vessel is known, the absolute blood velocity in centimetres per second can be determined. However, velocity has not been used much in obstetrics, except in assessing the rhesus-affected fetus when high blood velocities are associated with fetal anaemia. Most studies have looked at resistance to flow, which is reflected in the diastolic component. A small amount of diastolic flow implies high resistance downstream to the vessel being studied and implies low perfusion. A high diastolic component indicates low downstream resistance and implies high perfusion (Figure 6.6). A measure of the amount of diastolic flow relative to systolic is provided by several indices, such as the pulsatility index (PI) or resistance index (RI), which essentially compare the amount of diastolic flow to systolic flow. When these indices are high, this indicates high resistance to flow; when the indices are low, resistance to flow is low.

Pre-eclampsia and IUGR are associated with increased resistance in the uteroplacental circulation, and is identifiable in Doppler waveforms. Abnormal uterine artery waveforms retain an early pregnancy appearance, low flow at diastole and diastolic notching after 20 weeks (Figure 6.7). Diastolic notching indicates that the spiral arteries, which are downstream from the uterine artery, remain muscular and compliant and, therefore, that trophoblast invasion of these arteries is incomplete or inadequate. The use of uterine artery Doppler as a screening tool to identify women at

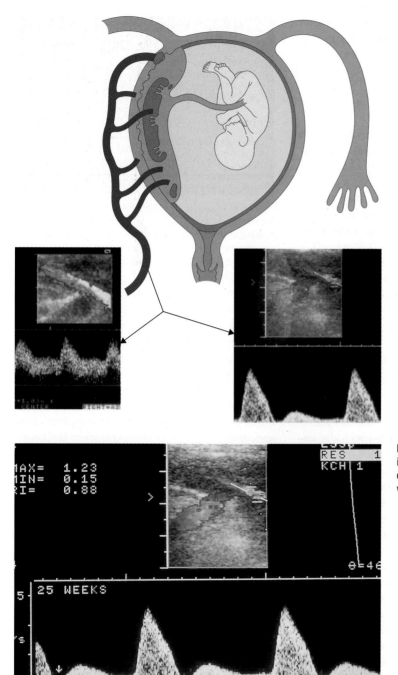

**Figure 6.6** Left: a low-resistance waveform from the uterine artery; note the abundance of diastolic flow. Right: a high-resistance waveform from the uterine artery; note the notches and reduced diastolic flow.

**Figure 6.7** The uterine artery is easily identified crossing medial to the external iliac vein. A high-resistance waveform is demonstrated.

risk of pre-eclampsia or IUGR prior to the development of clinical symptoms has been investigated. High-resistance waveform patterns are associated with adverse outcomes; 60–70 per cent of women with bilateral uterine artery notches at 20–24 weeks' gestation will subsequently develop pre-eclampsia, IUGR or placental abruption. However, a systematic review of 27 studies found uterine artery Doppler had low value in predicting pre-eclampsia, IUGR and perinatal death in low-risk women (Chien et al. 2000) and routine uterine artery Doppler screening is not currently recommended [National Institute for Clinical Excellence (NICE) 2003].

## Measurement of cervical length

Studies using transvaginal ultrasound indicate a strong association between cervical length and preterm delivery. A study of 2500 women screened at 24 and again at 28 weeks demonstrated that the risk of preterm delivery increased as length of the cervix decreased. In this study, the sensitivity of cervical length screening in identifying those women destined to deliver preterm was low: 54 per cent at 24 weeks and 70 per cent at 28 weeks (Iams et al. 1996). Current evidence suggests that routine antenatal cervical assessment for risk of preterm delivery by transvaginal ultrasound does not improve outcomes and it is not generally advocated for healthy pregnant women.

## Issues in routine scanning

Although the early and mid-pregnancy scans are now widely accepted as part of standard antenatal care, routine ultrasound screening of all pregnancies has generated controversy. The value of routine ultrasound has been debated in terms of clinical and cost effectiveness, and the potential psychological impacts on women and their families. The clinical impact of the mid-pregnancy routine scan is illustrated by the meta-analysis shown in Figure 6.8: eight studies evaluating random allocation of antenatal patients to routine scanning or scanning on indication are compared. In the routine scan group, there was a significant reduction in the numbers of multiple pregnancies undiagnosed at 26 weeks and of inductions of labour for post-term pregnancy. No definite benefit could be demonstrated in terms of perinatal mortality, the incidence of low birth weight or neonatal condition between the two groups.

A principal aim of the mid-pregnancy scan is to detect fetal anomaly, which is advocated on the basis of allowing parents to choose termination if a major anomaly is suspected, or appropriate plans for delivery or referral to be made if a condition requiring specialist antenatal or early neonatal intervention (e.g. an abdominal wall defect) is detected. Anomaly screening only lowers perinatal mortality rates if parents choose termination of pregnancy.

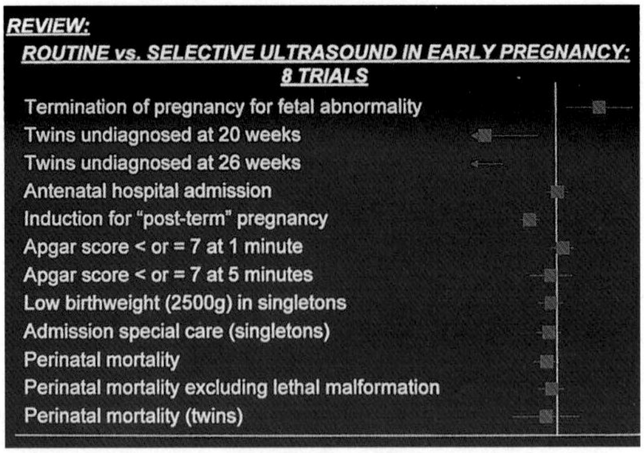

**Figure 6.8** Meta-analysis of eight studies comparing routine and selective scanning. Routine ultrasound reduces the number of undiagnosed twins and unnecessary inductions of labour and increases the number of terminations of pregnancy for fetal anomalies, but has not been shown to reduce prenatal mortality or morbidity.

Routine ultrasound is also advocated on the basis of positive effects on pregnant women and their families. Ultrasound has been credited with reducing anxiety, increasing bonding and encouraging women to comply with health education advice. Scans are attractive to parents and seen as an opportunity to 'meet the baby' and gain reassurance that all is well with the pregnancy. Perceptions of the experience are undoubtedly influenced by the attitude of the sonographer: communication and feedback is very important in making the scan a positive experience.

Even when no adverse findings are reported, a number of women report being worried about something they saw or heard. Research on the psychological impact of ultrasound in pregnancy has been limited. There is little evidence to support the contention that ultrasound reduces anxiety; this effect is just as likely to be caused by increased anxiety prior to the scan. Similarly, the evidence that ultrasound promotes bonding or positively affects health-related behaviours, such as smoking, is inconclusive. Further research is required to determine whether these effects are real.

Ultrasound is a screening procedure and requires the woman's informed consent. Current evidence suggests that many women do not receive sufficient information regarding the purpose and limitations of routine scans to facilitate informed choice (Kohut et al. 2002). A proportion of women will experience a poor pregnancy outcome despite a 'normal scan'; psychological adjustment may be affected, if they felt the problem should have been identified by the scan. In some situations, ultrasound can engender increased anxiety for parents: failed scans do not provide reassurance expected and mean that the woman has to attend for a repeat. The scan may indicate a possible problem necessitating further investigation (e.g. finding of a low-lying placenta or soft markers for chromosomal abnormality). Uncertain findings have been reported to have a negative impact on women's feelings regarding their pregnancy, even when these are not confirmed by later tests. In a small number of cases, routine ultrasound scanning identifies clearly defined bad outcomes. Fetal death may be diagnosed in the early pregnancy scans, and mid-pregnancy scans may identify serious abnormalities, raising the possibility of termination of pregnancy or neonatal intervention. The impact of these findings is likely to be similar whether ultrasound or another screening technique is used; however, parents may feel less prepared for bad news from a scan perceived as routine.

## Clinical applications of ultrasound

### Ultrasound in the third trimester

Ultrasound is used selectively in the third trimester when there are specific clinical indications:
- to assess fetal growth;
- to assess fetal well-being.

#### Assessing fetal growth and estimating fetal weight

External dimensions can be used to chart the growth rate of the fetus *in utero*. The standard measurements used in the assessment of fetal growth/weight are the biparietal diameter, head circumference, abdominal circumference (AC) and femur length (Figure 6.3). It is customary now to measure all these parameters when assessing fetal size, as it provides information about fetal symmetry. In addition, when combined in an equation, these measurements provide a more accurate estimate of fetal weight (EFW) than any of the parameters taken singly. All measurements can be immediately compared with a normal reference range taken from an unselected population.

In pregnancies at high risk of IUGR, serial measurements are plotted on the normal reference range. Growth patterns are helpful in distinguishing between different types of growth restriction (symmetrical and asymmetrical). Asymmetry between head measures (BPD, HC) and abdominal measure (AC) can be

identified in IUGR, where a brain-sparing effect will result in a relatively large head circumference compared with the abdominal circumference. The opposite may occur in a diabetic pregnancy, where the abdomen is disproportionately large owing to the effects of insulin on the fetal liver and fat store. Cessation of growth is an ominous sign of placental failure. However, the importance of serial measurements has lessened with more dynamic tests of fetal well-being, such as umbilical and fetal Doppler and the antenatal cardiotocograph (see later).

Of all the parameters measured, the AC is the most accurate predictor of fetal weight because it is reduced in both symmetric and asymmetric IUGR. However, equations combining several parameters will reduce the random variation in the accuracy of the predictions. For example, by combining BPD, HC, AC and FL, fetal weight will be predicted to within 150 g/kg of true weight. This is especially valuable in predicting the weight of small fetuses, such as growth-restricted preterm infants, to provide information as to their potential viability. For example, an estimated birth weight of less than 600 g would generally be considered non-viable. Birth weight assessments, however, are less accurate with larger babies and, above 3 kg; ultrasound assessments are little better than estimates made by abdominal palpation. Routine ultrasound in the third trimester to assess fetal size is not advocated; the detection rate of the late SGA fetus on a single ultrasound scan is little better than that obtained by serial measurements of the symphysis–fundal height.

#### Placental appearance

The appearance of the placenta in the second and early third trimesters is one of a fairly uniform texture (echogenicity). Towards the end of the third trimester, the placenta develops a mature appearance, being distinctly lobular with white echoes demarcating the cotyledons. While there is some evidence that premature maturation of the placenta is associated with impaired function, this is not strong enough to make it a useful test.

### Ultrasound in the assessment of fetal well-being

#### Amniotic fluid volume

The amount of amniotic fluid in the uterus is a guide to fetal well-being in the third trimester. A precise evaluation cannot be made by ultrasound, as the fluid gathers in irregular pockets around the fetus; this is demonstrated on ultrasound as echo-free spaces. Two relatively crude methods are used as indicators of volume. The maximum vertical pool is measured after a general survey of the uterine contents. Measurements of less than 2 cm suggest oligohydramnios and measurements greater than 7 cm suggest polyhydramnios. The amniotic fluid index (AFI) is the sum of all the maximum vertical pool measurements from the four quadrants of the uterus, and provides a more useful measurement. The AFI alters throughout gestation but, in the third trimester, it should be between 10 and 25 cm; values below 10 cm indicate a reduced volume and below 5 cm indicate oligohydramnios, while values above 25 cm indicate polyhydramnios. Amniotic fluid volume is decreased in fetal growth restriction, in association with redistribution of fetal blood away from the kidneys to vital structures, such as the brain and heart; there is a consequent reduction in renal perfusion and urine output.

## Cardiotocography

Antenatal cardiotocography (CTG) uses external (and, therefore, indirect) methods of monitoring the fetal heart rate. The most widely used method for obtaining this information is ultrasound fetal CTG. This utilizes the Doppler principle to detect fetal heart motion. Signals can also be obtained from antenatal fetal electrocardiography but this is more prone to failure. The interval between successive beats is measured, thereby allowing a continuous assessment of fetal heart rate. Antenatal CTG may be indicated in the presence of specific risk factors, but is not recommended as a routine part of antenatal care, as there is little evidence that it improves outcomes (NICE 2003) and may increase the rate of obstetric intervention.

The woman should be comfortable and in a left lateral or semirecumbent position (avoiding compression of the maternal vena cava). An external ultrasound transducer for monitoring the fetal heart and a tocodynometer (stretch gauge) for recording uterine activity are secured overlying the uterus. Recordings are then made for at least 30 minutes, and the output from the CTG machine is conventionally consists of an ink tracing of fetal heart rate and a second tracing of uterine activity (Figure 6.9).

Fetal cardiac physiology
Fetal cardiac behaviour is regulated through sympathetic and parasympathetic signals and by vasomotor,

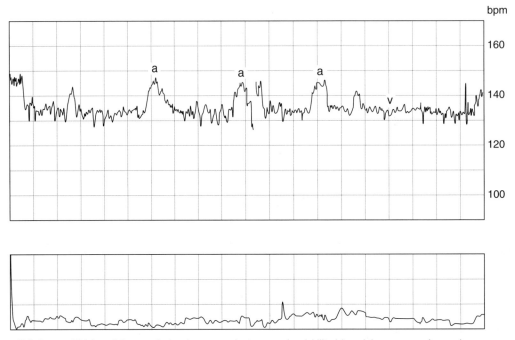

**Figure 6.9** A normal fetal cardiotocograph showing a normal rate, normal variability (v), and the presence of several accelerations (a).

chemoceptor and baroreceptor mechanisms. Pathological events, such as fetal hypoxia, modify these signals and also the fetal cardiac response.

Fetal heart rate variability

Under normal physiological conditions, the interval between successive heartbeats (beat-to-beat) varies. This is called 'short-term variability' and increases with increasing gestational age. It is not visible on standard CTG (although this information can be obtained from fetal electrocardiograms; see later). In addition to these beat-to-beat variations in heart rate, there are longer-term fluctuations in heart rate occurring between 2–6 times per minute. The preferred term for this variation in fetal heart rate is 'baseline variability'. Normal baseline variability reflects a normal fetal autonomic nervous system. As well as gestational age, baseline variability is modified by fetal sleep states and activity, and also by hypoxia, fetal infection and drugs suppressing the fetal central nervous system, such as opioids, and hypnotics (all of which reduce baseline variability). Baseline variability is considered abnormal when it is less than 10 beats per minute (bpm; Figure 6.10). As fetuses display deep sleep cycles of 20–30 minutes at a time, baseline variability may be normally reduced for this length of time, but should be preceded and followed by a period of trace with normal baseline variability, if the CTG is continued for a sufficient duration.

Baseline fetal heart rate

The baseline fetal heart rate falls with advancing gestational age as a result of maturing fetal parasympathetic (vagal) tone. It is best determined over a period of 5–10 minutes. The normal fetal heart rate at term is 110–150 bpm, whilst prior to term, 160 bpm is taken as the upper limit of normal. A rate lower than 110 bpm is termed a fetal bradycardia. If all other features of the CTG are normal, this is unlikely to represent fetal hypoxia unless the rate is less than 100 bpm. Fetal heart rates between 150 and 170 bpm are again unlikely to represent fetal compromise, if the trace is otherwise normal (normal baseline variability in the presence of accelerations and in the absence of decelerations) and there are no antenatal risk factors. Fetal tachycardias can be due to congenital tachycardias and are also associated with maternal or fetal infection, acute fetal hypoxia, fetal anaemia and drugs such as adrenoceptor agonists (ritodrine).

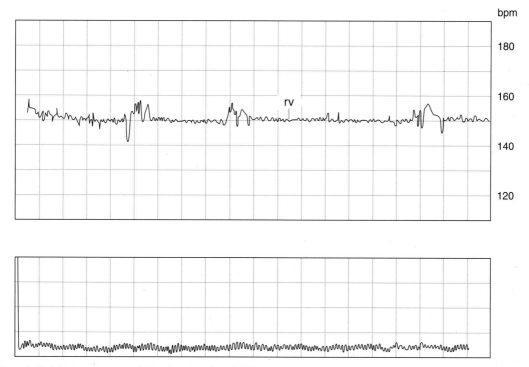

**Figure 6.10** A fetal cardiotocograph showing a baseline of 150 beats per minute (bpm) but with reduced variability.

## Fetal heart rate accelerations

These are increases in the baseline fetal heart rate of at least 15 bpm, lasting for at least 15 seconds. The presence of two or more accelerations on a 20–30-minute CTG defines a reactive trace. The presence of acceleration is important as they are only observed very rarely in the presence of fetal hypoxia (i.e. they are normally suggestive of fetal health). Accelerations can be so frequent as to suggest a fetal tachycardia (Figure 6.11) and this emphasizes the need to interpret CTG tracings carefully in the light of the overall clinical picture.

## Fetal heart rate decelerations

These are transient reductions in fetal heart rate of 15 bpm or more, lasting for more than 15 seconds. Occasional decelerations are frequently seen on otherwise normal CTG tracings. Decelerations that occur in the presence of other abnormal features (see box), such as reduced variability or baseline tachycardia, are more likely to reflect fetal hypoxia. When baseline variability is reduced, decelerations can be less than 15 bpm from the baseline and still be highly significant (Figure 6.12).

In summary, a normal antepartum fetal CTG can be defined as having a baseline of 110–150 bpm, with baseline variability exceeding 10 bpm, and with more than one acceleration being seen in a 20–30-minute tracing. Reduced baseline variability, absence of accelerations and the presence of decelerations are all suspicious features. A suspicious antenatal CTG must be interpreted in clinical context. If multiple antenatal risk factors have already been identified, a suspicious CTG may warrant delivery of the baby, although when no other risk factors are present, a repeated investigation later in the day may be more appropriate.

### The computerized CTG

The basis of fetal CTG is pattern recognition and this leads to differences in interpretation between different clinicians. Computerized CTG interpretation packages have been developed. These packages have been thoroughly field tested in comparison with human experts and have been shown to be equal, or superior, to human interpretation in differentiating normal from abnormal outcome.

One commonly used package relies on the computer's ability to calculate heart rate variability by measuring the variation in frequency of individual heartbeats and assessing increased variability with fetal movements. In this way, fetal heart rate accelerations are identified by a reduced interval between beats and decelerations are identified from an increased interval. A sinusoidal trace can be recognized by short-term variation of more than two standard deviations below the mean value expected for a given gestation.

Several potential advantages of a computerized interpretation seem to exist. The computer is often able to declare a CTG normal after 10 minutes (rather than the more standard 30-minute tracing normally performed manually). Second, if signal contact is lost during the tracing, it triggers an alarm, requiring the Doppler transducer to be repositioned. The interactive nature of this monitoring also reduces the total duration of CTG recording and aids interpretation.

### Biophysical profile

In an effort to refine the ability of fetal CTG to identify antenatal hypoxia, investigators have looked at

---

### Cardiotocography: a summary of fetal heart rate patterns and their implications

**Normal**
- Baseline rate 110–150 bpm
- Variability 10–25 bpm
- Two accelerations in 20 minutes
- No decelerations

**Suspicious**
- Absence of accelerations (important), +
- Abnormal baseline rate (<110 or >150 bpm)
- Reduced variability (<10 bpm)
- Variable decelerations

**Abnormal**
- No accelerations and two or more of the following:
  - Abnormal baseline rate
  - Abnormal variability
  - Repetitive late decelerations
  - Variable decelerations with ominous features (duration >60 seconds, late recovery baseline, late deceleration component, poor variability between/during decelerations)

**Others**
- Sinusoidal pattern
- Prolonged bradycardia
- Shallow decelerations with reduced variability in a non-reactive trace

+, absence of accelerations alone may not be suspicious

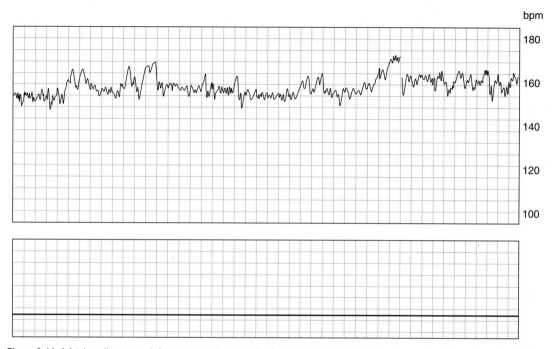

**Figure 6.11** A fetal cardiotocograph from a term pregnancy. The true baseline is about 150 beats per minute (bpm), as seen at the start of the trace. This baby was very active and the apparent raised baseline rate for the majority of the tracing is due to almost continuous accelerations.

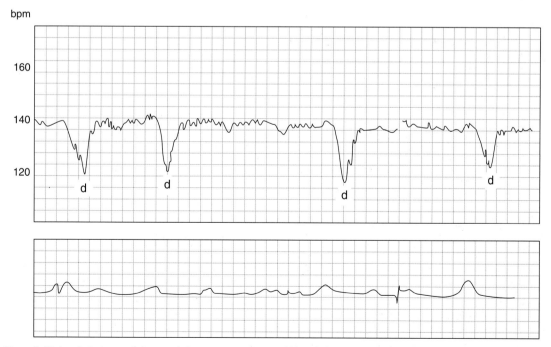

**Figure 6.12** An admission cardiotocograph from a term pregnancy. Although the baseline fetal heart rate is normal, there is reduced variability, an absence of fetal heart rate accelerations and multiple decelerations (d). The decelerations were occurring after uterine tightenings and are, therefore, termed 'late'.

**Table 6.1** – Biophysical profile scoring

| Biophysical variable | Normal (score 2) | Abnormal (score 0) |
| --- | --- | --- |
| Fetal breathing movements | >1 episode for 30 seconds in 30 minutes | Absent/<30 seconds in 30 minutes |
| Gross body movements | >3 body/limb movements in 30 minutes | <3 body/limb movements in 30 minutes |
| Fetal tone | >1 episode body/limb extension followed by return to flexion, open–close cycle of fetal hand | Slow, or absent extension–flexion of body or limbs |
| Reactive fetal heart rate | >2 accelerations with fetal movements in 30 minutes | <2 accelerations, or 1 + deceleration in 30 minutes |
| Qualitative amniotic fluid | >1 pool of fluid, at least 1 cm × 1 cm | Either no measurable pool, or a pool <1 cm × 1 cm |

additional fetal parameters. In studies, exposure of pregnant animals to hypoxic gas mixtures induced fetal hypoxia; under these conditions, fetal biophysical variables, such as breathing movements and forelimb movements, are abolished. This reduction in movement may persist even after the normal fetal oxygenation has been re-established. Similar changes in those active biophysical variables controlled by the central nervous system have been noticed in acutely hypoxic human fetuses, including reduction in breathing movements, gross body movements, flexor tone and accelerations in fetal heart rate related to movements. If chronic fetal hypoxia occurs, there is an associated reduction in amniotic fluid volume and fetal growth restriction is seen. By assigning each of the active variables, and also amniotic fluid volume and the CTG scores of either 2 (=normal) or 0 (=suboptimal), it is possible to assign an individual fetus a score of between 0 and 10. This is the basis of fetal biophysical profiling (Table 6.1).

Initial observational studies demonstrated a strong association between low biophysical profile scores and increased perinatal mortality; delivery when scoring below <6 was advocated to reduce perinatal mortality. A subsequent Cochrane systematic review of four randomized controlled trials failed to substantiate early optimism regarding the usefulness of biophysical profile (Alfirevic and Neilson 2000). When compared with conventional fetal monitoring (cardiotocography) in high-risk pregnancy, biophysical profiling had no effect on pregnancy outcome (either beneficial or harmful). The reviewers concluded that the trials considered had serious limitations, reducing their values in assessing the merits of biophysical profiling, particularly with regard to the small number of women studied (<3000) and low perinatal mortality rates reported. Moreover, the impact of biophysical profiling on other factors, such as rates of obstetric intervention, hospitalization, neonatal morbidity and women's satisfaction, was not considered. Larger randomized-controlled studies are required before any definite conclusions regarding the efficacy of biophysical profiling can be reached.

### Doppler investigation

The principles of Doppler have already been discussed. The umbilical artery has been the most extensively studied vessel because signals can be obtained with inexpensive continuous wave Doppler equipment. It should be regarded as a placental vessel, however, and only by studying fetal vessels with the more expensive colour Doppler machines can important information on the fetal response to hypoxia be made.

### Umbilical artery

Umbilical artery waveforms provide information on fetoplacental blood flow and are used to assess placental function in high-risk pregnancies (e.g. with hypertension, or where there is an SGA fetus, or an elevated uterine artery resistance index or notch). Normally diastolic flow in the umbilical artery increases (i.e.

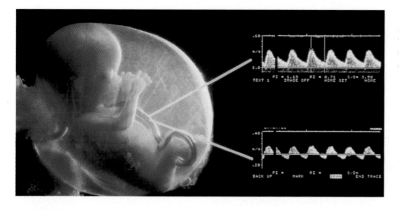

**Figure 6.13** Normal (top) and abnormal (bottom) Doppler signals from the umbilical artery. Reversed flow in diastole indicates poor placental function and impending fetal demise.

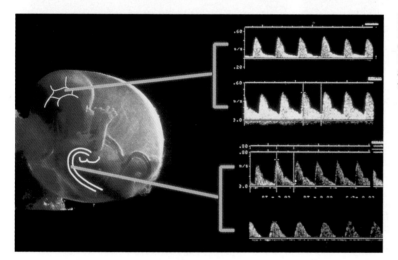

**Figure 6.14** Normal and abnormal Doppler signals from the middle cerebral artery and thoracic aorta. Increasing flow in the middle cerebral artery and absence of diastolic flow in the aorta indicate fetal acidaemia.

placental resistance falls) throughout gestation. If the resistance index in the umbilical artery rises above the 95th centile of the normal graph, this implies faulty perfusion of the placenta, which may eventually result in fetal hypoxia. Absent or reversed end-diastolic velocity in the umbilical artery is a particularly serious development with a strong correlation with fetal distress and intrauterine death (Figure 6.13). Meta-analysis of several randomized studies shows that umbilical Doppler monitoring reduces perinatal mortality in high-risk pregnancies (Neilson and Alfirevic 2000).

### Fetal vessels

Falling oxygen levels in the fetus result in a redistribution of blood flow to protect the brain, heart, adrenals and spleen, and vasoconstriction in all other vessels. Several fetal vessels have been studied and reflect this 'centralization' of flow. The middle cerebral artery will show increasing diastolic flow (falling pulsatility index) as hypoxia increases, while a rising resistance in the fetal aorta reflects compensatory vasoconstriction in the fetal body. When diastolic flow is absent in the fetal aorta, this implies fetal acidaemia (Figure 6.14). Perhaps the most sensitive index of fetal acidaemia and incipient heart failure is demonstrated by increasing pulsatility in the central veins supplying the heart, such as the ductus venosus and inferior vena cava. When late diastolic flow is absent in the ductus venosus, then delivery should be considered, as fetal death is imminent (Figure 6.15).

## Developments in imaging

### Magnetic resonance imaging

This technique utilizes the effect of powerful magnetic forces on spinning hydrogen protons, which

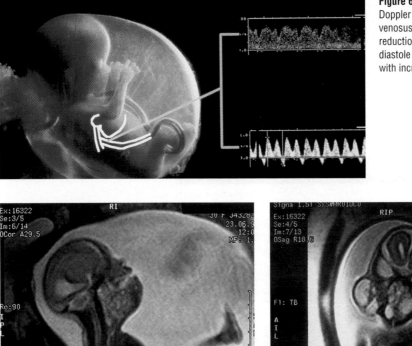

**Figure 6.15** Normal and abnormal Doppler signals from the ductus venosus. There is progressive reduction of flow to the heart in late diastole (i.e. with atrial contraction), with increasing fetal acidaemia.

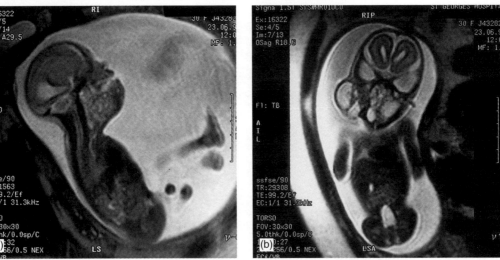

**Figure 6.16** (a) and (b) Magnetic resonance imaging scan of fetus showing thyroid tumour.

when knocked off their axis by pulsed radio waves, produce radiofrequency signals as they return to their basal state. The signals reflect the clinical composition of tissue (i.e. the amount and distribution of hydrogen protons) and thus the images provide significant improvement over ultrasound in tissue characterization. The technique also has the advantage of providing sectional images in any plane. The main disadvantage is that magnetic resonance imaging (MRI) is many times more expensive than ultrasound and images are more likely to be affected by movement artefacts. Some centres sedate the woman prior to an examination to reduce fetal movement.

Magnetic resonance imaging provides superb images of fetal anatomy and is extremely useful when ultrasound images are not diagnostic or when they are suboptimal because of maternal obesity. An example of a fetal MRI scan is given in Figure 6.16.

## Three-dimensional ultrasound

This technique may transform ultrasound imaging in the future. In conventional scanning, the ultrasound beam is swept electronically in a single plane across a flat transducer. In three-dimensional scanning, the beam is swept in two orthogonal planes to capture a block or volume of echoes, which are digitally stored. The aim of the operator is to capture a volume from the region of interest and this is normally completed in 5–15 seconds, depending on the required volume for diagnosis. After this, the volume of echoes can be resliced in any plane to provide the appropriate two-dimensional image. Furthermore, by surface or volume rendering, lifelike three-dimensional reconstructions of surface features of the fetus, or particular organs, can be made and surface or volume rendering can remove artefacts or structures that obscure the image.

The advantages are that the scanning time can be drastically shortened and volumes can be stored for later analysis. In the future, volumes will be transferred electronically to tertiary centres for expert diagnosis. There is evidence that three-dimensional imaging improves the diagnosis of certain fetal abnormalities, such as cleft lip and palate, and it is likely to be popular with parents because the images are very lifelike (Figure 6.17).

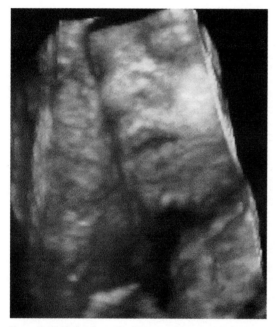

**Figure 6.17** Three-dimensional ultrasound scan of fetal face.

consequent reduction in blood flow to other organs. This will lead to asymmetrical growth with relative brain sparing and oligohydramnios owing to reduced renal perfusion.
  - Reduction of fetal activity to conserve oxygen and reduce anaerobic metabolism. This will result in a reduction of general body and breathing movements.
  - Modification of the autonomic control of the fetal heart with a reduction in baseline variability.
- Ultimately, as fetal acidaemia develops as a result of anaerobic glycolysis, there will be abnormal Doppler waveforms in the ductus venosus as a consequence of right heart failure, and decelerations in the fetal heart trace as a result of increased vagal tone.
- Most of these changes can now be documented by means of Doppler ultrasound and antenatal cardiotocography. A brief summary of the sequence of events is given in Figure 6.18.

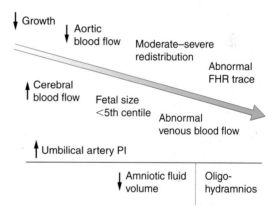

**Figure 6.18** Sequential changes in tests of fetal well-being in uteroplacental failure. FHR, fetal heart rate; PI, pulsatility index.

- Abnormalities of fetal well-being are usually the result of impaired transfer of nutrients and oxygen across the placenta leading to the development of intrauterine growth restriction and fetal hypoxia.
- The fetal responses to placental insufficiency are:
  - Reduction of growth rate in response to impaired transfer of nutrients and to conserve oxygen.
  - Redistribution of the circulation to preferentially perfuse the brain, myocardium and adrenal gland with a

- The decision when to deliver the baby will be taken by the obstetrician on the basis of an evaluation of several of these antenatal tests together with the maternal condition, such as the presence of pre-eclampsia or diabetes mellitus. For example, after 32 weeks, the decision to deliver might be based on an SGA infant with oligohydramnios and evidence of circulatory redistribution. Before 32 weeks, delivery may be delayed in order to achieve greater fetal maturity; in this situation, tests of fetal cardiac function (ductus venosus and cardiotocography) become critical.

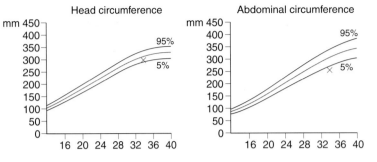

**Figure 6.19** Plot of fetal head circumference and fetal abdominal circumference for case history.

BB, an 18-year-old in her first pregnancy, attends for review at the community clinic at 34 weeks' gestation. Her dates had been confirmed by ultrasound at booking (12 weeks). She is a smoker. The midwife measures her fundal height at 30 cm; all other observations are within normal limits. The midwife refers the woman to the maternity day unit at the local hospital. An ultrasound scan is performed because of her concern that the fetus is small for gestational age and the measurements are plotted (Figure 6.19).

### Do the ultrasound findings support the midwife's suspicion that the fetus is SGA?

Yes, because the fetal abdominal circumference is on the fifth centile for gestation. This finding does not give an indication of the well-being of the fetus and is compatible with intrauterine growth restriction secondary to placental insufficiency or a healthy constitutionally small baby.

### What additional features/measures on ultrasound assessment could give an indication of fetal well-being?

*Liquor volume*
Amniotic fluid volume is decreased in fetal growth restriction associated with fetal hypoxia, with redistribution of fetal blood flow away from the kidneys to vital structures such as brain and heart, with a consequent reduction in renal perfusion and urine output.

*Biophysical profile*
In the presence of fetal hypoxia associated with IUGR, fetal biophysical variables, such as gross body movements, flexor tone and fetal breathing movements are abolished. These can be observed using ultrasound.

*Doppler ultrasound*
*Umbilical artery*: Waveforms from the umbilical artery provide information on fetoplacental blood flow and placental resistance. Diastolic velocity in the umbilical artery increases (i.e. placental resistance falls) throughout gestation. If the resistance index in the umbilical artery rises above the 95th centile of the normal graph, this implies faulty perfusion of the placenta, which may eventually result in fetal hypoxia. Absent or reversed end-diastolic velocity in the umbilical artery is a particularly serious development with a strong correlation with fetal distress and intrauterine death.

*Fetal vessels*: Falling oxygen levels in the fetus result in a redistribution of blood flow to protect the brain, heart, adrenals and spleen, and vasoconstriction in all other vessels. The middle cerebral artery will show increasing diastolic flow as hypoxia increases, while a rising resistance in the fetal aorta reflects compensatory vasoconstriction in the fetal body. When diastolic flow is absent in the fetal aorta, this implies fetal acidaemia. Increasing pulsatility in the central veins supplying the heart, such as the ductus venosus and inferior vena cava are indicators of fetal acidaemia and impending heart failure; when late diastolic flow is absent in the ductus venosus, fetal death is imminent.

*Cardiotocography*
Fetal tachycardia, reduced variability in heart rate, absence of accelerations and presence of decelerations identified on a cardiotocograph are associated with fetal hypoxia.

# References

Alfirevic Z, Neilson JP. Biophysical profile for fetal assessment in high risk pregnancies. *Cochrane Database of Systematic Reviews* 2000; Issue 2:CD000038.

Bricker LJ, Garcia J, et al. Ultrasound screening in pregnancy: a systematic review of the clinical effectiveness, cost-effectiveness and women's views. *Health Technology Assessments* 2000; **4**(16):i–vi, 1–193.

Chien PF, Arnott N, et al. How useful is uterine artery Doppler flow velocimetry in the prediction of pre-eclampsia, intrauterine growth retardation and perinatal death? An overview. *British Journal of Obstetrics and Gynaecology* 2000; **107**(2):196–208.

Iams JD, Goldenberg RL, et al. The length of the cervix and the risk of spontaneous premature delivery. National Institute of Child Health and Human Development Maternal Fetal Medicine Unit Network. *New England Journal of Medicine* 1996; **334**(9):567–72.

Kohut RJ, Dewey D, et al. Women's knowledge of prenatal ultrasound and informed choice. *Journal of Genetic Counselling* 2002; **11**(4):265–76.

Neilson JP, Alfirevic Z. Doppler ultrasound for fetal assessment in high risk pregnancies. *Cochrane Database of Systematic Reviews* 2000; Issue 2:CD000073.

Newnham JP, Evans SF, et al. Effects of frequent ultrasound during pregnancy: a randomised controlled trial. *Lancet* 1993; **342**(8876):887–91.

National Institute for Clinical Excellence. *Antenatal care: routine care for the healthy pregnant woman.* London: RCOG Press, 2003.

Ziskin MC. Update on the safety of ultrasound in obstetrics. *Seminars in Roentgenology* 1990; **25**(4):294–8.

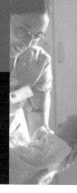

# Prenatal diagnosis

## OVERVIEW

Prenatal diagnosis aims to detect fetal malformation as early as possible during pregnancy, so that health professionals can supply parents with sufficient objective information to allow informed decision-making regarding the subsequent management of the pregnancy. Congenital abnormalities are malformations or disorders present at birth. They are caused by a variety of factors including those that are inherited, placental, environmental or due to incidents related to birth. Congenital abnormality occurs in approximately 2 per 100 pregnancies. Table 7.1 shows the classification and incidence of common congenital abnormalities.

**Table 7.1** – Classification and prevalence of common congenital abnormalities

| Congenital abnormality | Example | Incidence per 1000 births |
|---|---|---|
| Structural | Congenital heart disease | 4–6 |
| | Neural tube defects | 2–6 |
| | Cleft lip/palate | 1–2 |
| | Talipes equinovarus | 1 |
| Chromosomal | Trisomy 21 (Down's syndrome) | 1.5 |
| | Monosomy X (Turner's syndrome) | 0.3 |
| | Other trisomies (13 and 18) | 0.3 |
| Genetic | Cystic fibrosis | 0.5 |
| | Sickle cell disease | Depends on ethnicity |
| Miscellaneous | Viral infection | 0.2 |

The prenatal diagnosis of congenital abnormality has become an integral and important part of antenatal care, coordinated nationally by the UK National Screening Committee. Prenatal diagnosis has two parts – screening and diagnosis, the differences of which are set out in Table 7.2. All women are offered screening to identify those pregnancies at risk of congenital abnormality in order to target diagnostic services appropriately, as diagnostic tests are expensive, invasive and carry a risk of inducing miscarriage. Should the fetus be affected, the parents will need sufficient, realistic and empathetic information to facilitate decision-making. If the fetal condition is untreatable, not compatible with extrauterine life or associated with significant handicap, the parents may decide to terminate the pregnancy. Alternatively, they may decide to continue with the pregnancy, research the realities of living with a child with the diagnosed disability and make suitable plans for the birth to occur at the most appropriate venue where expertise is available to ensure optimal treatment and prognosis for their child.

**Table 7.2** – Differences between prenatal screening and diagnostic tests

|  | Screening | Diagnostic tests |
| --- | --- | --- |
| Population tested | All women | Women at 'high risk' |
| Purpose of test | Select a 'high-risk' group | To diagnose abnormality |
| Usual method of testing | Maternal history | Ultrasound |
|  | Maternal biochemistry | Amniocentesis |
|  | Maternal virology | Chorion villi sampling |
|  | Ultrasound | Cordocentesis |
| Prerequisite to test | Diagnostic test available | Patient aware of potential risks |
| Risk of test | Anxiety of a 'screen-positive' result | Small risk of miscarriage from invasive test |

## Prenatal screening and diagnostic tests

### Psychological implications

An essential consideration within the sphere of prenatal diagnosis is the resulting psychological effects on the parent(s). In a society where the majority of children are planned, with normality and health the expectation, fetal abnormality and the prospect of terminating a wanted pregnancy can result in grief and devastation for the parent(s). Questioning a woman's capability to produce normal children can cause increased stress, which can potentially result in two interlinking and damaging psychological outcomes – increased anxiety levels and disordered antenatal attachment. It is suggested that pregnancy itself provokes higher anxiety levels and a heightened sensitivity to stressors; any compounding stress may lead to severe anxiety and disordered coping mechanisms. Severe anxiety in pregnancy has been associated with both psychological and physical consequences, including increased dependency on smoking and drugs; spontaneous abortion; and preterm labour. It has also been found that severe anxiety regarding fetal normality leads to the woman withholding emotional attachment to the developing fetus, afraid to invest too much emotional energy in a pregnancy that may be terminated.

A further consideration within prenatal screening is the psychological harm caused by false-positive results. When screening suggests the possibility of fetal abnormality, parental concerns and anxiety for the future of their pregnancy are instigated. Even following further conclusive tests which exclude abnormality, doubt regarding fetal normality persists, causing further anxiety throughout the pregnancy and, in some cases, this continues throughout the child's early years.

However, the facility to screen and diagnose congenital abnormality provides reproductive choices and autonomy for parents. It is particularly beneficial for those parents with the risk of inherited abnormality, providing them with the opportunity to have their desired family.

### Informed consent

Paramount within prenatal diagnosis is the concept of informed consent. All parents should be given accurate, relevant and understandable information about the effects and prognosis of the condition, and the effectiveness and limitations of the proposed tests in order that they can make a reasoned decision. Several studies have shown that there are inherent difficulties with ensuring that information given to parents is assimilated, particularly when offering screening tests. Women and their partners often envisage screening tests as routine and innocuous, a scientific method of confirming their fetus is healthy. As a result, they are often unaware of the possible devastating consequences of screening. It is essential, therefore, that sufficient time is taken when offering screening tests to discuss the full implications of screening, including the possibility of false-negative and false-positive results; the possibility of further more invasive tests and the decisions regarding the management/termination of pregnancy should the test diagnose fetal abnormality.

It is essential that health professional have an in-depth knowledge of prenatal diagnosis in order to provide parents with adequate information to make informed choices.

## Invasive diagnostic tests

A number of different tests exist to enable sampling material of fetal origin (Table 7.3). The sample obtained can be used for cytogenetic, biochemical, enzymatic or DNA analysis to give a prenatal diagnosis.

Generally, these tests are invasive in nature and carry a small risk of miscarriage.

### Chorion villi sampling

A thin needle is passed transabdominally or transcervically under ultrasound guidance into the placenta (chorionic plate) (Figure 7.1). Chorionic villi, which are the same genetic material as the fetus, are aspirated or biopsied through this needle. This test is usually performed at or after 10 weeks' gestation. Although the miscarriage rate after chorion villi sampling (CVS) is relatively high at 2–3 per cent, this is due to the higher rate of spontaneous miscarriage at this gestation. The

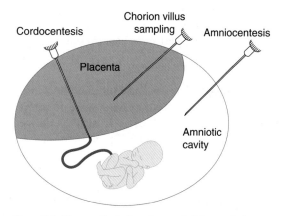

**Figure 7.1** Diagram illustrating placement of the needle for amniocentesis, chorion villi sampling and cordocentesis.

**Table 7.3** – Details of prenatal diagnostic procedures

|  | Amniocentesis | Chorion villi sampling | Cordocentesis |
|---|---|---|---|
| Gestation | 15–40 weeks | 10–40 weeks | 20–40 weeks |
| Route | Transabdominal | Transabdominal/ transcervical | Transabdominal |
| Cells sampled | Fetal fibroblasts | Trophoblast cells | Fetal white blood cells |
| Procedure-related 1% risk of miscarriage | 1% | 1% | 1% |
| Direct karyotype result | FISH for chromosomes 13, 18, 21 and XY – 24–48 hours | Not needed | 24–48 hours |
| Culture karyotype result | 2–3 weeks | 1–2 weeks | 24–48 hours |
| Mosaicism rate on karyotype | None | 1% | None |

FISH, fluorescence *in-situ* hybridization.

procedure-related miscarriage rate is the same as amniocentesis (1 per cent). Although it is technically possible to do CVS at earlier gestations, this is generally avoided, as it is associated with a higher rate of cleft lip/palate and digital amputation abnormalities.

### Amniocentesis

A thin needle is passed transabdominally under ultrasound guidance into the amniotic cavity (Figure 7.1). A small amount of amniotic fluid that contains fetal cells is removed. This test is usually performed at or after 15 weeks' gestation. The procedure-related miscarriage rate for this test is 1 per cent. Although it is technically possible to perform amniocentesis at earlier gestations, this is generally avoided, as it is associated with a higher cell culture failure rate, higher rate of miscarriage, neonatal talipes and respiratory difficulties.

### Cordocentesis

A thin needle is passed transabdominally under ultrasound guidance into the umbilical cord to sample fetal blood (Figure 7.1). This test is usually performed at or after 20 weeks' gestation. The procedure-related miscarriage rate for this test is 1 per cent. Although it is technically possible to do this test at earlier gestations, this is generally avoided, as it is associated with a higher rate of miscarriage.

## Laboratory analysis

### Cytogenetic analysis

Cells obtained from invasive prenatal diagnostic tests are cultured until sufficient cells in mitosis are available to make a cytogenetic diagnosis. The more rapidly the tissue divides, the quicker the results are available. Hence the time for diagnosis is 2–3 weeks for amniocentesis, 1–2 weeks for CVS and 24–48 hours for cordocentesis.

With CVS, the sampled chorionic villi have so many cells already in mitosis that a 'direct' result may be available in 24–48 hours. In this instance, the quality of the diagnosis is adequate to exclude an aneuploidy (abnormal number of chromosomes). The direct preparation is usually not of sufficient quality to permit G-banding; hence chromosomal aberrations, such as deletions or inversions, cannot be effectively excluded.

The use of fluorescence in-situ hybridization (FISH) can facilitate rapid results with amniocentesis. The technique detects and localizes specific DNA sequences directly in interphase or metaphase, and hence cell culture is not required. It allows the rapid (24–48 hours) prenatal diagnosis of major aneuploidies for chromosomes 13, 18, 21 and XY.

### DNA analysis

Fetal DNA obtained from invasive tests can be used for DNA probe (sickle cell disease and cystic fibrosis), polymerase chain reaction (PCR) (fragile X syndrome, congenital toxoplasmosis and cytomegalovirus) or linkage analysis (fragile X syndrome).

### Biochemical and enzymatic analysis

When DNA analysis is not possible, biochemical or enzymatic assays can be performed for specific diseases (congenital adrenal hypoplasia and mucopolysaccharidoses).

## Diagnosis of structural abnormalities

Structural abnormalities constitute the majority of congenital abnormalities encountered in clinical practice. There are established screening programmes for fetal neural tube and cardiac defects; these are discussed in detail in this section. Other fetal structural malformations occur less commonly and are sporadic in nature.

The Royal College of Obstetricians and Gynaecologists has recommended a two-stage ultrasound scan (USS) programme for screening for structural abnormalities: an initial USS at booking (11–14 weeks) and a further USS at or around 20 weeks. Details of these routine USS are provided in Chapter 6 along with details of the features that should be identified on the later scan.

## Neural tube defects

Neural tube defects (NTDs) are among the most common major abnormalities. NTDs occur due to defects in the formation of the neural tube during embryogenesis. The aetiology is multifactorial with well-defined environmental, genetic, pharmacological and geographical factors implicated.

Neural tube defects affecting the cranial vault present on ultrasound as anencephaly or encephalocoele. Anencephaly is universally lethal, while the prognosis for encephalocoele is related to the size of the defect.

The remainder of the NTDs, termed spina bifida, can occur at any point along the spinal cord; however, the most common site is usually at the caudal end. The local effects of spina bifida (paralysis of the legs, urinary and faecal incontinence) depend on the spinal level and the number of spinal segments affected in the lesion. Spina bifida has previously been associated with impaired intellect due to progressive hydrocephalus and infection of ventriculoperitoneal shunts. With modern imaging techniques and antibiotics, the intellectual prognosis for this condition is much improved.

### Prenatal screening and diagnosis of neural tube defects

When a parent or previous sibling has had an NTD, the risk of recurrence is 5–10 per cent. Mid-trimester maternal serum alpha-fetoprotein (AFP) levels are increased in pregnancies affected by open NTDs. These were once used as the established screening tests for NTDs, with screen-positive women being referred for amniocentesis. The presence of acetyl cholinesterase, a central nervous system (CNS) neurotransmitter, in amniotic fluid was taken as being diagnostic of an open NTD.

The need for a two-step screening/diagnosis process was quickly superseded by the development of high-resolution ultrasound. Anencephaly and encephalocoeles are detectable on first trimester ultrasound (Figure 7.2). Spina bifida on the other hand requires the systematic detailed examination of the fetal spine (Figure 7.3) at the routine 20-week anomaly scan. The diagnosis may be suspected from the visualization of the 'lemon' (shape of the skull) and 'banana' (absent cerebellum) signs in the fetal brain at this examination (Figure 7.4). The sensitivity of ultrasound for both open and closed NTDs is greater than 95 per cent. Other CNS abnormalities (not strictly NTDs), such as hydrocephalus, can also be detected at the 20-week scan (Figure 7.5 and Table 7.4).

### Prevention of neural tube defects

Folate deficiency and drugs that interfere with folate metabolism (i.e. antiepileptics) are implicated in about 10 per cent of NTD cases. Periconceptual folate supplementation of the maternal diet reduces the risk of developing these defects by about half. Folic acid should be given for at least 3 months prior to conception and for the first trimester of pregnancy. The dosage of folic acid is 400 μg for primary prevention and 4 mg for women wishing to prevent a recurrence of an NTD or for women with Type I diabetes mellitus.

## Congenital heart defects

Abnormalities of the heart and great arteries are another common group of congenital abnormalities.

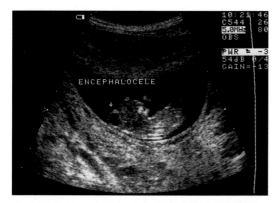

**Figure 7.2** Fetal encephalocoele detected at 12 weeks' gestation.

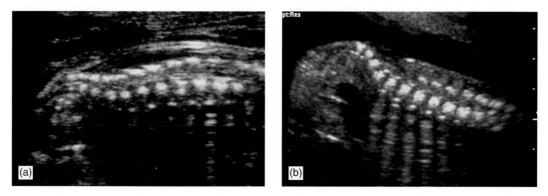

**Figure 7.3** (a) Normal fetal spine showing posterior spinous process. (b) Abnormal fetal spine with spinous process absent in the sacral and fifth lumbar segments.

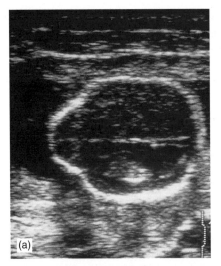 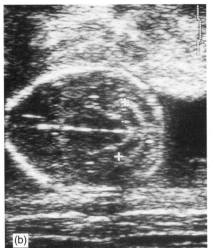

**Figure 7.4** (a) Lemon-shaped skull, and (b) curved (banana) cerebellum, which are typical cranial signs of spina bifida.

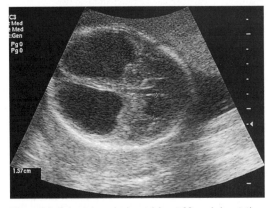

**Figure 7.5** Enlarged cerebral ventricles at 22 weeks' gestation, diagnostic of hydrocephalus.

About half are either lethal or require major surgery, with the remainder being asymptomatic. The aetiology of congenital heart defects (CHDs) is heterogeneous and includes genetic factors, environmental factors (e.g. diabetes mellitus), drugs (e.g. lithium) and viral infections (e.g. rubella). Gene mutations and chromosomal abnormalities account for less than 5 per cent of cases.

*Prenatal screening for congenital heart defects*
When a previous sibling or father is affected by CHD, the risk is 2 per cent. When two siblings or the mother has CHD, the recurrence risk is 10 per cent. The second major group considered to be at high risk are women with Type I diabetes mellitus, where the incidence of CHD is doubled. However, more than 90 per cent of fetuses with CHD occur in pregnancies without such risk factors.

**Table 7.4** – Some major structural abnormalities detectable by ultrasound at the mid-trimester scan

| Body system | Example |
| --- | --- |
| Cranium | Anencephaly* |
| | Encephalocoele* |
| | Hydrocephalus |
| Skeleton | Spina bifida |
| | Kyphoscoliosis |
| Thorax | Congenital heart disease |
| | Cystic adenomatoid malformation |
| | Diaphragmatic hernia |
| Abdomen | Gastroschisis |
| | Exomphalos* |
| | Renal agenesis |
| | Multi/polycystic disease |
| | Hydronephrosis |
| Limbs | Talipes equinovarus |
| | Polydactyly* |

*The abnormalities with an asterisk can frequently be detected at the first trimester scan.

*Prenatal diagnosis of congenital heart defects*
Although 90 per cent of major CHDs may be detected antenatally in specialist centres, in most units performing routine 20-week anomaly scans, this figure is closer to 30 per cent. As specialist fetal echocardiography cannot be performed on all pregnancies, the limiting

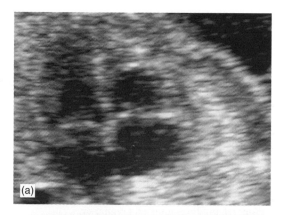

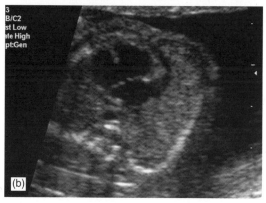

**Figure 7.6** (a) Normal four-chamber fetal heart, and (b) abnormal heart with atrioventricular and septal defect.

factor in diagnosis is selection of cases for referral to these specialist units (Figure 7.6).

## Gastrointestinal abnormalities

### Bowel obstruction
Bowel obstruction above the ileum (e.g. duodenal and oesophageal atresia) usually result in polyhydramnios and is easily visualized with ultrasound. Duodenal atresia is characteristically associated with a 'double-bubble' appearance on ultrasound. One-third of cases will be associated with Down's syndrome and amniocentesis to allow karyotyping should be considered.

### Abdominal wall defects
Omphaloceles are due to a midline abdominal wall defect through which the peritoneal sac herniates. This sac will contain varying amounts of abdominal contents, including small bowel and liver. Approximately 50 per cent of omphaloceles have associated cardiac

or chromosomal abnormalities. In gastroschisis, the insertion of the umbilical cord is intact but there are free loops of bowel in the amniotic cavity. In the majority of cases, the anomaly is isolated and there is no increased incidence of chromosomal anomalies.

## Renal tract abnormalities

Major abnormalities of the renal tract, such as renal agenesis, will normally be detected by 20 weeks because of the associated oligohydramnios.

### Renal pelvis dilatation
The commonest abnormality seen in the renal tract and identified on ultrasound is mild pelvic calyceal dilatation. This abnormality is found in approximately 2 per cent of fetuses on the second trimester scan, and the significance of the finding is controversial. Pelvic calyceal dilatation may be physiological or result from mild reflux or pelviureteric junction obstruction. Postnatal renal ultrasonography is required to assess progression or regression. Failure of resolution increases the risk of urinary tract infections.

## Other structural abnormalities

### Cleft lip/palate
The typical cleft lip appears as a linear defect extending from the lip to the nostril, with the majority of cases (75 per cent) being unilateral. In about 50 per cent of cases, both the lip and palate are defective, in the remainder, either the lip or palate is involved. Cleft lip (with or without cleft palate) is identifiable on ultrasound, whereas the diagnosis of isolated cleft palate is difficult. Associated abnormalities are found in about 15 per cent of fetuses with cleft lip/palate, usually because genetic or chromosomal abnormalities are implicated in the aetiology. Cleft lip/palate is also associated with some anticonvulsant drugs. Postnatally, because of cosmetic, feeding and respiratory problems, early surgical correction is usually advocated.

### Talipes equinovarus
In talipes equinovarus, also known as clubfoot, the forefoot is supinated and the ankle is plantar flexed. The deformity is bilateral in 50 per cent of cases and affects twice as many males as females. The aetiology is sporadic and the condition is neurological in origin, with the skeletal malformation being secondary. The

diagnosis is reliably established on ultrasound, except in positional talipes, a temporary malformation secondary to oligohydramnios. Talipes equinovarus is lethal in about 20 per cent of cases because of associated malformations, most commonly spina bifida.

## Chromosomal abnormality

The most common chromosomal abnormalities can be classified as either aneuploidies (usually trisomies) or sex chromosome abnormalities.

### Aneuploidies

Trisomies occur in the majority of cases due to non-disjunction in meiosis. This abnormality of gametogenesis is known to occur more frequently with advancing maternal age. Rarely, trisomies may occur owing to unbalanced translocations (6 per cent) or mosaicism (4 per cent). Although any chromosome may be affected, it is usually only trisomies 13 (Patau's), 18 (Edwards') and 21 (Down's) that are seen at birth, as most other trisomies spontaneously miscarry within the first trimester. Down's syndrome is associated with 500 possible documented features; this result in characteristic mental and physical features. Trisomies 13 and 18 are associated with such major structural defects that their diagnosis is usually suspected on antenatal ultrasound. Since trisomies 13 and 18 are associated with intrauterine death (90–95 per cent), screening programmes are geared mainly towards the antenatal detection of Down's syndrome, which is the commonest chromosomal abnormality at birth.

### Sex chromosome abnormalities

Unlike trisomies, the prevalence of sex chromosome abnormalities does not change with maternal age. The cumulative prevalence of Turner's (monosomy X or 45XO), Klinefelter's (47XXY) and other sex chromosome abnormalities is greater than Down's syndrome. Turner's syndrome individuals are infertile females of normal intellect and short stature. Klinefelter's syndrome individuals are infertile males with slightly reduced IQ, testicular dysgenesis and tall stature. As many of the characteristics of these conditions are mild, many affected individuals remain undiagnosed throughout their lifetime. Routine screening for these conditions is not available and the diagnosis is often made incidentally.

### Fragile X

Fragile X syndrome is the most common inherited cause of mental retardation, explaining the excess of males affected by non-specific mental retardation in the population. The fragile X gene (FMR1) becomes hypermethylated and inactivated multiple (>200) repeats. The estimated prevalence of the condition is 1 in 4000 males. Prenatal diagnosis is possible using PCR and Southern analysis, but only on male fetuses at present. As screening for fragile X in pregnancy is not feasible, prenatal testing is reserved for families where one of the parents is known to be a carrier by virtue of a previous affected pregnancy.

## Screening tests for Down's syndrome

### Maternal age and history

The prevalence of Down's syndrome increases with advancing maternal age (Figure 7.7). Because of this, historically, women over the age of 35 were offered diagnostic testing for Down's syndrome. However, 90 per cent of pregnant women are younger than 35 years and, despite being at lower risk, they give birth to 75–80 per cent of Down's syndrome babies. Women who have already had a pregnancy affected by Down's syndrome are routinely offered prenatal diagnosis, based on their background risk for trisomy being slightly increased.

### Maternal serum biochemistry

Measurement of maternal serum hormones during the second trimester (14–22 weeks' gestation) offers an alternative method of screening. The two main hormones of fetal origin that are commonly assayed are alpha-fetoprotein and human chorionic gonadotrophin (hCG). In pregnancies complicated by a

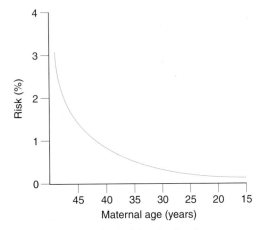

**Figure 7.7** Down's syndrome risk and maternal age.

fetus with Down's syndrome, these levels are decreased and increased respectively. Based on maternal age, gestation and variation in hormone levels, an algorithm predicts the individual's risk for a Down's syndrome pregnancy: the current standard provides a detection rate of 60 per cent and a false-positive rate of less than 5 per cent. This is not diagnostic, but identifies a group at high risk (1:250) who should be offered a diagnostic test, such as amniocentesis [National Institute for Clinical Excellence (NICE) 2003]. It is also important to remember that being assessed as low risk, based on biochemical screening, does not exclude an affected pregnancy.

First trimester screening uses two biochemical markers, pregnancy-associated plasma protein (PAPP-A; which is lowered in Down's syndrome) and beta-hCG (which is elevated) in addition to maternal age, to provide an individual risk in a similar fashion to second trimester biochemical screening. The advantage of early screening is that the termination of pregnancy, if required, may be performed as a day-case surgical procedure rather than by induction of labour.

## Ultrasound

### Nuchal translucency

A newer screening test for Down's syndrome involves the sonographic measurement of the subcutaneous collection of fluid in the nuchal (behind the neck) region of the fetus at 10–13 weeks' gestation. The nuchal translucency (NT) measurement is increased in the majority of aneuploid fetuses in the first trimester

of pregnancy (Figure 7.8 and Table 7.5). Based on maternal age, gestation and NT measurement, an algorithm predicts the individual's risk for Down's syndrome in a similar way to the biochemical screening.

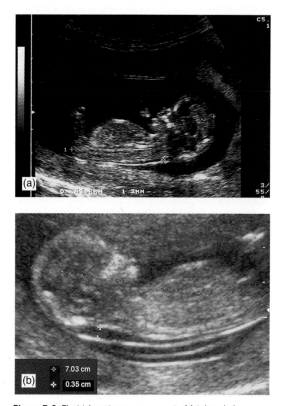

**Figure 7.8** First trimester measurement of fetal nuchal translucency. (a) Normal, and (b) 3.5 mm (increased), suggestive of chromosome abnormality.

**Table 7.5** – Screening tests for Down's syndrome

| Method | Maternal age (History) | Maternal serum biochemistry (Blood test) | Nuchal translucency (Ultrasound scan) |
|---|---|---|---|
| Gestation | Any | 10–14 weeks (PAPP-A, beta-hCG) 15–22 weeks (AFP, hCG) | 10–14 weeks |
| Sensitivity | 25% | 60–75% | 75–80% |
| Advantages | Simple, cheap | Operator-independent Screens for neural tube and  abdominal wall defects | Early test Screens for all aneuploidy Applicable in multiple pregnancy |
| Disadvantages | Poor sensitivity | Late test Specific for Down's Requires dating scan | Operator-dependent |

AFP, alpha-fetoprotein; hCG, human chorionic gonadotrophin; PAPP-A, pregnancy-associated plasma protein.

Combining NT measurement with maternal serum biochemical markers increases the sensitivity of the tests. The Guidelines for Antenatal Care from NICE (2003) recommend that, by April 2007, all pregnant women should be offered screening tests for Down's syndrome that provides a detection rate above 75 per cent with a false-positive rate of less than 3 per cent. Tests that currently meet this standard are, at 11–14 weeks' gestation, the combined test (NT, hCG and PAPP-A) and, at 14–20 weeks' gestation, the quadruple test [NT, PAPP-A, unconjugated oestriol (uE3) and inhibin A].

Other ultrasound anomalies

In addition to increased NT, other common abnormalities detected by ultrasound in Down's syndrome include brachycephaly and ventriculomegaly in the skull and brain, cardiac defects, echogenic chordae tendineae in the heart, echogenic bowel, mild hydronephrosis, short femur, and abnormal hands and feet. At later gestations, fetuses may be small for gestational age.

## Genetic disorders

There are numerous congenital abnormalities that exhibit a classical Mendelian pattern of inheritance. The commonest of these, cystic fibrosis and the haemoglobinopathies, are discussed below. Additionally numerous genetic syndromes exist; the majority of these are sporadic, but some have recessive, dominant or sex-linked patterns of inheritance. The majority of conditions with recessive, dominant or sex-linked inheritance patterns have a relatively low frequency and are only screened for in families with a known history. These families should have genetic counselling regarding the disease, likelihood of recurrence and discussion of the possible implications of diagnostic testing prior to testing.

### Cystic fibrosis

Cystic fibrosis is an autosomal recessive condition and the most common lethal genetic disease in Caucasians. The cystic fibrosis gene has been isolated to the long arm of chromosome 7 and there are over 700 mutations identified to this region that are responsible for the disease. The commonest of these mutations is δF508, which is present in 68 per cent of cases. Multiple gene mutations and the cost of DNA testing

for the population are the major reasons why effective prenatal screening has not been effective to date. At present, prenatal diagnosis is offered only to parents who are known carriers, usually because they have had an affected child already.

### Haemoglobinopathies

Sickle cell anaemia and thalassaemia are both autosomal recessive conditions with considerable disease heterogeneity. The carrier frequency may be as high as 20 per cent, especially in African (sickle cell disease) and Mediterranean (thalassaemia) populations. Screening of at-risk populations is possible by haemoglobin electrophoresis. Sickle cell mutations are limited in number and fairly well characterized, hence prenatal diagnosis is usually possible. As there are numerous thalassaemia mutations, parental studies are a prerequisite to establish whether a fetal diagnosis is possible. Prenatal diagnosis is made on fetal DNA, which can be obtained by any of the invasive techniques. As the risk of an affected pregnancy is high (25 per cent) for parents who are carriers, early testing through CVS is advocated.

## Congenital viral and parasitic infections

Fetal infection with rubella, cytomegalovirus (CMV), toxoplasmosis and parvovirus are known to have potentially serious deleterious effects (Table 7.6) and these are discussed in detail in Chapter 13. Maternal viral infections in pregnancy are relatively infrequent, with the likelihood of transplacental transfer and fetal infection increasing with gestational age. Most infected fetuses (>95 per cent), however, remain unaffected. The risk of a congenitally infected fetus being affected is inversely proportional to the gestational age. Hence, although the chance of fetal infection is low in early pregnancy, if infected, the fetus is likely to be seriously affected and the pregnancy is doomed to miscarriage. Therefore, the most susceptible pregnancies are those infected at 12–18 weeks' gestation, when infected fetuses are likely to be seriously affected and yet survive.

### Screening for congenital viral and parasitic infections

There is an established screening programme for rubella in pregnancy. Rubella-susceptible women are

**Table 7.6** – Characteristics of congenital viral infection

|  | Rubella | Cytomegalovirus | Toxoplasmosis | Parvovirus |
|---|---|---|---|---|
| Source | Infected individuals | Infected individuals | Cat litter, undercooked meat | Infected children |
| Features of congenital infection | Cataracts | Microcephaly | Microcephaly | Aplastic anaemia |
|  | Ventriculomegaly | Ventriculomegaly | Hydrops |  |
|  | Cerebral calcification | Cerebral calcification |  |  |
|  | Heart defects | Heart defects | Heart defects |  |
|  | Growth restriction | Growth restriction | Growth restriction |  |
|  | Hepatomegaly | Hepatomegaly | Hepatomegaly |  |
|  | Thrombocytopenia | Thrombocytopenia | Thrombocytopenia |  |
|  | Mental retardation | Mental retardation | Mental retardation |  |

advised to avoid antenatal exposure to the virus and are vaccinated in the puerperium. Screening is not advocated for maternal CMV or toxoplasmosis infections in pregnancy because of the low incidence, the high false-positive rates, and the risk of miscarriage consequent on the invasive prenatal diagnostic tests necessary to confirm fetal infection. Additionally, confirming fetal infection does not necessarily indicate that the fetus has been affected.

## Prenatal diagnosis of congenital viral and parasitic infections

In cases of confirmed maternal viral infection, regular fetal ultrasound to detect the characteristic features of congenital infection is advocated. There is limited evidence that treatment of toxoplasmosis-infected mothers with spiramycin may prevent congenital fetal infection. Congenital parvovirus infection may result in a temporary fetal aplastic anaemia and hydrops. Supportive therapy with intrauterine fetal blood transfusions in these cases dramatically improves the prognosis.

## Future developments in prenatal diagnosis

## Fetal cells in the maternal circulation

The presence of fetal cells in maternal blood is an established phenomenon. The methods for their isolation,

identification and genetic analysis continue to be refined. Most investigators are focused on the isolation of fetal nucleated red blood or trophoblastic cells. The validation of a reliable technique for the safe, non-invasive acquisition of fetal cells will revolutionize prenatal diagnosis.

## Pre-implantation genetic diagnosis

Couples at high risk of having pregnancies with inherited diseases may benefit from pre-implantation genetic diagnosis (PGD) in the early stages of human zygote/embryo development. The development of PGD allows parents to avoid the decision to terminate a pregnancy. PGD has evolved from the development of safe and effective techniques for embryo biopsy and the appropriate methods of genetic diagnosis by FISH or PCR.

## Three-dimensional ultrasound

Advanced imaging technology has permitted the real-time three-dimensional reconstruction of data acquired by specially adopted ultrasound machines. This technology permits the increased resolution required for certain fetal malformations, such as cleft lip/palate. Routine two-dimensional ultrasound requires the sonographer to 'reconstruct' the third dimension in a mental image. The real practical value of three-dimensional ultrasound technology is the potential to allow the remote acquisition of ultrasound data by technicians that can latter be analysed by appropriate experts.

## Fetal magnetic resonance imaging

The uses of prenatal magnetic resonance imaging (MRI) are being evaluated increasingly. The development of ultrafast MRI sequences to overcome fetal movement artefact has resulted in significant improvement in the quality and usefulness of the image. MRI has the potential to become a powerful adjunct to the evaluation of the abnormal fetus discovered on ultrasound.

---

### 🔍 Key Points

- Although there are numerous congenital abnormalities, the overall prevalence of disorders is approximately 2 per 100 pregnancies.
- Tests for fetal abnormality fall into two groups, namely screening and diagnostic. Screening tests are not diagnostic but enable the selection of pregnancies to which diagnostic tests can be applied, enabling the early detection of conditions to allow appropriate management.
- It is important to consider the psychological implications of prenatal screening and to ensure that sufficient information and time has been given to allow the parents informed choices.
- A number of different tests exist to enable sampling material of fetal origin (Table 7.3). The sample obtained can be used for cytogenetic, biochemical, enzymatic or DNA analysis to give a prenatal diagnosis. Generally, these tests are invasive in nature and carry a risk of miscarriage.
- Ultrasound plays a major role in screening for a wide range of structural abnormalities of the fetus.

- Periconceptual folate supplementation of the maternal diet given for at least 3 months prior to conception and for the first trimester of pregnancy reduces by about half the risk of the fetus developing neural tube defects.
- In screening for Down's syndrome, an age-modified individual maternal risk can be calculated by the gestation-corrected assessment of second trimester maternal serum levels of AFP and hCG, and by first trimester maternal serum levels of PAPP-A and hCG.
- The sonographic measurement of the subcutaneous collection of fluid in the nuchal region of the fetus (NT) at 10–13 weeks' gestation offers another approach to screening for Down's syndrome. Based on maternal age, gestation and NT measurement, an algorithm predicts the individual's risk of a Down's syndrome pregnancy in a similar way to the biochemical screening. NT can be combined with first trimester biochemical screening to improve the detection rate of Down's syndrome fetuses.

---

### CASE HISTORY

A 24-year-old primigravida at 10 weeks' gestation attends the booking clinic. She has a friend who has a Down's syndrome child and is particularly anxious about knowing the chances of her baby having the condition. She has read about a 'blood test' for Down's syndrome in a magazine and wishes to discuss this along with other options for screening and diagnosis of Down's syndrome.

**What issues would you wish to discuss with her to ensure she has sufficient information to make an informed decision?**

*Discussion regarding Down's syndrome*
- Find out what she already knows.
- Explanation of the cause of the congenital abnormality.
- How the baby could be affected.

- That the severity of the disease cannot be diagnosed, and that there is a considerable range.
- Explore personal risk factors.

*Details of the 'blood test'*
- When biochemical screening for Down's syndrome can be performed: (a) first trimester; and (b) second trimester (14–26 weeks).
- A scan needs to be performed prior to the blood test to confirm gestation (AFP, HCG and PAPP-A are gestation related)
- When, where and how much maternal venous blood will be taken.
- How long the results take to be returned (usually within 24–48 hours).
- How she will receive the results.

*What the test does*

- It measures levels of pregnancy-associated hormones in the maternal circulation. In the first trimester, PAPP-A and beta-hCG and, in the second trimester, AFP and beta-hCG (AFP is typically low, hCG high and PAPP-A low compared to the population median in affected pregnancies).
- Combined with her age and gestation, an algorithm will give a personal risk of her having a Down's syndrome baby. It should be emphasized that this only gives a risk analysis and is not diagnostic.
- This can be categorized as high when the risk is 1:250.

*What the test does not do*

- It does not diagnose Down's syndrome.
- If the blood result shows she is in the high-risk category, she will require further investigation to confirm the diagnosis (i.e. amniocentesis or CVS).
- Both of these diagnostic tests are invasive procedures associated with a 0.5–1 per cent risk of miscarriage.

*Additional points*

- If she is in the low-risk category, she can still have a baby with Down's syndrome.
- Measurement of nuchal thickness by ultrasound in the first trimester either on its own or in combination with first trimester biochemical screening is another option to screen for Down's syndrome. If used in conjunction with biochemical serum markers, it provides a higher chance of detection (75 per cent) and a lower false-positive rate (3 per cent).
- A detailed anomaly scan at 18–20 weeks may identify associated anomalies (e.g. cardiac abnormalities or other 'soft markers' in an affected fetus).
- She needs to consider the implications of positive diagnostic testing – would she consider termination of pregnancy or wish to continue with the pregnancy with the provision of appropriate advice regarding the development of a child with Down's syndrome.
- If she wishes to continue with the pregnancy regardless of outcome, she may wish to decline testing.

## Reference

National Institute for Clinical Excellence. *Antenatal care: routine care for the healthy pregnant woman.* London: RCOG Press, 2003.

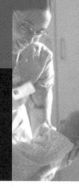

# Antenatal complications

## OVERVIEW

There are a variety of maternal and fetal complications that can arise during pregnancy. Regular antenatal examinations beginning in early pregnancy assist in preventing many complications from developing. This chapter discusses some of the common complications associated with pregnancy and the role the midwife can play in the diagnosis, treatment and care of women who may experience such conditions.

Whenever the midwife detects a deviation from the norm in the health of the woman or fetus, she must refer the woman to a qualified health practitioner as may be reasonably expected to have the necessary skills and expertise to assist her. However, it is expected that the midwife continues to play a fundamental role in providing information, advice and physical and psychological support to these women and their families to enable them to cope with pregnancy and its complications, and any lifestyle changes in the best way possible.

## MATERNAL COMPLICATIONS

### Hyperemesis gravidarum

A small proportion of women (0.3–2 per cent) who experience nausea and vomiting will develop a more serious condition known as hyperemesis gravidarum, which requires urgent medical referral. In this situation, admission to hospital is advised and antiemetics, such as metoclopramide or prochlorperazine, are prescribed. In addition, intravenous hydration support should be administered as long as the woman is vomiting. In the severest cases, total parenteral nutrition (TPN) is given, and parenteral B complex

vitamins including thiamine (to prevent Wernicke's encephalopathy) are reported to reduce the mortality of the condition.

Oesophageal tears (Mallory Weiss syndrome) and haematemesis may also occur in women with severe and persistent vomiting. A sliding scale course of steroids has been used with encouraging results in uncontrolled studies. In the very worst cases, termination of pregnancy may be considered if the woman becomes malnourished and dehydrated such that there are signs of major organ failure. Some studies have found that a diet with a high total fat content, particularly saturated fat, increases the risk of severe hyperemesis. It is, therefore, important that midwives encourage women to eat a well-balanced diet containing all the food groups in adequate proportions prior to conception/in early pregnancy in order to reduce the incidence of this disorder.

## Pruritus gravidarum (cholestasis of pregnancy)

Pruritus gravidarum is intense itching that occurs without a rash and can affect up to 20 per cent of pregnant women. The itching may be attributed to scabies, pediculosis, urticaria, atopic eczema, candidiasis, trichomonal infections or related to drug therapy. Should these causes be ruled out, about 0.2–0.4 per cent of women will continue to experience pruritus owing to an alteration in hepatic function. Normal levels of oestrogen and progesterone may interfere with hepatic secretion of bile acids, which then accumulate in the skin to cause pruritus in susceptible women.

Liver function tests should always be performed to exclude obstetric cholestasis (see Chapter 12). Serum alkaline phosphatase and transaminase levels may be raised and bilirubin levels may be normal or slightly increased. Should the midwife suspect cholestasis of pregnancy, she should refer the woman for consultant care, as maternal and perinatal morbidity/mortality may be increased. The condition may necessitate the birth of the fetus being expedited. Pruritus gravidarum may be generalized or localized to the abdomen. Calamine lotion may help to relieve the itching in mild cases, with antihistamine tablets being prescribed for the more severe cases. The condition may resolve following the baby's birth, but may recur in subsequent pregnancies or with the use of some oral contraceptive pills.

## Symphysis pubis dysfunction

Symphysis pubis dysfunction (SPD) usually occurs in the third trimester of pregnancy and can be an excruciatingly painful condition. The symphysis pubis joint becomes unstable, causing the two halves of the pelvis to rub on one another when walking or moving. It has been suggested that SPD develops as a result of ovarian and placental hormonal effects in pregnancy relaxing the pelvic ligaments and cartilages in preparation for labour and childbirth. This may increase the normal 4 mm gap between the ends of the symphysis pubis to as much as 9 mm. It is considered abnormal should the joint widening exceed 10 mm,

and this is defined as symphysis pubis diastasis or symphysial separation. Although the incidence of diastasis is variable in the literature (ranging from 1:300 to 1:20 000), long-term morbidity can result and may necessitate surgical fixation of the symphysis pubis.

It is essential that midwives have the skills to recognize SPD and how it may affect the woman both physically and psychologically, so that appropriate advice and support with its management may be given. This will involve resting the symphysis pubis joint as much as possible, avoiding prolonged weight-bearing, the climbing of stairs and seeking help with essential activities such as housework, childcare and shopping. Abduction of the hips should be avoided as much as possible and the woman should be advised to keep her legs as close together as is comfortable, particularly when getting in and out of a car and turning in bed. A pillow placed between the legs to keep the knees in apposition when resting may also help to ease some of the discomfort.

If symptoms do not subside, the midwife should refer the woman to a physiotherapist for a full pelvis and back assessment, and treatment of any pelvis misalignment. Although a pelvic support belt or a trochanteric support belt may give some relief, these belts will not correct any underlying pelvic asymmetry. In addition, the use of elbow crutches can maintain mobility while reducing strain in the pelvis, if the woman experiences pain when weight-bearing. Analgesia should also be offered to help the pain and discomfort.

Where a vaginal birth is anticipated, it is important that the range of hip abduction is measured and recorded in the woman's notes in advance of labour. However, in severe cases, an elective Caesarean section may be undertaken. Water can be effective as an analgesic as it relieves weight bearing and allows a change in position with maximum ease. However, wherever possible the midwife should encourage the woman to be mobile and upright, adopting positions in which she is most comfortable and where any hip movement is pain free. The midwife should also consider undertaking vaginal examinations with the woman in a lateral position. Should the woman choose an epidural (or if a spinal anaesthesia is required), it is important that the midwife ensures that the woman does not exceed her range of pain-free hip abduction while the anaesthesia is effective.

In the second stage of labour, a supported 'all fours' or lateral position will help in reducing strain on the symphysis pubis. Should the lithotomy position be required for a ventouse extraction, forceps delivery or suturing the perineum, the hips should be abducted simultaneously within the pain-free range of movement and maintained in this position for only a minimal amount of time as possible. *It is essential that midwives refrain from the practice of encouraging women to push with their feet placed on the midwives' hips as this forcibly abducts the hips and could lead to diastasis of the symphysis pubis.*

During the postnatal period, the woman should be referred to the physiotherapist for assessment, advice and treatment. It may be necessary for her to be on complete bed rest for 24–48 hours or until the acute pain subsides. Assistance and support may be required to care for herself and baby, and consequently improve the quality of life. In such a situation, the woman may feel especially inadequate and socially isolated, putting her at risk of developing postnatal depression. It is, therefore, important for community midwives to continue visiting the woman at home for as long as is felt necessary [Nursing and Midwifery Council (NMC) 2004] to provide both physical and emotional support in order to reduce any longer term maternal morbidity.

## Complications associated with abnormalities of the reproductive system

The incidence of anomalies associated with the reproductive system is unknown and many defects remain asymptomatic. While structural abnormalities of the uterus are likely to cause complications in pregnancy and labour, there may be other conditions such as fibroids or uterine displacement also affecting pregnancy and labour outcome.

### Developmental anomalies

The majority of the female reproductive system develops from the müllerian ducts that form during embryonic life. Should one of the ducts fail to develop, a *unicornuate* uterus is likely to arise, which is a rare anomaly. The müllerian ducts fuse and the median septum eventually breaks down to form a single uterus. If this process fails, then abnormalities such as *double uterus* (with/without a double cervix and vagina; *uterus didelphys*), *bicornuate* uterus or *subseptate* uterus may occur. Furthermore, as the müllerian ducts develop closely together with the wolffian ducts in embryonic life, there may also be malformations of the kidneys and ureters. It is, therefore, important that an assessment of the renal system be included in the care of women with müllerian duct anomalies. However, structural anomalies are often discovered incidentally at the time of a pelvic operation, such as a laparoscopy, or an ultrasound scan.

The presence of a uterine malformation is associated with a four-fold increase in the risk of spontaneous miscarriage and preterm labour, as the underdeveloped myometrium is unable to stretch and develop to accommodate the growing fetus. There is also an increased incidence of Caesarean sections as a consequence of abnormalities of lie and presentation of the fetus.

A vaginal septum may either be longitudinal or transverse, complete or partial. Although it may be detected on vaginal examination, as the tissue is usually soft and easily deflected by the examining fingers, the diagnosis is often overlooked. A high vaginal septum usually prevents cervical dilatation and can obstruct the descent of the fetus during labour. In instances where the breech presents, the fetus may sit astride a longitudinal septum. In the second stage of labour, the septum may become visible in front of the presenting part as it advances. Consequently, the septum may need to be divided in order to allow the birth of the fetus.

## Abdominal pain in pregnancy

Abdominal pain is a common complaint in pregnancy and is experienced by most women at some stage. It consequently presents a problem for the midwife of how to distinguish between the physiologically normal (indigestion) and the pathological pains requiring urgent medical referral, such as appendicitis or pyelonephritis. It is important that the midwife takes a detailed history and performs a physical examination in order to make a decision about whether to refer the woman, such that her observations and decision-making may be crucial to a successful pregnancy outcome. The care and management will depend on the cause (p. 96), and the maternal and fetal condition. For many of these conditions, abdominal pain is one of the many, but not necessarily, an overriding symptom.

## Causes of abdominal pain in pregnancy

**Pregnancy specific**

*Physiological*
- Heartburn
- Vomiting
- Constipation
- Round ligament pain
- Braxton–Hicks contractions

*Pathological*
- Ectopic pregnancy
- Miscarriage
- Uterine fibroids
- Placental abruption
- Preterm labour
- Severe pre-eclampsia
- HELLP syndrome
- Uterine rupture

**Incidental causes**

*Common pathology*
- Urinary tract infection/ pyelonephritis
- Appendicitis
- Intestinal obstruction
- Cholecystitis
- Inflammatory bowel disease
- Peptic ulcer
- Renal disease
- Ovarian torsion (cysts)
- Acute pancreatitis
- Pneumonia: lower lobe
- Tuberculosis (associated with HIV infection)
- Malaria

*Rare pathology*
- Rectus haematoma
- Pulmonary embolism
- Sickle cell crisis
- Arteriovenous haemorrhage
- Malignant disease

HELLP, haemolysis, elevation of liver enzymes and low platelets; HIV, human immunodeficiency virus.

## Retroversion of the gravid uterus

Approximately 15 per cent of women have a retroverted uterus where the long axis of the uterus is directed backwards during pregnancy. In most cases, it corrects spontaneously as the pregnancy develops, with the uterus rising out of the pelvis into the abdomen as an anteverted uterus would. In a small proportion of cases, the uterus remains in retroversion and eventually by 12–14 weeks gestation, the uterus fills up the entire pelvic cavity becoming confined beneath the sacral promontory. This is known as *incarceration of the retroverted gravid uterus*. The base of the bladder and the urethra consequently become stretched causing retention of urine. This is not only very painful for the woman, but it may cause

long-term damage, if the bladder becomes overdistended. Urinary stasis can also lead to infections developing, including pyelonephritis. In this situation, the midwife may seek advice from an obstetrician or a senior midwife and, with the woman's consent, undertake catheterization of the bladder to relieve the retention. It is usual for an indwelling catheter to be used to keep the bladder empty while enabling the uterus to rise out of the pelvis.

## Ovarian cysts

Ovarian cysts are common in pregnancy but the incidence of malignancy is uncommon in women of childbearing age. The most common types of pathological ovarian cyst are serous cysts and benign *teratomas*. Physiological cysts of the corpus luteum may grow to several centimetres but rarely require any treatment, should the woman remain asymptomatic. However, it is usual for such cysts to be regularly reviewed following pregnancy by clinical and ultrasound examination. On the other hand, large cysts, such as *dermoids*, may require surgery in pregnancy.

Surgery is usually delayed until the late second or early third trimester, when there is the potential that, if the baby were born, it would be able to survive. The major problems in pregnancy are of large (>8 cm) ovarian cysts, which may undergo torsion, haemorrhage or rupture, causing acute abdominal pain. The resulting pain and inflammation may lead to a miscarriage or preterm labour. Symptomatic cysts, most commonly as a result of torsion, will require an emergency laparotomy and ovarian cystectomy, or even oophorectomy, if the cyst becomes twisted.

## Fibroids (leiomyomas)

Fibroids are firm, benign compact masses of smooth muscle and fibrous tissue that lie in the cavity of the uterus (submucous), within the uterine muscle (intramural) or on the outside surface of the uterus (subserous). The incidence of detectable fibroids in pregnancy is 1 per cent with the lowest risk being in Caucasian women. However, the risk increases in Afro-Caribbean woman and women over 35 years of age. The size of fibroids varies and, although they are known to increase in size during pregnancy, this tends to be limited and mainly in the first trimester.

Consequently, the outcome of pregnancy is dependent on the position of the fibroid and, in some instances, obstruction may occur.

A large fibroid at the cervix or in the lower uterine segment may prevent descent of the presenting part, causing malpresentation and obstructed labour (Figure 8.1). Caesarean section is most likely if the fibroid is situated in the lower segment. Should fibroids prevent the complete separation of the placenta, severe postpartum haemorrhage may result, necessitating urgent blood transfusion. Removal of fibroids during Caesarean section may also result in excessive haemorrhage, so these should be left in place and details recorded in the woman's medical notes.

Red degeneration is one of the commonest complications of fibroids in pregnancy. Should the growth of a fibroid be rapid, it may exceed its blood supply and thus become ischaemic where the central core necroses and bleeding occurs into the middle. The fibroid subsequently takes on a reddish appearance. The woman experiences severe acute abdominal pain with tenderness over the fibroid, frequent vomiting and pyrexia. If these symptoms are severe, uterine contractions may be precipitated, causing miscarriage or preterm labour. Other causes of pain need to be excluded, such as appendicitis or placental abruption. Red fibroid degeneration requires admission to hospital where an ultrasound scan can be performed to aid differential diagnosis of the pain, as the relationship between the placental site and the focus of the pain can be established. The degeneration can be seen clearly on

ultrasound scan. The pain is usually relieved by analgesia and rest, and the symptoms tend to settle within a few days without any further treatment.

Torsion may occur in a subserous pedunculated fibroid in the same way that a large ovarian cyst can become twisted. When this happens, acute abdominal pain and tenderness may make the two conditions difficult to distinguish from one another. In this situation, a detailed and accurate history by the midwife followed by either a transvaginal or transabdominal ultrasound scan will confirm the diagnosis.

## Bleeding in pregnancy

Vaginal bleeding in pregnancy is abnormal and is a cause of concern for women, especially those who have had a previous experience of fetal loss. The midwife should take any reports of bleeding seriously. Prior to referring the woman to medical colleagues, it is vital the midwife takes a detailed history from the woman and makes an accurate initial assessment in order to determine what effect the blood loss has had on the health and well-being of the woman and fetus.

### Implantation bleeding

During implantation of the blastocyst when the trophoblast erodes the endometrial epithelium, the woman may experience a small vaginal blood loss. As this tends to occur around the time of menstruation, the bleed may be mistaken for a period, although it tends to be much lighter. If the expected date of birth is to be calculated from the menstrual history, midwives should be aware of the significance of implantation bleeding.

### Cervical eversion (erosion/ectropion)

This condition is commonly and erroneously known as cervical erosion (see Chapter 4). Hypersensitivity of the endocervical cells increases the quantity of vaginal discharge and, as the cells are vascular, it may also cause intermittent blood-stained loss or spontaneous bleeding. Bleeding following sexual intercourse is common with cervical eversion. Eversion tends to require no treatment during pregnancy and usually it will disappear during the postnatal period.

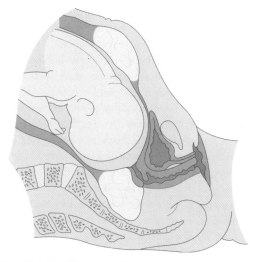

**Figure 8.1** Fibroids complicating pregnancy.

## Cervical polyps

Polyps are small pedunculated growths attached to the cervix and, during pregnancy, there is a risk that they may bleed. They can be visualized on speculum examination and, unless the bleeding is profuse or a cervical smear indicates malignancy, there is usually no treatment required during pregnancy.

## Carcinoma of the cervix

The incidence of cancer in pregnancy is 1:6000 live births. Carcinoma of the cervix is the most frequently diagnosed cancer in pregnancy. Good preconception screening includes ensuring that a woman has had a cervical smear (Papanicolaou smear) within the preceding 3–5 years prior to conception. *Cervical intraepithelial neoplasia* (CIN) is the precursor to invasive cancer of the cervix. If the condition is detected at this stage, treatment can be given and the cytology subsequently reverts to normal.

Approximately 80 per cent cases of carcinoma of the cervix are diagnosed in the first and second trimesters of pregnancy. However, cervical abnormalities are much more difficult to deal with in pregnancy, as the cervix can be difficult to visualize at colposcopy, as well as there being a risk that any biopsy will cause considerable bleeding and can induce miscarriage. Risk factors associated with cervical cancer include:

- early age of sexually activity;
- many sexual partners;
- unprotected intercourse;
- human papilloma virus (HPV);
- smoking;
- manual social classes;
- early first pregnancy;
- increased parity.

Although the disease may be asymptomatic, a common presenting feature is vaginal bleeding. Speculum examination may reveal a friable or ulcerated lesion with bleeding and purulent discharge. As these symptoms may be mistaken for symptoms of pregnancy, there may sometimes be a delay in diagnosis of the carcinoma. Treatment depends on the stage of the disease and gestation, and can evoke complex ethical and moral dilemmas for the woman, her family and those involved in her care and management. Laser treatment or cryotherapy can be carried out following colposcopy on an outpatient basis and will result in the destruction of the abnormal area of the cells. Should a cone biopsy to remove cervical tissue be necessary, and the woman has been found to have early changes in cervical cytology, treatment is usually delayed until the end of pregnancy to avoid the risk of haemorrhage and miscarriage.

However, if the cervical changes are advanced and diagnosis is made in the first or second trimester, the woman may be faced with the difficult choice as to whether to terminate the pregnancy in order to undergo treatment. Should the diagnosis be made later on in pregnancy, a decision to expedite the baby's birth may be made in order for the woman to commence treatment. Usually this is by Caesarean section followed by a radical hysterectomy (Wertheim's hysterectomy). A vaginal birth is associated with a poorer prognosis for the woman, as cervical dilatation may cause dissemination of malignant cells, such that metastases have been found in episiotomy sites. Midwives can play a vital role in informing all women of the importance of regular smear tests in respect of national and local guidelines, and to ensure that maternity records reflect the most recent cytology result. This may mean that the midwife recommends the woman to have a cervical smear taken at the 6 weeks postnatal examination.

## Spontaneous miscarriage/abortion

In the UK, as in most other countries, there is no formal record of miscarriages, and so the exact incidence is unknown. However, it is estimated that 15 per cent of all confirmed pregnancies result in a miscarriage (some texts use the term 'abortion'), the majority of which occur during the first trimester and are classified as *early* miscarriages. However, 1–2 per cent of spontaneous miscarriages do not occur until the second trimester of pregnancy, between 12 and 24 weeks' gestation and are consequently known as *late* or *second trimester miscarriages*. Furthermore, as the fetus is potentially viable from 24 weeks' gestation, the midwife is legally responsible to notify all births occurring after this time (NMC 2004). If the birth of a baby occurs after 24 weeks and prior to 37 weeks of pregnancy, it is referred to as preterm (see Chapter 11).

Should a miscarriage occur during the second trimester, it is particularly distressing to the woman, as not only may the pregnancy have become noticeable abdominally, but also she may have begun to experience fetal movements. In addition, miscarriage can be associated with major haemorrhage and sepsis and, although maternal death is a recognized consequence, it is rare. Nevertheless, infective sequelae may also lead to subsequent morbidity and the impairment of future fertility.

The causes of miscarriage in most cases remain unknown but may include the following.

- *Fetal*: 50 per cent are due to chromosomal abnormalities of the conceptus.
- *Maternal:*
  - advancing maternal age;
  - structural abnormalities of the reproductive system – bicornuate uterus, fibroids;
  - defective implantation;
  - endocrine abnormalities – deficits in the corpus luteum, low progesterone levels;
  - infections – rubella, chlamydia, listeria, bacterial vaginosis;
  - maternal disease – diabetes, renal disease, thyroid dysfunction;
  - environmental factors – excessive alcohol, coffee, smoking;
  - multigravidae and previous history of spontaneous miscarriage;
  - cervical weakness – laceration or stretching from previous childbirth/abortion;
  - immunological factors;
  - poor socioeconomic status;
  - stress and anxiety.
- *Paternal*: Poor sperm quality and possible source of chromosomal abnormalities.

A specific risk factor for late miscarriage is mid-trimester amniocentesis. This procedure, commonly performed at 16–18 weeks' gestation, is associated with a 0.5 per cent chance of subsequent pregnancy loss. However, in the majority of cases, despite detailed investigations, no cause for the spontaneous miscarriage is ever found.

There are a number of types of spontaneous miscarriage, as highlighted in Figure 8.2. However, as with any condition, the presenting symptoms of second trimester miscarriage are diverse and may vary between individuals. It is important that midwives are familiar with the range of signs and symptoms that may present with each type of miscarriage as shown in Table 8.1. Commonly, there may be uterine cramping and bleeding, and the membranes may be intact or ruptured. However, events may progress rapidly without significant pain, with the woman complaining of relatively minor backache or abdominal discomfort.

## Threatened miscarriage

Any vaginal bleeding in pregnancy should be considered to be a threatened miscarriage until a diagnosis has been confirmed. Slight bleeding usually occurs during the first 3 months of pregnancy that may be painless or associated with lower abdominal pain or backache resembling period pains. However, there is no cervical dilatation and the uterus remains soft with no tenderness when palpated. Although the symptoms may continue over a period of time, the presence of a fetal heart using a hand-held Doppler device (sonicaid) with a closed cervix is often reassuring. A total of 70–80 per cent of women diagnosed with a threatened miscarriage in the first trimester continue with their pregnancies to term.

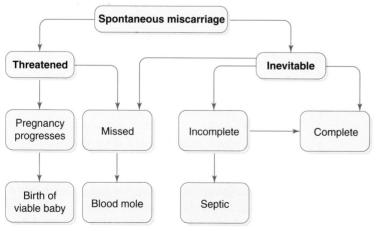

**Figure 8.2** Classification of spontaneous miscarriage.

**Table 8.1** – Signs and symptoms of miscarriage

| Signs and symptoms | Threatened miscarriage | Inevitable miscarriage | Incomplete miscarriage | Complete miscarriage | Delayed miscarriage | Septic miscarriage |
|---|---|---|---|---|---|---|
| **Bleeding** | Scanty | Heavy/clots | Heavy/profuse | Minimal/ none | Some spotting; possible brown loss | Variable; may smell offensive |
| **Pain** | Variable | Severe/ rhythmical | Severe | Diminishing/ none | None | Severe/ variable |
| **Cervical os** | Closed; intact membranes | Open (>3 cm); ruptured membranes | Open | Closed | Closed | Open |
| **Uterus (if palpable)** | Soft; no tenderness | Tender; may be smaller than expected | Tender/painful | Firm; contracted | Smaller than expected | Bulky/tender/ painful |
| **Additional signs and symptoms** | | | Tissue present in cervix; shock | | Fetal death on ultrasound scan | Maternal pyrexia, tachycardia, hypotension |

In the past, women have been advised to rest but there is a lack of evidence to prove this is effective in preserving such a pregnancy. Furthermore, vaginal examinations should not be undertaken nor should aperients/enemas be given, as this may induce uterine contractions. After taking a detailed history and making an assessment of vital signs such as temperature, pulse and blood pressure, the midwife should refer the woman for medical attention straight away, where she may be admitted to hospital or seen as an outpatient in an early pregnancy unit (if available). A pregnancy test would be carried out followed by an ultrasound scan to ensure viability of the fetus. Assessment of fetal growth is important in order to ensure that there is no restriction of fetal size as a consequence of poor placental function. However, should the bleeding persist, the pain may become rhythmical and the uterus contracts to expel the contents as the miscarriage becomes *inevitable*.

## Inevitable miscarriage

The main feature of an inevitable miscarriage is cervical dilatation with evidence of the membranes bulging or amniotic fluid draining through the external os diagnosed on speculum examination or transvaginal ultrasound scan. As the name indicates, the pregnancy loss is unavoidable. The bleeding becomes more severe with clots or the gestation sac containing the embryo or fetus, and the woman may consequently collapse from the blood loss and pain as the uterus begins to contract to expel its contents. The gestation sac may be expelled complete (*complete miscarriage*) or in part, where placental tissue is usually retained (*incomplete miscarriage*). Digital vaginal examinations should be avoided in order to prevent further stimulation of uterine activity or exacerbation of any infection that may be present. It is, therefore, important that a vaginal swab is taken via a speculum examination, especially if the membranes have ruptured.

There is currently no place for tocolysis in the prevention of second trimester pregnancy loss. Even in later pregnancy, tocolytics are only used to secure short-term prolongation of the pregnancy of up to 48 hours. Furthermore, once the membranes have ruptured, the situation becomes more difficult, with a consequential poor prognosis that is dependent on the gestation of the pregnancy. As the interval between membrane rupture and the birth of the baby can occasionally be measured by weeks, some inevitable second trimester miscarriages may result in preterm births. However, if contractions and the birth of the fetus do not ensue for some time, membrane rupture with oligohydramnios in the second trimester carries a significant risk of fetal lung hypoplasia. Depending on the blood loss and if there is no uterine activity or signs of infection, there is no urgency to intervene. However, it is important that the parents are counselled about the poor prognosis and that any intervention only takes place when they are ready. Whilst some may want to wait for nature to take its course, others may want more immediate action. In both cases, continuing support from the midwife and obstetrician is important.

Careful observation of any signs of infection is vital; the woman may assess her own temperature at home with advice about reporting any changes in vaginal discharge or the development of lower uterine tenderness. Chorioamnionitis usually manifests with the onset of uterine contractions and consequent birth. Although vaginal infection may be difficult to identify, there is some evidence that empirical antibiotics, such as erythromycin with metronidazole, should be given, particularly with membrane rupture near viability. However, care must be exercised if there is already clinical evidence of chorioamnionitis, as any delay in terminating the pregnancy may lead to worsening infection and consequent maternal morbidity. In such cases, augmenting the uterine contractions may be the most appropriate management.

When a woman presents with an open cervical os and bulging membranes, an emergency cervical cerclage to close it may be considered. However, the results are poor and are related to the cervical dilatation at insertion. A dilatation of more than 3 cm with an effaced cervix poses extreme difficulties even for the most experienced obstetrician. Bleeding, contractions or infection are all contraindications to cervical cerclage. Depending on the initial dilatation of the cervix, the prospect of the pregnancy proceeding beyond 26 weeks may be less than 50 per cent.

Should a midwife be called to attend a woman experiencing an inevitable miscarriage at home, it is vital that the extent of the blood loss is assessed by inspection of a sanitary towel or undergarments and baseline observations of temperature, pulse and blood pressure are undertaken. If the fetus has been expelled and the woman is bleeding, an oxytocic drug should be given. Any products of conception that have been expelled should be saved for inspection. The midwife should then arrange transfer to the local hospital by ambulance. If the woman is showing signs of shock, the support of paramedics must be sought to assist with resuscitating her and stabilizing her condition before transfer.

It is important that the woman is offered adequate analgesia, as the pain experienced may be as intense as contractions during labour; this may include epidural anaesthesia, although patient-controlled subcutaneous anaesthesia (PCA) has been found useful in such situations. Depending on the woman's condition upon arrival at hospital, expectant management or medical management using prostaglandins, such as cervagem or cytotec followed by a high-dose oxytocin intravenous infusion, may be considered. A blood transfusion may also be administered if the blood loss has been severe. Owing to its relatively small size, the fetus will almost always be born vaginally even if there is a transverse lie or fetal malformation. Unfortunately, retention of the placenta either total or partial, is more common, and surgical evacuation of retained products of conception (ERPC) under anaesthesia may be required. Should there be evidence of any uterine surgery, such as a previous Caesarean section, then special care should be taken when emptying the uterus by either medical or surgical means. It is important the midwife keeps the woman and her partner informed of what is happening, and prepares them for every eventuality to avoid unnecessary distress. Depending on the gestation, an identifiable body or complete embryo may be born vaginally. However, in some instances, nothing is identifiable.

There may be cases of the baby being born alive should an inevitable miscarriage occur late in the second trimester. Rapid assessment of the baby at birth is required by the midwife as, depending on the gestation and place of birth, the baby may breathe and survive, albeit for only a short time. It is, therefore, important that the midwife acknowledges such signs of life, informs the parents and swiftly seeks the assistance of the paediatrician, especially if there is any uncertainty as to the gestation or the pregnancy is close to 24 weeks. Immediate transfer to a neonatal intensive care unit may be required should the baby be considered viable. Alternatively, the midwife should encourage the woman to touch or hold her baby, and comfort care be given to the baby. In this event, the midwife is responsible for notifying the baby's birth and, should the baby die, the death is also registered (NMC 2004).

Once the uterus is empty, the pain ceases and signs of pregnancy regress. The uterus is firmly contracted when the abdomen is palpated and an empty uterus is seen, if visualized on ultrasound scan. No further medical intervention is usually necessary, but midwives should advise women to seek advice if bleeding recurs or a pyrexia develops. Vulval hygiene is particularly important to reduce the risk of infection and women who have experienced a surgical ERPC should also be screened for chlamydial infection. Prophylactic broad-spectrum antibiotics may also be prescribed in such cases.

If the woman begins to experience signs of lactation, the midwife should advise her to wear a well-fitting brassiere in order to minimize any discomfort. In addition, cabergoline may be prescribed to suppress lactation. Should the woman be rhesus negative, anti-D gammaglobulin is given within 72 hours of the miscarriage to prevent isoimmunization and potential rhesus problems in future pregnancies. Whatever the outcome of an inevitable miscarriage, the midwife must ensure that the woman not only receives appropriate physical care, but also that she and her family receive the psychological support they require, be it by professionals or from support groups, such as the Stillbirth and Neonatal Death Society (SANDS) or the Miscarriage Association, in order to come to terms with their situation. In addition, follow-up by a senior obstetrician and specialist midwife may be appropriate for some families so they have an opportunity to discuss the outcome of the pregnancy and their prospect of future pregnancies. Most hospitals and maternity units offer a funeral or memorial service for pre-viable fetuses and burial facilities; all must offer respectful disposal. The hospital chaplain may be a valuable source of advice and support in this respect.

## Delayed miscarriage (missed abortion/ silent miscarriage)

A delayed miscarriage occasionally follows a threatened miscarriage and may also be known as a missed abortion or silent miscarriage. In this situation, bleeding occurs between the gestation sac and the uterine wall, and the embryo consequently dies despite the presence of a viable placenta. As the cervix remains closed, the sac is retained. The uterus ceases to develop in size and, as the presence of the retained fetus appears to inhibit menstruation, the woman considers that her pregnancy is continuing. However, other signs of pregnancy may have disappeared. There may be variable bleeding from the vagina, ranging from nothing to a trickle of brownish discharge.

The diagnosis of a delayed miscarriage is confirmed by ultrasound scan. The uterus will eventually expel the fetus spontaneously but this may not occur for some time. Treatment is usually to evacuate the uterus either medically by the use of prostaglandins or surgically under general anaesthesia using a curette. As it can be very distressing to be faced with the prospect of surgical evacuation soon after receiving the news that the pregnancy is no longer viable, some women may decide upon expectant management. In such an instance, the woman returns home to await spontaneous expulsion of the fetus, thus giving her time to assimilate the bad news. However, these women should be given 24-hour access to telephone advice. If a well-formed dead fetus is retained *in utero*, it will become flattened and mummified rather than being reabsorbed; this is known as *fetus papyraceous* and is commonly associated with multiple pregnancies. Furthermore, there is a risk to the woman of hyperfibrinogenaemia when the fetus has been retained for some weeks.

## Septic miscarriage

This condition is most commonly a complication of incomplete miscarriage or induced termination owing to ascending infection. In the last triennium report into maternal deaths (2000–2002) there were two reported deaths in the UK from sepsis following spontaneous miscarriage (Lewis and Drife 2004). The causative organisms may include: *Staphylococcus aureus*, *Clostridium welchii*, *Escherichia coli* and group B haemolytic streptococci. In addition to the signs and symptoms of miscarriage, the woman also complains of feeling unwell and may present with a headache, pyrexia, tachycardia and nausea. The infection may be localized in the tubes and cavity of the uterus, or as generalized septicaemia with peritonitis. The damage caused by pelvic infection could result in adhesion formation, salpingitis and subsequent infertility.

It is important that the woman is admitted to hospital where blood cultures and vaginal swabs are taken to identify the cause of the infection and both broad-spectrum antibiotics and those effective against anaerobic infection are administered intravenously. When the woman's condition allows, she should be taken to theatre and the uterus emptied. Following the procedure, midwives should be aware of the signs of endotoxic shock as a result of severe infection, and the risk of disseminated intravascular coagulation, liver and renal damage. It is, therefore, important that the midwife makes careful observations to detect for organ damage, such as jaundice and oliguria, and seeks appropriate medical advice should the woman's condition deteriorate.

## Recurrent miscarriage

This term applies when three or more consecutive spontaneous miscarriages have occurred. The cause should be carefully investigated but, in some instances, there may not be a clear single factor, with the causative factors being different for each. The treatment will vary according to the cause. Should infection be a likely cause, then screening for genital tract pathogens with appropriate antibiotics may be prescribed in a future pregnancy. Where there is a weak cervix, a decision may be made to close it by the insertion of a suture (cervical cerclage). In this situation, the procedure is usually performed at 12–14 weeks' gestation either under a general or regional anaesthetic. By this gestation, the risk of first trimester miscarriage has passed. The suture is removed at 37 weeks' gestation, or when the woman presents in labour or whenever the membranes spontaneously rupture prior to term. Other investigations prior to the next pregnancy may include karyotyping of the woman and her partner, a detailed ultrasound examination of the woman's pelvic cavity and blood tests to exclude the presence of antiphospholipid antibodies.

## Termination of pregnancy

Termination of pregnancy (abortion) may become necessary in some pregnancies and, in the second trimester, this may be as a result of a fetal malformation, fetal death or where the life of the woman is at risk should the pregnancy continue. In the UK, a termination of pregnancy is undertaken within the legislation of the Abortion Act (1967). Amendments to this Act under the Human Fertilisation and Embryology Act 1990 came into force in 1991, and made the termination of pregnancies legal in certain circumstances *after* 24 weeks. Midwives are in a vital position to give women accurate factual information about the purpose of the antenatal screening or diagnostic tests offered, the possible anomalies that may be detected and the options available locally to enable an informed choice to be made about termination of pregnancy. Furthermore, all women who choose to terminate their pregnancy require adequate support and counselling, before and after the procedure. Social, medical and psychological factors will all contribute to the decision.

There are two options to terminate a pregnancy using either medical or surgical means and, ideally, both procedures should be available and explained to the woman so she can make an informed choice. Medical termination usually requires at least a day in hospital. As a legal termination should not result in a live birth, feticide may be carried out as part of or prior to the procedure if it is undertaken late in the second trimester. The progesterone antagonist, mifepristone, is administered over 48–72 hours to enable the uterus to become more responsive to prostaglandins and thus significantly shortens the induction–delivery interval. The woman is usually admitted to hospital 2–3 days following the administration of mifepristone, and then receives oral or vaginal prostaglandins, such as cytotec. In most cases, this stimulates uterine contractions and induces a miscarriage within 12–18 hours. In some instances, however, a large-dose oxytocin infusion may be administered intravenously. Adequate pain relief should be maintained throughout the labour either by epidural anaesthesia or by a PCA opiate pump.

Ideally, the woman should be cared for in a single room to protect her privacy within a transitional ward between the maternity and gynaecology areas. In such circumstances, it may be appropriate for the named midwife to care for the woman during the termination. However, *all* midwives, regardless of personal opinion and belief, have a professional duty to provide physical and psychological care to women undergoing termination of pregnancy. Where there are issues concerning conscientious objection towards participating in termination of pregnancies, the midwife should discuss these with her manager and supervisor of midwives, so that the parameters of her involvement are clearly defined and understood (Marshall and Raynor 2002, Raynor and Marshall 2002, NMC 2004). The woman and her partner should participate as in a labour and should be encouraged to see and hold the baby if they wish.

In some areas, a surgical termination of pregnancy may not be available, as it is a hazardous procedure requiring highly specialized skills and is usually only undertaken in pregnancies of up to 18 weeks' gestation.

Although it is a short procedure requiring only a few hours in hospital, it can present increasing hazards proportionate to the gestational age. This is because the fetal parts are bigger, and the risk of tearing the cervix or damaging the uterus is greater. Consequently, the family cannot see the fetal parts after the termination. The cervix should be prepared with a prostaglandin preparation or with Dilapan that absorbs moisture and swells up over 8–12 hours. The cervix is then already 12–14 mm dilated before the surgical procedure commences. The procedure should be performed with ultrasound available to confirm the gestational age and guide the insertion of the first instruments. It is also used at the end of the procedure to verify that the uterus is empty. Syntocinon is used to ensure the uterus is contracted after the termination.

Placental expulsion may be delayed when second trimester termination is undertaken and the woman may require a manual removal of the placenta. Following termination, prophylactic antibiotics may be given as well as anti-D immunoglobulin to non-sensitized rhesus-negative women.

## Antepartum haemorrhage

This is defined as bleeding from the genital tract in late pregnancy from 24 weeks and before the birth of the baby. Bleeding that occurs during labour is referred to as *intrapartum* bleeding. Antepartum haemorrhage is a serious complication of pregnancy that may place the life of the woman and baby at significant risk should it be from the placental site. Fetal mortality and morbidity are significantly increased, and include stillbirth and neonatal death. In addition, as a result of premature separation of the placenta and consequent hypoxia, severe neurological damage may occur in the baby. Furthermore, the woman may develop shock and disseminated intravascular coagulation with possible death (although rare in the UK) as a result of severe antepartum haemorrhage.

The two main types of antepartum haemorrhage involving premature separation of the placenta are *abruptio placentae* and *placenta praevia*. However, there may have been instances of incidental bleeding from other parts of the genital tract, known as *extraplacental* bleeding, during late pregnancy. Such bleeding can arise from local lesions, such as cervical polyps, cervical eversion, cervicitis, vaginal infection or carcinoma of the cervix (as discussed earlier in this chapter).

## Abruptio placentae (placental abruption)

This is accidental bleeding from the premature separation of a normally situated placenta. The bleeding is maternal and/or fetal and, consequently, the situation is acutely dangerous for both the woman and fetus. The bleeding can be *revealed* in two-thirds of cases (Figure 8.3) and, in the remaining third of cases, is *concealed* where no blood loss is seen per vaginam (Figure 8.4).

The cause of the placental separation cannot always be explained and in 40 per cent of cases no cause is ever found. The following risk factors, however, have been associated with the condition:

- hypertensive disease;
- sudden decompression of the uterus (e.g. spontaneous rupture of the membranes in cases of polyhydramnios);
- preterm prelabour rupture of the membranes;
- trauma resulting from external cephalic version, road traffic accident, a fall or blow to the abdomen;

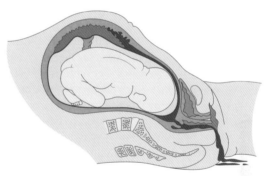

**Figure 8.3** Placental abruption with revealed haemorrhage.

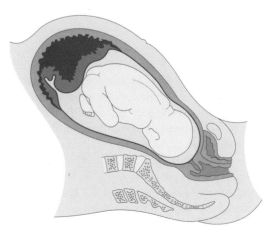

**Figure 8.4** Placental abruption with concealed haemorrhage.

- smoking;
- illegal drug misuse.

## Placenta praevia

In this situation, the bleeding occurs from the separation of an abnormally situated placenta. The placenta lies partly or wholly in the lower uterine segment (see Figure 8.5), and bleeding is inevitable when labour begins and the cervix dilates. However, the bleeding may be also be provoked. In this situation, the bleeding is from the maternal not fetal circulation and consequently is more likely to compromise the woman than the fetus.

The cause of placenta praevia is unknown but the following are known to be associated:

- multiparity;
- increasing maternal age;
- multiple pregnancy;
- assisted conception;
- scarred uterus: previous caesarean section;
- placental abnormality: bipartite, succenturiate placentae;
- uterine structural anomaly;
- smoking.

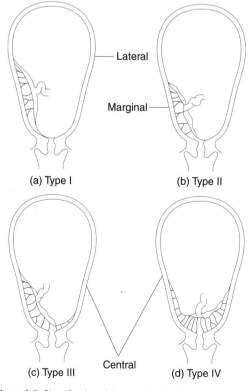

(a) Type I

(b) Type II

(c) Type III   Central   (d) Type IV

**Figure 8.5** Classification of degrees of placenta praevia.

Antepartum haemorrhage must always be taken seriously, and any woman presenting with a history of fresh vaginal bleeding should be admitted to hospital for prompt and proper investigations. It is, therefore, important that the midwife makes an accurate initial assessment of the maternal and fetal condition, and attempts to establish whether the bleeding is placental or from a local lesion. Referral to the obstetrician is necessary in all cases of antepartum haemorrhage no matter what the extent or cause of the bleeding. At the one extreme, the woman may present with pallor, tachycardia, a painful firm abdomen, underwear soaked in fresh blood and reduced fetal movements and, consequently, requires emergency assessment and management for a possible placental abruption (see Chapter 16). However, a woman having had a small postcoital bleed with no systemic signs or symptoms represents the other extreme, which is not as life-threatening or urgent.

The midwife should ascertain the degree of the blood loss and whether there was any trigger to have caused it, such as an injury or sexual intercourse. Any pain or contractions accompanying the bleeding will also be noted along with the extent of fetal movements since the bleeding commenced. Furthermore, it is also useful that details of the last cervical smear and its results are recorded in order to exclude possible carcinoma of the cervix.

Clinical examination should include assessing the woman's pulse and blood pressure, an abdominal examination to determine whether the uterus is soft or tender and firm, including auscultation of the fetal heart and undertaking a cardiotocograph (CTG). Only once it has been established by ultrasound scan that the placenta is not a praevia should a speculum vaginal examination be undertaken to visualize the cervix.

Depending on the degree of bleeding and maternal shock, venepuncture should be undertaken for a full blood count and clotting studies. If either abruptio placentae or placenta praevia are suspected, then it is important that at least 6 units of blood are crossmatched and made ready for emergency use. An ultrasound scan to assess fetal size, presentation, volume of amniotic fluid, placental position and morphology would also be undertaken before the obstetrician decides on subsequent management.

If the condition of the woman and fetus becomes compromised by the antepartum haemorrhage, decisions may have to be made to expedite the birth of the baby irrespective of gestation. In this situation, maternal steroid injection should still be given to assist fetal lung maturity. However, should the bleeding continue, the midwife should be alert for the woman developing signs of shock and whether emergency measures, such as intravenous fluid and oxygen therapy, are warranted (see Chapter 16). If the bleeding settles, then the woman must be admitted to hospital for at least 48 hours for observation, as the risk of the antepartum haemorrhage recurring is high within this time scale. In cases where the woman is rhesus negative, the midwife should undertake a further venepuncture for a Kleihauer test. This will determine whether any, and how much, fetal blood has leaked into the maternal circulation and, as a result, if an injection of anti-D is required to prevent rhesus isoimmunization. Where the bleeding is minimal and the cause is clearly extraplacental, once there is a reasonable certainty that cervical carcinoma is excluded by the woman's smear history and direct visualization of the cervix, then symptomatic management may be undertaken, such as antifungal preparations for candidiasis.

## Venous thromboembolism

Haemostasis is dependent on the mechanism of blood coagulation and the counterbalancing effect of fibrinolysis, the latter ensuring that the blood vessels are reopened in order to maintain patency of the circulation. Blood clotting is a complex process involving a large number of clotting factors and occurs in three main stages:

- thromboplastin is released in response to tissue damage and platelet breakdown;
- prothrombin is converted into thrombin (a proteolytic enzyme) in the presence of calcium ions;
- fibrinogen is converted into fibrin by the action of thrombin.

Consequently, fibrin forms a network of long sticky strands that entrap blood cells to form a clot. This coagulated material contracts and expels serum (plasma depleted of its clotting factors). The coagulation process is counterbalanced by the presence of heparin that is produced in the liver. Fibrinolyis, therefore, is the breakdown of fibrin and occurs as a response to clot formation. Clotting will continue unless fibrinolysis occurs. This is achieved by the activation of a series of enzymes ending with the proteolytic enzyme plasmin. This breaks down the fibrin into clots to form fibrin degradation products (FDPs). This clot dispersal is a protective mechanism to prevent capillary blockage. Occasionally tissue damage is so severe or widespread

that there is a massive release of thromboplastin into the general circulation causing widespread clotting throughout the body. This is known as disseminated intravascular coagulation (DIC) (see Chapter12).

In pregnancy, there is an alteration in the thrombotic and fibrinolytic mechanisms owing to an increase in clotting factors (VIII, IX and X), and in fibrinogen levels with a reduction in protein S and antithrombin III concentrations. The possible purpose of these changes is to reduce the likelihood of haemorrhage following childbirth. However, these physiological changes also present a risk to the woman of thromboembolism (the obstruction of a blood vessel by a blood clot) and any underlying prevalence to thrombosis may be unmasked in pregnancy (for risk factors, see box, below). High levels of circulating oestrogen are associated with changes in clotting factors; the situation is in some ways comparable to that of women developing a deep vein thrombosis (DVT) while taking the combined oral contraceptive pill. Furthermore, venous stasis in the lower limbs due to the weight of the gravid uterus placing pressure on the inferior vena cava compounded by immobility presents an additional risk factor to the pregnant woman. Whilst pregnancy itself increases the risk of DVT by five times, the risk is increased by ten times should the woman have a Caesarean section. However, in the postnatal period, the risk of DVT following a Caesarean section is probably around 1 per cent.

### Risk factors for thromboembolic disorders

| Pre-existing factors | Pregnancy-specific factors |
|---|---|
| • Maternal age >35years | • Hypertensive disorders |
| • Thrombophilia | • Multiple pregnancy |
| • Obesity >80 kg | • Grand multiparity |
| • Previous thromboembolism | • Caesarean section (greater if emergency) |
| • Severe varicose veins | • Damage to the pelvic veins |
| • Smoking | • Sepsis |
| • Malignancy | • Prolonged bed rest |

### Thrombophilia

Some women are predisposed to thrombosis through changes in the coagulation–fibrinolytic system. These factors may be inherited or acquired. Inherited thrombophilias include protein C, protein S and antithrombin (AT) III deficiency. However, the discovery of new thrombophilias continues at an alarming rate. Acquired thrombophilia is most commonly associated with antiphospholipid syndrome (APS), which is the combination of lupus anticoagulant with or without anticardiolipin antibodies Such women can also present with a history of recurrent miscarriage and/or thrombosis. APS may be associated with other autoantibody disorders, such as systemic lupus erythematosus (SLE); however, this is rare.

It is, therefore, crucial that women with a history of thrombotic events are screened for thrombophilia. However, it should be acknowledged that, should this screening be initially undertaken in pregnancy, the interpretation of results may be complicated by the physiological decrease in protein S and antithrombin III levels. The presence of thrombophilia, with a history of thrombotic episode(s), means that prophylaxis should always be considered during pregnancy.

## Deep vein thrombosis

The commonest symptoms of deep vein thrombosis are pain in the calf, with varying degrees of redness or swelling. In pregnancy, a woman's legs frequently swell, therefore, the midwife should be alert to recognize the significance of unilateral symptoms. Although physical signs are few, except that the calf may frequently be tender to gentle touch, it is important that the midwife seeks details from the woman about symptoms of pulmonary embolus (PE), such as breathlessness and chest pain. This is because most women who develop a PE initially present with DVT. The midwife, therefore, is responsible to refer the woman to the obstetrician for further investigation. Where there is any suspicion of DVT, heparin or a low-molecular-weight heparin is administered until the diagnosis is confirmed or refuted. A firm diagnosis is usually made by either venography or Doppler ultrasound, the latter being the preferred choice, as it is a non-invasive assessment of the deep veins between the knee and the iliac veins. Calf veins are often poorly visualized; however, it is known that a thrombus confined purely to the calf veins with no extension is very unlikely to give rise to a PE.

## Pulmonary embolus

It is crucial that the midwife is able to recognize the signs of pulmonary embolus, as missing the diagnosis could have fatal implications. The most common presentation in pregnancy is of mild breathlessness, or inspiratory chest pain, slight tachycardia (pulse >90/minute) and a mild pyrexia (temperature >37.5°C). However, the pregnant woman does not usually present with cyanosis. In rare instances, the woman may present with sudden cardiorespiratory collapse typical of a massive PE that requires the midwife's prompt assessment and execution of emergency measures including basic life support (see Chapter 16).

Clinical suspicion, together with risk factors for PE, makes immediate full anticoagulation and confirmation of the diagnosis not merely advisable, but essential and preferable within 24 hours. Ventilation–perfusion imaging can be safely performed in pregnancy, as the radiation to the fetus is minimal. A positive diagnosis of PE has major implications for long-term anticoagulants.

## Anticoagulants and thromboprophylaxis

Heparin prolongs the activated partial thromboplastin time (APTT; otherwise known as kaolin cephalin time; KCT). The activity of low-molecular-weight heparin derivatives is assessed by factor X assay. Both are given intramuscularly or intravenously. They do not cross the placenta, are not teratogenic and the effect can be stopped within hours by discontinuing further administration. Although they are regarded as relatively safe, maternal thrombocytopenia can be a distinctive but rare reaction and, if treatment is prolonged for more than 6 months, there is also a risk of osteoporosis.

Warfarin is another anticoagulant that is given orally and its effect is to prolong the prothrombin time (PT). However, as warfarin crosses the placenta should it be given in the first trimester, it can cause limb and facial defects in the fetus. Furthermore, fetal intracerebral haemorrhage can also result owing to its administration in the second and third trimesters. Consequently, the use of warfarin is largely confined to women at highest risk of thromboembolism requiring full anticoagulation, with limited exposure to the second and third trimesters.

Thromboprophylaxis is, therefore, a controversial issue in pregnancy to the extent that the Royal College of Obstetricians and Gynaecologists (RCOG) (2004) has issued a recommendation with respect to thromboembolism and, in particular, its associated risk with Caesarean sections. The details are included in the box on p. 108, and include the use of subcutaneous heparin and the wearing of elasticated thromboembolic disorders stockings, known as TED stockings. If prophylaxis

## Risk assessment for factors associated with thromboembolism at Caesarean section and recommendations for thromboprophylaxis (RCOG 2004)

| Low risk | Medium risk | High risk |
|---|---|---|
| *(a) Factors associated with thromboembolism at Caesarean section* | | |
| • Elective Caesarean section | • Age >35 years | • Three or more moderate risk factors |
| • Uncomplicated pregnancy | • Weight >80 kg | • Extended surgery (Caesarean section, hysterectomy) |
| • No other risk factors | • Para 4 or more | • A personal history of thrombosis, thrombophilia, DVT, PE |
| | • Gross varicose veins | • A family history of thrombosis, thrombophilia, DVT, PE |
| | • Current infection | • Antiphospholipid antibody |
| | • Pre-eclampsia | |
| | • Immobility prior to surgery >4 days | |
| | • Major current illness | |
| | • Emergency Caesarean section in labour | |
| *(b) Recommendations for thromboprophylaxis (RCOG 2004)* | | |
| Early mobilization and hydration | Subcutaneous heparin **or** thromboembolic stockings (TED stockings) | Heparin **and** full-length thromboembolic stockings |

is considered appropriate in the management of women who have a significant risk of thromboembolism following Caesarean section, then it is recommended this should continue until the fifth postoperative day.

## FETAL COMPLICATIONS

### Disorders of the amniotic fluid

The main features of amniotic fluid are discussed in Chapter 3.

### Oligohydramnios

Oligohydramnios is an abnormally small amount of amniotic fluid – around 300–500 mL at term, although amounts may vary. The midwife may suspect oligohydramnios antenatally when, upon inspection of the abdomen, the uterus appears smaller than expected for the period of gestation and the woman may also complain of reduced fetal movements. Reduced amniotic fluid volume may also present following a history of preterm prelabour rupture of the membranes (PPROM; see Chapter 11). When the abdomen is palpated, the uterus feels small and compact, and

fetal parts are easily felt. Auscultation of the fetal heart is clearly audible and usually within the normal classification. Breech presentation may also be detected. In cases of oligohydramnios, referral to the obstetrician would always be expected.

An ultrasound scan and placental function tests should be undertaken to differentiate oligohydramnios from intrauterine growth restriction. However, both may occur in cases where there is also placental insufficiency. The scan would attempt to estimate the amniotic fluid volume (AFV) that is the single deepest pool of amniotic fluid. However, a more accurate diagnosis may be obtained by measuring the amniotic fluid index (AFI). This is a measurement derived by adding together the deepest vertical pools of amniotic fluid in each of the four quadrants around the fetus. Oligohydramnios is defined as an AFI (i.e. <5th centile for the gestation). In addition, structural defects, such as renal anomalies, may be visible on the scan. The possible causes of oligohydramnios and anhydramnios (no amniotic fluid) are highlighted below in Table 8.2.

The fetal prognosis in respect of perinatal morbidity and mortality depends on the cause of oligohydramnios. When diagnosed in the first trimester, it is often found to be associated with renal agenesis (absence of kidneys) or Potter's syndrome in which the fetus also has pulmonary hypoplasia. Renal agenesis and bilateral

**Table 8.2** – Possible causes of oligohydramnios and anhydramnios

| Too little production | Diagnosed by: |
|---|---|
| Renal agenesis | Ultrasound: no renal tissue, no bladder |
| Multicystic kidneys | Ultrasound: enlarged kidneys with multiple cysts, no visible bladder |
| Urinary tract abnormality/obstruction | Ultrasound: kidneys may be present, but urinary tract dilatation |
| IUGR and placental insufficiency | Clinical: reduced symphysis fundal height, reduced fetal movements, possibly abnormal CTG |
| | Ultrasound: IUGR, abnormal fetal Dopplers |
| Maternal drugs (NSAIDs) | Withholding NSAIDs may allow amniotic fluid to reaccumulate |
| Post-dates pregnancy | |

| Leakage | Diagnosed by: |
|---|---|
| Preterm prelabour rupture of the membranes (PPROM) | Speculum examination: pool of amniotic fluid on posterior blade |

CTG, cardiotocograph; IUGR, intrauterine growth restriction; NSAIDs, non-steroidal anti-inflammatory drugs.

multicystic kidneys carry a fatal prognosis as extrauterine life is impossible without functioning kidneys. Furthermore, chronic oligohydramnios can cause compression deformities, such as flattening of the nose, micrognathia (deformity of the jaw) and talipes. The skin also appears dry and leathery.

If oligohydramnios develops as a result of intrauterine growth restriction/uteroplacental insufficiency, it is usually in the post-term pregnancy where, as a result, the perfusion to the fetal organ systems, including the kidneys, also reduces. However, in this situation, the oligohydramnios is of a less severe degree and rarely causes limb and lung complications. In some cases, amnioinfusions with normal saline or 5 per cent glucose have been undertaken in order to prevent fetal compression deformities and hypoplastic lung disease, whilst also prolonging the pregnancy. To date, there have been no studies undertaken to determine the benefits and hazards of this intervention in the second trimester. However, studies have reported that when undertaken during labour, amnioinfusions have been found to reduce the Caesarean section rates and improve fetal outcome.

The management of oligohydramnios in a post-term pregnancy (up to 42 weeks gestation) remains controversial as it is a poorly understood phenomenon. It has been suggested that the AFI should be measured twice weekly as amniotic fluid can reduce very quickly and is highly suggestive of placental insufficiency. Although in such a situation, it may also be considered useful for regular 20–30 minutes CTG recordings to be undertaken, neither of these tests can totally guarantee fetal well-being and subsequent outcome.

Labour may occur spontaneously or be induced, and this will be determined by the condition of the fetus. As a consequence of diminished amniotic fluid volume, uterine contractions can be exceptionally painful for the woman and so it may be appropriate for the midwife to offer her adequate analgesia, such as epidural anaesthesia during labour. There is also a risk of cord compression and impairment of the placental circulation resulting in fetal hypoxia. Should this become apparent, it is important that the midwife undertakes continuous monitoring of the fetal heart during labour. Furthermore, if the fetus passes meconium during labour, it will tend to be more concentrated and consequently presents an increased risk to an already asphyxiated baby during birth. In rare cases, the membranes may adhere to the fetus. Ideally, a paediatrician should be present for the birth of the baby, especially in cases where the fetus has shown signs of compromise during labour and to undertake an initial examination, observing for any physical abnormalities resulting from the oligohydramnios.

# Polyhydramnios

Polyhydramnios is known to be present in a pregnancy when there is an excess of amniotic fluid. On ultrasound examination, the AFV exceeds 8 cm and the calculated AFI is more than 24 cm (i.e. >95th centile for gestation). Some writers further categorize polyhydramnios into *mild* (AFI 25–30 cm), *moderate* (AFI 30.1–35 cm) and *severe* (AFI more than 35 cm). *Chronic polyhydramnios* is a gradual accumulation of amniotic fluid from about the 30th week of pregnancy and is the most common type that presents. *Acute polyhydramnios* is less common and is sudden on onset, presenting at about 20 weeks of pregnancy. The uterus reaches the xiphisternum in about 3 or 4 days.

Polyhydramnios may be caused by maternal, placental or fetal factors, and is often associated with monozygotic twins and the consequential twin-to-twin transfusion syndrome, and severe fetal abnormality, although in some cases, the cause may be unknown. Maternal factors include diabetes mellitus, whereas associated placental factors include chorioangioma (a rare tumour of the placenta). However, the fetal factors leading to polyhydramnios are mainly associated with malformations that subsequently have an effect on the ability of the fetus to swallow and absorb amniotic fluid. These include oesophageal atresia/ tracheo-oesophageal fistula, duodenal atresia, anencephaly and open neural tube defect. In rare cases, polyhydramnios has also been associated with rhesus isoimmunization.

Polyhydramnios may present as severe abdominal swelling and discomfort, including breathlessness. The condition may also exacerbate the symptoms of pregnancy, such as indigestion, heartburn and constipation. In addition, oedema and varicosities of the lower limbs and vulva may be present. On examination, the abdomen will appear distended and globular in shape with an increased symphysis–fundal height (SFH) to that expected for the period of gestation. The abdominal skin appears stretched and shiny with noticeable striae gravidarum and superficial blood vessels. Furthermore, the abdomen may be tense, tender and the fetal poles will be hard to palpate. A fluid thrill may be felt from one side of the abdomen to the other when one side is gently tapped. In cases of acute polyhydramnios, it may be useful to measure the abdominal girth in order to establish the rate of increase. Auscultation of the fetal heart can be extremely difficult owing to the quantity of fluid allowing increased mobility of the fetus. An ultrasound scan is used to confirm the diagnosis. In addition to calculating the AFV and AFI to determine the severity of the polyhydramnios, the scan may also reveal multiple pregnancy or fetal abnormality.

Midwives should also be aware of possible complications associated with polyhydramnios in order to advise the woman accordingly so that appropriate assessment and management be carried out in the likelihood they may occur. Such *complications* include the following:

- maternal ureteric obstruction;
- increased fetal mobility leading to unstable lie and malpresentation;
- cord presentation and cord prolapse;
- preterm and prelabour rupture of the membranes;
- placental abruption when the membranes rupture;
- increased perinatal mortality rate;
- increased incidence of Caesarean section;
- postpartum haemorrhage.

The management of polyhydramnios may involve admitting the woman to hospital under consultant care, but this will depend on her condition and that of the fetus. It is directed towards establishing the cause and determining the fetal prognosis, relieving the discomfort of the woman if necessary by amnio-drainage, and assessing the risk of preterm labour due to uterine overdistension. Polyhydramnios due to maternal diabetes needs urgent investigation, as it often suggests high maternal blood glucose levels. In this context, polyhydramnios should correct itself when the woman's glycaemic control is optimized. However, twin-to-twin transfusion syndrome is a rare cause of acute polyhydramnios in the recipient sac of monochorionic twins. It is associated with oligohydramnios and a fetus that is growth restricted in the other sac. The condition may be rapidly fatal for both twins. In such cases, amnio-drainage and removing the placental vascular connections by laser may be undertaken to help improve the discomfort for the woman as well as improve the prognosis for the twins. This is further discussed in Chapter 9.

In cases of mild asymptomatic polyhydramnios, the woman is not usually admitted to hospital, but should be advised to rest as much as possible and to seek admission once she suspects her membranes have ruptured. In women with symptoms associated with polyhydramnios, recommending an upright position to relieve any dyspnoea and antacids for heartburn and nausea may be suggested. If the discomfort is severe, then the short-term temporary measure of amnio-drainage may be considered whereby no more than 500 mL amniotic fluid is drained off at any one time. However, this procedure is not without the risk of introducing infection and inducing labour. There is also the likelihood of the fluid rapidly reaccumulating and the procedure needing to be repeated. Owing to the rapid increase of amniotic fluid, the membranes usually rupture spontaneously and the fetus (or fetuses) are born, very premature in a stream of amniotic fluid.

The presence of any fetal abnormalities will determine the mode and timing of the birth of the baby. If gross fetal abnormality is detected, then labour may be induced. If the fetus has an operable condition, such as oesophageal atresia, the woman should be transferred to a hospital with a neonatal surgical unit.

If induction is contemplated in order to relieve symptoms, it is important that it is undertaken when the fetus is lying longitudinally in the uterus. When an artificial rupture of membranes is undertaken, the process should be done cautiously, allowing the amniotic fluid to drain out slowly to avoid altering the lie, preventing cord prolapse and placental abruption that can be caused by a sudden reduction in uterine size. However, labour usually commences spontaneously and progresses without any further complications. The midwife should be prepared for the possible change of fetal position and prolapsed cord should the membranes rupture spontaneously. There is also a greater risk of postpartum haemorrhage owing to the overdistension of the uterine muscles. The baby should be carefully examined for any abnormalities following its birth and the patency of the oesophagus assessed by passing a nasogastric tube.

## Malpresentations and unstable lie at term

### Malpresentations of the fetus

A malpresentation of the fetus is any presentation other than the vertex and thus can be a face, brow shoulder or breech. Such presentations can present the midwife with a challenge with both the recognition and diagnosis in pregnancy (and also during labour) for failure to do so could lead to serious complications, such as obstructed labour, uterine rupture including fetal and maternal death. However, it is rare

to diagnose a *face* or *brow* presentation in pregnancy since these tend to develop during labour in most cases. Such presentations would only become significant should they persist once labour has commenced. A cephalic presentation in a known anencephalic fetus may be presumed to be a face presentation.

### Transverse or oblique lie

The midwife should always be aware that any woman presenting at term with a transverse or oblique lie is at potential risk of cord prolapse following spontaneous rupture of the membranes, and prolapse of the hand, arm or shoulder once in labour. In most cases, the

| Predisposing factors associated with malpresentations of the fetus | |
|---|---|
| **Uterine** | **Fetal** |
| • Fibroids | • Multiple pregnancy |
| • Placenta praevia | • Congenital abnormality, e.g. anencephaly or hydrocephalus |
| • Structural anomalies of the uterus | • Neuromuscular conditions |
| • Uterine surgery | |
| • Oligohydramnios | |
| • Polyhydramnios | |

woman is a multigravida with lax uterus and abdominal wall musculature.

The midwife may suspect a transverse or oblique lie by abdominal inspection where the abdomen often appears broad and asymmetrical. The symphysis–fundal height may be less than expected, and on pelvic and fundal palpation, neither fetal head nor buttocks are felt. The free moving head is found on one side of the abdomen and the breech at a slightly higher level on the other. Consequently, it is the shoulder that presents. The lie and presentation are confirmed on ultrasound scan while any cause such as placenta praevia or uterine anomoly is excluded at the same time. Following this, an external cephalic version (ECV) may be attempted. Should this fail or the fetus be in a transverse lie at the next antenatal visit, the woman is admitted to hospital for further investigations. She may remain in hospital until the baby is born because of the risk of cord prolapse and possible arm prolapse when the membranes rupture. Shoulder presentations account for approximately 1:300 pregnancies, but only 17 per cent of these cases remain as a transverse lie at the onset of labour, the majority being multigravidae.

Should the woman go into labour with a transverse lie, a vaginal birth would be impossible. This is one situation where it is important the woman is made fully aware that a Caesarean section is undertaken otherwise both she and the fetus are at considerable risk of morbidity and mortality. The only exemption to this is for an exceptionally preterm or small fetus, where vaginal birth may occur irrespective of lie or presentation.

## Breech presentation

The fetus presents by the breech in 40 per cent of pregnancies at 26 weeks, 20 per cent at 30 weeks and 3 per cent by term. Consequently, a breech presentation only becomes a problem if the fetus (or first presenting fetus in a multiple pregnancy) is not cephalic by 37 weeks. There are three types of breech; the commonest is *extended* (frank) breech (Figure 8.6). Less common is a *flexed* (complete) breech (Figure 8.7) and least common is a *footling* breech, where a foot presents at the cervix. The breech may also present by the *knee*, but this is extremely rare. Prolapse of the cord and foot are risks associated of breech presentation.

The diagnosis of a breech presentation may be more difficult in primigravidae because of their firm abdominal muscles. On palpation, the lie would be noted as longitudinal with a soft presentation. The fetal head can usually be felt in the fundus as a hard round mass. However, depending whether or not the legs are extended with the feet splinting the head, as a consequence this will prevent the ballottement of the fetal head. If the breech is anterior and well flexed, the head may be difficult to palpate abdominally. The woman may complain of discomfort under her ribs especially at night, owing to the pressure of the head on the diaphragm. The auscultation of the fetal heart may be heard above the umbilicus if the breech has not passed through the brim of the pelvis (more common in pregnancy with a flexed breech). If the legs are extended, the breech can descend into the pelvis more easily and so

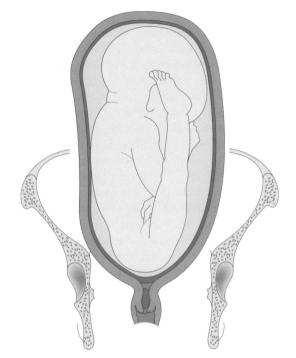

**Figure 8.6** Frank breech (also known as extended breech) presentation with extension of the legs.

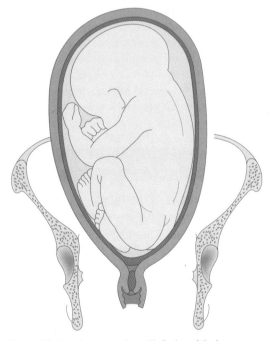

**Figure 8.7** Breech presentation with flexion of the legs.

the fetal heart is usually heard at a lower level. An ultrasound scan may be performed to confirm the findings and make a decision about subsequent intrapartum management. This is discussed in detail in Chapter 15.

---

**Factors strengthening the likelihood of a vaginal breech birth versus planned Caesarean section**

| Vaginal breech birth | Caesarean section |
|---|---|
| • Fetal size 2.5–3.5 kg | • Fetal size <2.5 kg and >3.5 kg |
| • Adequate pelvic size on pelvimetry | • Small pelvis on pelvimetry or very flat sacrum |
| • Flexed attitude: neck | • Primigravida |
| • Multigravida | • Previous Caesarean section |
| • Breech deeply engaged | • Extended neck |
| • Positive mental attitude of woman and partner | |
| • Midwives and obstetricians familiar and competent with vaginal breech technique | |

---

## External cephalic version (ECV)

The most common situation arises when a woman, with an otherwise uncomplicated pregnancy, presents in the antenatal clinic at 36 weeks' gestation and the midwife discovers the presentation is breech. If there are no contraindications (see box), an external cephalic version as shown in Figure 8.8, may be performed at 36–37 weeks by a skilled senior obstetrician or specially trained midwife under the guidance of an ultrasound transducer. ECV is a relatively straightforward and safe technique, and has been shown to reduce the number of Caesarean sections due to breech presentations. The technique is easier to perform in multigravida women where the uterus is already relatively lax. Alternatively, it can be performed following the administration of tocolytics, such as nifedipine. ECV is much more difficult in women who are overweight or have fibroids. Furthermore, deep engagement of the breech makes any manipulation more difficult. A fetal heart rate trace (CTG) must be performed before and after the procedure. If the procedure fails, or becomes difficult, it is abandoned.

Approximately two-thirds of breech presentations can be turned to cephalic using ECV.

---

**Contraindications and risks of external cephalic version (ECV)**

| Contraindications to ECV | Risks of ECV |
|---|---|
| • Placenta praevia | • Placental abruption |
| • Oligohydramnios and polyhydramnios | • Premature rupture of the membranes |
| • History of antepartum haemorrhage | • Cord accident |
| • Previous Caesarean or myomectomy scar on the uterus | • Transplacental haemorrhage (? administer anti-D) |
| • Multiple pregnancy | • Fetal bradycardia |
| • Pre-eclampsia or hypertension | |
| • Decision already made for elective Caesarean section | |

---

## Unstable lie

After 36 weeks of pregnancy, the lie is considered to be unstable when instead of remaining longitudinal, it varies from one examination to the other between longitudinal, transverse and oblique. Any condition in late pregnancy that increases the mobility of the fetus or prevents the head from entering the brim of the pelvis may cause this (e.g. lax uterine muscles in multigravidae, contracted pelvis, polyhydramnios and placenta praevia).

It may be advised that the woman is admitted to hospital to prevent an unsupervised onset of labour should the lie be other than longitudinal. An alternative management plan would be for the woman to admit herself as soon as labour commences. However, the midwife should stress the risks associated with possible rupture of the membranes and cord prolapse should she choose to remain at home. Ultrasonography can be undertaken to exclude placenta praevia and attempts may then be made to correct the lie and malpresentation by undertaking an ECV. Should this not be possible, or attempts are unsuccessful, then Caesarean section is then considered. Nevertheless, an unstable lie will often correct itself in early labour in a multigravida providing the membranes are intact.

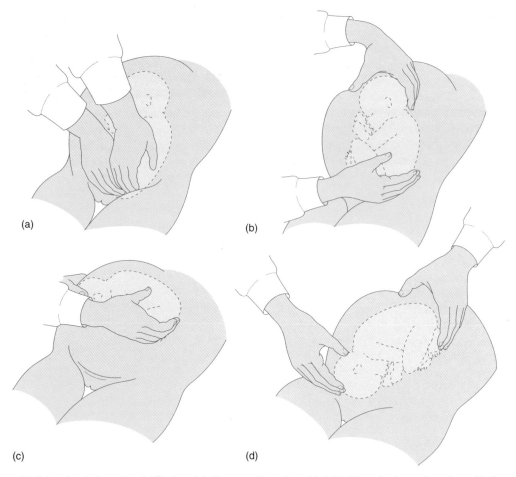

**Figure 8.8** External cephalic version. (a) The breech is disengaged from the pelvic inlet; (b) version is usually performed in the direction which increases flexion of the fetus and makes it do a forward somersault (c); on completion of the version, the head is often not engaged for a time (d).

## Post-term (prolonged) pregnancy

By definition, term is the end of pregnancy and is the period of time between the 37th and 42nd week. A pregnancy that exceeds 294 days from the first day of the last menstrual period is considered to be post-term or prolonged. (The terms are used interchangeably in most text.) However, this would occur in <5 per cent of pregnancies, if no intervention was undertaken. It is, therefore, vital that the definition of post-term pregnancy depends on the accuracy of the woman's dates and a first trimester ultrasound estimation of crown–rump length.

At 40 weeks of pregnancy, perinatal mortality is lowest, but then increases after 42 weeks. Where the perinatal mortality and morbidity in post-term pregnancies are increased, this may be as a result of labour and birth and not antenatal events. There may be an association with the fetal condition known as postmaturity, characterized by reduction in subcutaneous fat, absence of lanugo and vernix caseosa and meconium staining. Macrosomia (a birth weight of >4 kg) also occurs in about 10 per cent of post-term pregnancies with 1 per cent of babies weighing over 4.5 kg. This has an effect on pregnancy outcome by contributing to cephalopelvic disproportion and shoulder dystocia.

It is now thought that the morphological changes attributed to placental ageing may be a maturation process increasing the efficiency of the villi rather than decreasing it. As a result the placenta continues to grow and develop beyond term. However, post-term pregnancy may be complicated by placental insufficiency, but this will have existed from earlier in the pregnancy rather than develop as a result of post-term prolonged pregnancy.

Currently there are no tests that can predict fetal outcome post-term. However, an ultrasound scan may give temporary reassurance that the AFV, AFI and fetal growth are within the normal range. CTG recordings should be carried out at least twice weekly from 42 weeks in conjunction with amniotic fluid volume measurements. Should the pregnancy be considered high risk, then biophysical profiles and Doppler ultrasound of the umbilical artery may also be carried out to assess fetal well-being. Immediate induction of labour should take place or the birth of the baby expedited in a post-term pregnancy if:

- there is reduced amniotic fluid on scan;
- fetal growth is reduced;
- there are reduced fetal movements;
- the CTG is not perfect;
- the woman is hypertensive or suffers from a significant medical condition.

When counselling the parents regarding waiting for labour to start naturally after 42 weeks, it is important that the woman is aware that no fetal surveillance test can guarantee the safety of her baby, and that perinatal mortality (stillbirth and neonatal death) is increased at least two-fold beyond 42 weeks. A labour induced post-term is more likely to require Caesarean section (see Chapter 15). This may partly be due to the reluctance of the uterus to contract properly, and the possible compromise of the postmature fetus, resulting in an abnormal CTG.

## Rhesus isoimmunization

All blood groups are defined in two ways. First of all there is the ABO group allowing four different permutations of blood group (O, A, B, AB) and, second, there is the rhesus system, which consists of C, D and E antigens. The importance of these blood group systems is that a mismatch between the fetus and woman mean that, when fetal red cells pass across to the maternal circulation, as they do to a greater or lesser extent during pregnancy, sensitization of the maternal immune system to the alien fetal red blood cells may occur.

ABO blood group isoimmunization may occur when the woman is blood group O and the baby is blood group A or B. Anti-A and anti-B antibodies are present in the maternal circulation naturally, hence do not require prior sensitization in order to be produced. This means that ABO incompatibility may occur in a first pregnancy. In this situation, anti-A or anti-B antibodies may pass to the fetal circulation, causing fetal haemolysis and anaemia. ABO incompatibility causes mild haemolytic disease of the baby, but can sometimes explain unexpected jaundice in an otherwise healthy term infant.

The rhesus system, however, is more commonly associated with severe haemolytic disease. Of all the antibodies (C, D and E), the D antigen is associated most commonly with severe haemolytic fetal disease, but this can *only* occur if the woman is D rhesus-negative and the baby is D rhesus-positive. Both anti-C and anti-E antibodies may also be associated with haemolytic disease requiring intrauterine fetal blood transfusion, but are much less commonly implicated. The spectrum of rhesus disease ranges from mild neonatal jaundice requiring phototherapy to the severely anaemic neonate requiring exchange blood transfusions. In the most severe of cases, however, stillbirth or neonatal death may occur.

Rare antibodies, such as those listed below, may unusually be associated with haemolytic disease:

- ABO;
- rhesus (C D E);
- anti Kell;
- anti Duffy;
- anti c (known as little c);
- anti S.

Rhesus disease is commonest among Caucasians, about 15 per cent of whom are rhesus negative, compared with 8 per cent of African and 1 per cent of Asian populations. Furthermore, rhesus disease is commonest in countries where anti-D prophylaxis is not widespread, such as in the Middle East and Russia. It does not affect a first pregnancy. It requires that the woman has had exposure to D rhesus-positive fetal cells in a previous pregnancy and then developed an immune response that has been lying dormant until a following pregnancy of a D rhesus-positive fetus. In the subsequent pregnancy, when maternal resensitization occurs, that is where rhesus-positive red cells pass from the fetus to the maternal circulation (Figure 8.9), IgG antibodies cross from the woman to the fetal circulation. Once a woman is sensitized to a fetal red cell antigen, the sensitization cannot be lost and the response will magnify with successive exposure, for instance in subsequent pregnancies.

The other two rhesus antigens (C and E) may also be associated with haemolytic disease of the fetus or

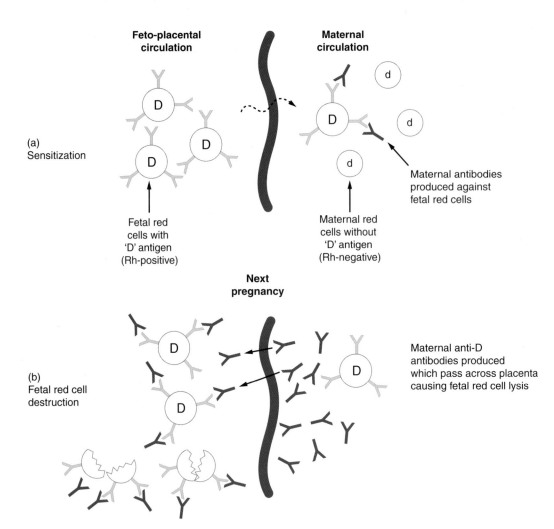

**Feto-placental circulation**

**Maternal circulation**

(a)
Sensitization

Maternal antibodies produced against fetal red cells

Fetal red cells with 'D' antigen (Rh-positive)

Maternal red cells without 'D' antigen (Rh-negative)

**Next pregnancy**

(b)
Fetal red cell destruction

Maternal anti-D antibodies produced which pass across placenta causing fetal red cell lysis

**Figure 8.9** The mechanisms of rhesus (Rh) sensitization and fetal red cell destruction.

neonate, and are inherited in exactly the same way as is rhesus antigen D. The genetic inheritance of rhesus disease is as follows and is represented diagrammatically in Figure 8.10:

- rhesus-negative mother, rhesus-negative father (homozygote) – *all* fetuses rhesus negative;
- rhesus-negative mother, rhesus-positive father (heterozygote) – 1:2 chance;
- rhesus-negative mother, rhesus-positive father (homozygote) – *all* fetuses rhesus positive.

If IgG antibodies are present in sufficient quantities, fetal haemolysis may occur, leading to such severe anaemia that the fetus may die unless an intrauterine exchange transfusion is undertaken. In such circumstances, the blood transfused should have a haemoglobin concentration of 22–24 g/dL, be cytomegalovirus negative, irradiated (to reduce the risk of graft versus host disease) and rhesus negative. Blood transfusions may be repeated every 7–10 days depending on the extent of the anaemia. Prior to 24 weeks intraperitoneal transfusions may be performed and then blood is transfused via cordocentesis However, after 34 weeks, the risks of cordocentesis (e.g. fetal bradycardia, cord tamponade or haemorrhage, fetal death) outweigh the risks of prematurity and the birth of the baby is usually expedited. Features of fetal anaemia do not become obvious unless the fetal haemoglobin is <6 g/dL. Such features include:

- polyhydramnios;
- cardiomegaly (enlarged fetal heart);

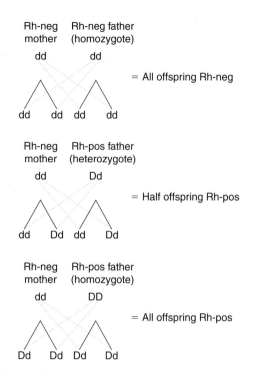

**Figure 8.10** Parental genotype determinants of rhesus (Rh) group.

- ascites and pericardial effusions;
- reduced fetal movements;
- abnormal CTG with reduced variability that may eventually develop into a sinusoidal trace;
- hyperdynamic fetal circulation (detected by Doppler ultrasound in the middle cerebral artery and aorta).

The midwife can play an important preventative role with families who have rhesus incompatibility to ensure they understand the significance it may have on them in subsequent pregnancies. This will include advising the woman about the frequent antibody assessment in pregnancy at booking, 24 and 36 weeks. An increasing titre to >10 iu/mL of atypical antibodies may suggest an impending problem and requires review by a specialist obstetrician/physician, if possible in a fetal medicine centre, so that early signs of fetal anaemia can be detected by ultrasound and, if appropriate, invasive assessment performed. It is important to note, however, absolute measurement of the antibodies does not correlate well with the degree of fetal anaemia. It is for this reason that invasive and non-invasive assessments of the fetus are indicated in risk situations to determine whether the fetus is developing anaemia.

The process of isoimmunization can be prevented by the intramuscular administration of anti-D immunoglobulins to a woman preferably within 72 hours of exposure to fetal red cells. Anti-D immunoglobulins soak up any circulating rhesus-positive cells before an immune response is triggered in the woman. The practical implications of this are that after any potential sensitising event such as:

- miscarriage;
- termination of pregnancy;
- antepartum haemorrhage;
- invasive prenatal screening (chorionic villus sampling, amniocentesis and cordocentesis);
- birth of the baby,

anti-D immunoglobulin must be given intramuscularly as soon as possible afterwards. It is normal practice to administer anti-D after any of these events; the exact dose is determined by the gestation at which sensitization has occurred and the size of the feto-maternal haemorrhage. If the sensitizing event occurred before 20 weeks, a dose of 250 iu anti D is administered and, beyond this gestation, a dose of 500 iu is given. However, larger doses may be given to suppress immunization from more extensive haemorrhage. A Kleihauer test should be performed on maternal blood to determine the proportion of fetal cells present and consequently calculate the amount of extra anti-D immunoglobulin required should a large transfusion have occurred.

Furthermore, in many countries, women who are rhesus negative are given anti-D at 28 and/or 34 weeks as prophylaxis. This is based on the finding that a small number of rhesus-negative women become sensitized during pregnancy despite the administration of anti-D following childbirth and without a clinically obvious sensitizing event. The likelihood is that a small feto-maternal haemorrhage occurs without any obvious clinical signs, therefore, prophylactic anti-D would reduce the risk of isoimmunization from this event. However, once sensitization has occurred, prophylactic anti-D is of little use.

If the fetus is known to be anaemic or has had multiple intrauterine transfusions, a neonatologist must be present at the birth should an exchange blood transfusion be required. Blood must, therefore, always be ready around the time the birth is expected. All babies born to rhesus-negative women should have cord blood taken at delivery for a full blood count, blood group and indirect Coombs test. It is, therefore, essential the woman and her family are kept fully informed of all aspects of care and management affecting the health and well-being of the baby once it is born. The midwife can play a vital role in supporting the woman both physically and psychologically; the extent of the latter will be determined by the outcome of pregnancy and the condition of the baby once it is born.

## REFLECTIVE ACTIVIY

Marie is 36 years old and is pregnant for the fifth time; she is expecting twins. Her four children range in age from 3 years to 12 years. She is a known smoker, although has reduced her intake during this particular pregnancy and has a history of varicose veins. She is blood group A rhesus negative.

She presents at the maternity assessment unit at 30 weeks with abdominal pain.

- As the midwife attending Marie, what further details would you wish to elicit from her to assist you making a differential diagnosis as to what the possible cause may be?
- What clinical observations would assist you?
- List the possible complications Marie may be presenting with.

- What are the risk factors pertinent to Marie's history that may have led you to this decision?
- For each complication listed, what further investigations may be undertaken to confirm the diagnosis?
- Consider one of these complications, and outline the subsequent care and management Marie may receive from the multidisciplinary team.
- What effect may the complication have on the health and well-being of the fetuses?
- What could be the potential outcome for Marie and her babies in this situation?

## Key Points

- The midwife should be fully aware of the physiology of pregnancy such that she can recognize when the pregnancy deviates from the norm and consequently refer to the appropriate practitioner.
- The midwife has a fundamental role in providing information, advice and physical and psychological support, including any lifestyle changes, to enable women and their families to cope with the physiological effects of pregnancy, and any complication that may arise.
- When the woman first presents with a potential complication in pregnancy, it is essential that the midwife takes a detailed history of the events and undertakes an accurate physical examination, as her observations and subsequent decision-making abilities may be crucial to a successful pregnancy outcome.
- In rare instances, the woman may present with sudden cardiorespiratory collapse typical of a massive pulmonary embolus that requires the midwife's prompt assessment and execution of emergency measures including basic life support.
- Where there are issues concerning conscientious objection towards participating in termination of

pregnancies, the midwife should discuss these with her manager and supervisor of midwives so that the parameters of her involvement are clearly defined and understood.

- Malpresentations of the fetus can present the midwife with a challenge with both the recognition and diagnosis in pregnancy (and also during labour) for failure to do so could lead to serious complications, such as obstructed labour and uterine rupture, including fetal and maternal death.
- Midwives should be fully conversant with local and national guidelines and recommendations for good practice in respect of the management of antenatal complications, in order that the best possible pregnancy outcome can be achieved for the woman and her baby.
- A collaborative, multidisciplinary approach to the care and management of women presenting with complications in pregnancy is fundamental to ensuring that maternal and fetal well-being is optimized.

# References and additional reading

Abortion Act 1967. London: HMSO.

Human Fertilisation and Embryology Act 1991. London: HMSO.

James DK, Steer PJ, Weiner CP, Gonik B (eds). *High risk pregnancy management options.* London: WB Saunders, 1999.

Lewis G, Drife J (eds). *Confidential Enquiry into Maternal and Child Health; why mothers die 2000–2002.* Sixth report of the confidential enquiries into maternal deaths in the UK. London: RCOG Press, 2004.

Marshall JE, Raynor MD. Conscientious objection 1: legal and ethical issues. *British Journal of Midwifery* 2002; **10:**388, 390–2.

Nursing and Midwifery Council. *Midwives rules and standards.* London: NMC, 2004.

Raynor MD, Marshall JE. Conscientious objection 2: professional responsibilities. *British Journal of Midwifery* 2002; **10:**574–7.

Royal College of Obstetricians and Gynaecologists. *Thromboprophylaxis during pregnancy, labour and normal vaginal delivery.* Guideline No. 37. London, RCOG, 2004 (available at www.rcog.org.uk).

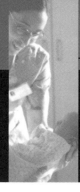

# Multiple pregnancy

## OVERVIEW

Multiple pregnancies consist of two (twins) or more fetuses (higher multiples). The majority are twin pregnancies (approximately 98 per cent). There are more risks for the mother and the fetuses with multiple pregnancy than with a singleton pregnancy, and the consequences of complications can lead to greater emotional, financial and practical difficulties for families.

## Prevalence

In the UK, twins currently account for approximately 1.5 per cent of all pregnancies. Higher multiples occur in approximately 1 in 2500 pregnancies. The causes of monozygotic twinning are unknown, but dizygotic twinning and higher multiples are associated with increasing maternal age, high parity, black race and increased maternal height and weight. Black races have the highest prevalence of twins, Japanese have the lowest.

Since the mid-1980s, the incidence of multiple pregnancy has been increasing. The reasons for this correspond to two related and overlapping trends. First, delay in childbearing results in increased maternal age at conception. Second, the increased use of infertility treatments, such as ovulation induction and *in-vitro* fertilization (IVF), often by older women,

further contributes. Currently in the UK with IVF, no more than two embryos are implanted and there is discussion as to whether this should be reduced to one embryo.

## Classification

The classification of multiple pregnancy is based on:
- number of fetuses – twins, triplets, quadruplets, etc.;
- number of fertilized ova – zygosity;
- number of placentae – chorionicity;
- number of amniotic cavities – amnionicity.

Non-identical/fraternal/dizygotic/binovular twins result from the fertilization of two separate ova, spontaneously released at ovulation, by two spermatazoa. Although they always have two functionally separate placentae (dichorionic), the placentae can become anatomically fused and appear to the naked eye as a

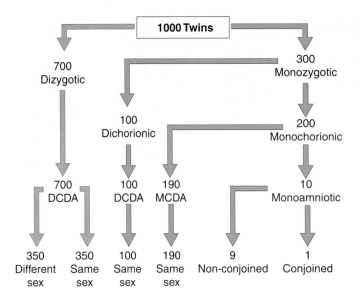

**Figure 9.1** Incidence of monozygotic and dizygotic twins. DCDA, dichorionic diamniotic; MCDA, monochorionic diamniotic; MCMA, monochorionic monoamniotic.

single placental mass. They always have separate amniotic cavities (diamniotic) and the two cavities are separated by a thick three-layer membrane (fused amnion in the middle with chorion on either side). The fetuses can be either same-sex or different-sex pairings.

Identical/monozygotic/uniovular twins develop from the fertilization of a single ovum by one spermatozoon that then splits into two identical structures; therefore, they are always same-sex pairings. They may share a single placenta (monochorionic) or have one each (dichorionic). The vast majority of monochorionic twins will have two amniotic cavities (diamniotic) but the dividing membrane will be thin, consisting of a single layer of amnion. Monochorionic twins may occasionally share a single sac (monoamniotic). If dichorionic, the placentae can become anatomically fused together and appear to the naked eye as a single placental mass.

Monochorionic placentae have the unique ability to develop vascular connections between the two fetal circulations. These anastamoses carry the potential for complications for the fetuses.

Figure 9.1 shows the relative distribution of the different types of twins in an hypothetical random selection of 1000 twin pairs.

The type of monozygotic twin depends on how long after conception the split occurs. When the split occurs within 3 days of conception, two placentae and

two amniotic cavities result, giving rise to a dichorionic diamniotic (DCDA) pregnancy. When splitting occurs between the fourth and eighth days, only the chorion has differentiated and a monochorionic diamniotic (MCDA) pregnancy results. Later splitting after the amnion has differentiated leads to both twins developing in a single amniotic cavity, a monochorionic monoamniotic (MCMA) pregnancy. If splitting is delayed beyond day 12, the embryonic disc has also formed and conjoined or 'Siamese' twins will result.

Monochorionic pregnancies have a 3–5 times higher risk of perinatal morbidity and mortality than dichorionic pregnancies.

## Ultrasound diagnosis

If ultrasound scanning facilities are available and the woman consents, multiple pregnancy can be diagnosed at 6 weeks. Because of the increased maternal and fetal risks with monochorionicity, determination of chorionicity is critical and is most reliably determined by ultrasound in the late first trimester (Moll 2003a). In dichorionic twins, there is a V-shaped extension of placental tissue into the base of the inter-twin membrane, referred to as the 'lambda' or 'twin-peak' sign. In monochorionic twins, this sign is absent and the inter-twin membrane joins the uterine wall in a T-shape (Figure 9.2).

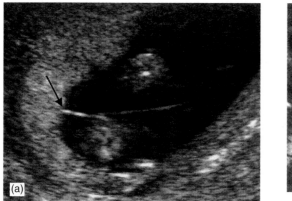 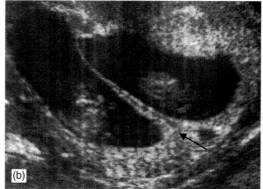

**Figure 9.2** Ultrasound appearance of monochorionic (a) and dichorionic (b) twin pregnancies at 12 weeks' gestation. Note that in both types there appears to be a single placental mass but in the dichorionic type there is an extension of placental tissue into the base of the inter-twin membrane forming the lambda sign.

Assessment of chorionicity later in pregnancy is less reliable and is based on the assessment of fetal gender, number of placentae and characteristics of the membrane between the two amniotic sacs. The 'lambda' sign becomes less accurate and membrane thickness must be utilized. Different-sex twins must be dizygotic and, therefore, dichorionic. In same-sex twins, two separate placentae means dichorionic, although the babies may still be monozygotic. However, monozygotic dichorionic twins do not carry the additional risks of vascular anastamoses.

## Diagnosis by the midwife

Where the technology is unavailable or the woman declines its use, the midwife can use other methods to determine a multiple pregnancy. These will include taking note of factors associated with multiple pregnancy to the woman's history, such as race, age, height, weight, parity, multiple pregnancy already in the family and any assisted reproduction techniques.

Examination of the abdomen can also be helpful. On inspection the uterus appears larger than expected for the length of the pregnancy, especially after the 20th week. Fetal movements may be seen over a wide area, the uterus may appear broad or round, and there may be excess striae gravidarum and amniotic fluid. On palpation, the fundal height may be greater than expected for the length of the pregnancy, more than one fetal pole may be felt in the fundus, and more than one fetal back and multiple limbs may be felt. The fetal heads may feel smaller than expected for the length of the pregnancy. Palpating three fetal poles is diagnostic of at least two fetuses.

To determine that more than one fetus is present, simultaneous auscultation for 1 minute of at least two fetal hearts, with a difference of at least 10 beats per minute (bpm), is required.

The differential diagnosis of a multiple gestation includes all the other cause of a 'large for dates' uterus, such as polyhydramnios, uterine fibroids, urinary retention and ovarian masses.

## Midwifery care

All the physiological changes of pregnancy, such as increased cardiac output, volume expansion, relative haemodilution, diaphragmatic splinting, weight gain and lordosis, are exaggerated in multiple pregnancy, with greater stresses placed on maternal reserves. In women with pre-existing health problems, such as cardiac disease or renal disease, a multiple pregnancy may substantially increase her risk of morbidity.

Because of this and the higher incidence of maternal and fetal complications, the woman will have increased surveillance prenatally, intranatally and postnatally. The midwife will work with the family doctor and the obstetrician to give care and monitor maternal and fetal well-being throughout the pregnancy.

### Breaking the news

Giving the news of a multiple pregnancy to parents has to be sensitively handled. Regardless of how much the pregnancy was planned or is wanted, most parents experience some shock and disbelief at the news. The midwife should be prepared to answer questions and give specific information, including referral to relevant support agencies and to a social worker, if appropriate, and if the woman chooses.

## Prenatal care

The possible variations in the usual prenatal care should be discussed with the mother. There should be opportunities for her to meet with the midwife more often during the pregnancy so that new and ongoing concerns can be addressed.

### Parent education

The parents should have access to detailed information about the pregnancy, its possible course, complications and outcomes. Discussion about the options for prenatal care and the birth should be offered, and the parents' wishes and concerns noted and addressed. A birth plan should be devised during the pregnancy.

As the risks of preterm birth and the need for the babies to be cared for in a neonatal unit (NNU) are increased, specific information/preparation should be available, including the option to visit the NNU.

Having to care for more than one baby can be a daunting proposition for parents, and the midwife should be able to give information, both verbal and written, to the parents to help prepare them for their parenting role. Practical information on feeding, clothing, equipment, organization and sources of help is valuable. Child development and coping with the needs of twins and higher multiples should also be addressed. Referral to support groups and/or the material they publish can be helpful for many parents.

### Folate supplementation

Multiple pregnancy brings an increased risk of fetal structural abnormalities; therefore, folate supplementation is recommended. However, the mother may already have been complying with the preconception and periconception folate supplementation recommended for all women about to embark on a pregnancy (Moll 2003a).

### Screening for congenital abnormalities

Variations in expected serum levels can help in the diagnosis of congenital abnormalities, but in multiple pregnancy the results may be too complex for a reliable diagnosis. Chorionic villus sampling is less often performed owing to the potential for fused placentae and the increased risk of pregnancy loss. Diagnosis of Down's syndrome by nuchal translucency can be accurate if the ultrasound scan is performed between 11 and 13 weeks. Dual needle insertion amniocentesis, ensuring each amniotic sac is sampled, between 15 and 20 weeks, can be undertaken. Echocardiography of monozygotic twins at 20 weeks is recommended as there is an increased risk of cardiac abnormalities.

Ultrasound scanning in the first trimester to determine chorionicity is recommended, as is scanning at 20 weeks for anomalies (Moll 2003a). Thereafter, 4-weekly scanning of dichorionic twins and 2-weekly scanning of monochorionic twins to assess fetal growth are recommended.

## Complications of multiple pregnancy

Multiple pregnancies bring increased risks of complications, although the incidence and degree varies depending on the woman and the classification of her pregnancy. Part of the midwife's role is to recognize the potential for complications, suggest preventive measures, refer as they occur and assist with management.

### Congenital abnormalities

Each twin in a dichorionic pregnancy has a risk of structural anomalies, such as spina bifida, that is similar to a singleton. Therefore, the chance of an anomaly in a dichorionic twin pregnancy is twice that of a singleton. In contrast, each twin in a monochorionic pregnancy carries a risk for abnormalities that is four times that of a singleton, possibly due to a higher risk of vascular events during embryonic development.

If one fetus has an anomaly, it can be managed expectantly or by selective fetocide of the affected twin. In cases where the abnormality is non-lethal but could result in handicap, the parents may need to decide whether the potential burden of a handicapped child outweighs the risk of loss of the normal twin from fetocide-related complications. These occur after

5–10 per cent of procedures. In cases where the abnormality is lethal it may be best to avoid such risk to the normal fetus, unless the condition itself threatens the survival of the normal twin. Fetocide in monochorionic pregnancies carries increased risk (Moll 2003b). Owing to the potential for twin-to-twin transfusion, a different technique is required and this is associated with a higher complication rate.

In twins, as in singletons, the risk for chromosomal abnormalities increases with maternal age. Monozygotic twins have the same genetic make-up, therefore chromosomal abnormalities such as Down's syndrome will affect neither fetus or both. The risk is based upon maternal age.

In dizygotic twins, the maternal age-related risk for chromosomal abnormalities for each twin remains the same as for a singleton pregnancy. Therefore, at a given maternal age, the chance that at least one of the twins will be affected is twice as high as in a singleton pregnancy.

## Minor disorders

The minor disorders of pregnancy, including morning sickness and heartburn, are usually more troublesome and may persist for longer owing to the increased levels of circulating hormones. As the pregnancy progresses, the increased uterine size and weight result in more pressure symptoms, such as ankle oedema, varicose veins, backache and dyspnoea, as well as tiredness. The midwife should be able to offer options to help the mother relieve/control these symptoms.

## Anaemia

Because of the extra demands for growth and fetal demands in a multiple pregnancy, iron and folate deficiency anaemia can occur. Additional iron and folate may be prescribed in the second trimester, although some doctors will not prescribe these unless there is a definite clinical need in the individual woman (Moll 2003a).

## Polyhydramnios

This condition is particularly likely to occur in a monochorionic twin pregnancy and/or when there are fetal abnormalities. The woman may suffer increased discomfort and pressure symptoms that can be difficult to relieve. Repeat therapeutic amniocentesis may help, although the associated risks of miscarriage and preterm birth may outweigh any possible symptom relief (Moll 2003a).

In the second trimester, acute polyhydramnios can occur. This condition can lead to miscarriage or preterm birth, therefore referral and urgent obstetric intervention are needed.

## Miscarriage, extreme preterm birth and mortality

Spontaneous preterm delivery is an ever-present risk in any twin pregnancy whose average gestation at birth is 37 weeks. Therefore, about half of all twins are born preterm. Most babies born from 32 weeks onwards have few problems. Almost all babies born at 23 weeks or less die. Rates of mortality and handicap steadily fall between 24 and 31 weeks.

In a dichorionic pregnancy, the chance of late miscarriage is 2 per cent, and 5 per cent will be born very preterm. With two babies resulting from each preterm twin birth, multiple gestations account for at least 10 per cent of NNU admissions. For monochorionic twins, the chance of early birth is increased even further, with 12 per cent born before viability, and 10 per cent being born between 24 and 32 weeks.

The overall perinatal mortality rate for twins is around six times higher than in singletons. The biggest contributor to this high rate is complications related to preterm birth. As preterm delivery is most common in monochorionic twins, their perinatal mortality secondary to this is twice as high as in dichorionic twins. Monozygotic twins also have both additional risks and unique complications that further increase their chance of death and handicap.

After the first trimester, intrauterine death of one fetus in a twin pregnancy may be associated with a poor outcome for the remaining twin. Maternal complications such as disseminated intravascular coagulation have been reported, but the incidence appears very low. In dichorionic twins, second or third trimester intrauterine death of one fetus may be associated with the onset of labour. However, in some cases, the pregnancy may continue uneventfully and even result in delivery at term. Careful fetal and maternal monitoring is required. By contrast, fetal death of one twin in a monochorionic twin pregnancy may result in immediate complications in the survivor. These include death or brain damage with subsequent neurodevelopmental handicap. Acute hypotensive episodes secondary to placental vascular anastomoses between the two fetuses result in haemodynamic volume shifts from the live to the dead fetus. Death or handicap of the co-twin occurs in up to 25 per cent of cases.

The midwife should give the parents the opportunity to discuss these risks, and give them specific information about the needs of babies born at these early gestations and the care they would require (Moll 2003a). A visit to the NNU should be arranged if the parents wish. Referral for genetic counselling should also be an option.

## Pregnancy-induced hypertension, pre-eclampsia and thromboembolism

These complications are more frequent in multiple pregnancies than in singleton pregnancies and the risk is higher in monozygotic than in dizygotic twin pregnancies. Management strategies are similar to those for women having singleton pregnancies.

## Twin-to-twin transfusion

In all monochorionic twin pregnancies, there are placental vascular anastamoses present that allow communication between the two fetoplacental circulations. In some monochorionic twin pregnancies, imbalance in the flow of blood across these arteriovenous communications results in twin-to-twin transfusion syndrome (TTTS). The development of mild, moderate or severe TTTS depends on the degree of imbalance. The donor fetus suffers from both hypovolaemia owing to blood loss and hypoxia owing to placental insufficiency, and may become growth restricted and oliguric. As fetal urine is the major component of amniotic fluid, this fetus develops oligohydramnios. The recipient fetus becomes hypervolaemic, leading to polyuria and polyhydramnios. Severe disease may become apparent at 18–24 weeks. The mother often complains of a sudden increase in abdominal girth associated with extreme discomfort. Clinical examination shows tense polyhydramnios and ultrasound scanning confirms the diagnosis.

More than 90 per cent of pregnancies complicated by TTTS end in miscarriage or severe preterm delivery, either due to the polyhydramnios or intrauterine death

of one or both fetuses. With treatment, one or both babies survive in about 70 per cent of pregnancies.

A common method of treatment is amniocentesis every 1–2 weeks with the drainage of large volumes of amniotic fluid. Exactly how this treatment improves the underlying pathophysiology is uncertain, but it appears to prolong the pregnancy and improve survival. More recently, some centres have used fetoscopically-guided laser coagulation to disrupt the placental blood vessels that connect the circulations of the two fetuses (Moll 2003a, b).

## Intrauterine growth restriction

Compared to singletons, the risk of poor growth is higher in each individual twin alone and substantially raised in the pregnancy as a whole. When a fetus is growth restricted, the main aims of prenatal care become prediction of the severity of impaired fetal oxygenation and selecting the appropriate time for birth. In singletons, this is a balance between the relative risks of intrauterine death, and the risk of neonatal death or handicap from elective preterm birth. The situation is much more complicated in twin pregnancies. The potential benefit of expectant management or elective birth for the small fetus must also be weighed against the risk of the same policy for the normally grown twin.

In a dichorionic pregnancy, each fetus runs twice the risk of a low birth weight and there is a 20 per cent chance that at least one of the fetuses will suffer poor growth. The chance of poor fetal growth for monochorionic twins is almost double that of dichorionic twins.

In dichorionic twin pregnancies where one fetus has intrauterine growth restriction (IUGR), elective preterm birth may lead to iatrogenic complications of prematurity in the previously healthy co-twin. In general, birth should be avoided before 32 weeks even if there is evidence of imminent intrauterine death of the smaller twin. However, this may not be applicable in the management of monochorionic twins. The death of one monochorionic twin may result in either death or handicap of the other because of acute hypotension secondary to placental vascular anastomoses between the two circulations (see 'Twin-to-twin transfusion' above). As the damage potentially happens at the moment of death of the first twin, the timing of birth may be a very difficult decision. Below

32 weeks' gestation, the aim is to prolong the pregnancy as far as possible without risking death of the growth-restricted twin.

## Antepartum haemorrhage

There are greater risks of antepartum haemorrhage from both placenta praevia and placental abruption in multiple pregnancies. The placental size is greater in multiple pregnancy; therefore, there is a greater chance of the placenta dipping into the lower uterine segment, resulting in placenta praevia. The size of the uterus is also larger and, if there is an abrupt change, such as when the membranes rupture, or where the placenta is affected by pregnancy-induced hypertension, placental abruption is more common.

## Umbilical cord entanglement

Because monoamniotic twins share a single amniotic cavity with no dividing membrane, they are at increased risk of cord accidents, predominantly through cord entanglement. Many clinicians advocate elective birth by Caesarean section at 32–34 weeks' gestation, as this complication is usually acute, fatal and unpredictable.

## Disrupted fetal growth and well-being

Measurement of fundal height and maternal reporting of fetal movements are unreliable, as the individual contribution of each twin cannot be assessed. Therefore, monitoring of growth and well-being is ideally by ultrasound scan. Each assessment should include fetal measurements, activity, lie and amniotic fluid volumes. In monochorionic twins, features of TTTS should be sought, including discordances between fetal size, activity, bladder volumes, amniotic fluid volumes and cardiac size. In any twin pregnancy, when one or both fetuses are small, additional information about well-being can be obtained from Doppler assessment of the circulations and from cardiotocography (CTG). Specialized twin monitors should be used to ensure both heart rates are sampled.

Ultrasound scans every 4 weeks in dichorionic twins and every 2 weeks in monochorionic pregnancies are appropriate, but should be modified to meet individual circumstances.

## Threatened preterm labour

As in singleton pregnancies, neither bed rest nor prophylactic administration of tocolytics are useful in preventing preterm birth in multiple pregnancy. However, screening for preterm birth may be worthwhile. Antenatal strategies in those women identified as high risk may include the following:

- screening for bacterial vaginosis (treatment may eliminate a co-factor for spontaneous preterm labour);
- screening for group B *Streptococcus* [intrapartum antibiotics reduce neonatal infection; Royal College of Obstetricians and Gynaecologists (RCOG) 2003];
- maternal steroid therapy to enhance fetal lung maturation (RCOG 2004);
- supplementary education as to the signs and symptoms of preterm labour (PTL);
- advance planning regarding intranatal care;
- additional medical and midwifery support.

Transvaginal ultrasound measurement of cervical length shows the most promise as a predictor of very preterm delivery and can be undertaken when other ultrasound examination is being performed (Moll 2003a). The woman should also be alert for the signs of PTL. Once PTL is diagnosed, NNU staff must be promptly involved. The use of tocolytic drugs in this situation, particularly the beta-agonists, carries risks of serious maternal morbidity.

## Intranatal care

Usually multiple pregnancies do not last until term. The average pregnancy lengths are 37 weeks for twins, 34 weeks for triplets and 32 weeks for quadruplets. Spontaneous onset of labour is preferred.

The birth should take place in a hospital with intensive care facilities for the woman and the babies (Moll 2003a). The woman should be introduced to the personnel who will care for her and her babies, including midwives, the obstetric team, the anaesthetist, and the NNU staff.

The complications of labour in multiple pregnancies can include the following (see Chapter 14):

- malpresentation;
- cord prolapse due to malpresentations;
- polyhydramnios, especially with premature rupture of the membranes, and the interval between each baby's birth;

- prolonged labour due to uterine muscle dysfunction associated with malpresentations and overdistension;
- locked twins owing to the first baby being born breech and locking the chin with the second twin's chin as it descends into the pelvis.

The mortality associated with all these complications is high; therefore, planned vaginal birth for multiple pregnancies is usually restricted to a diamniotic twin pregnancy when the first twin has a cephalic presentation (Moll 2003a). Caesarean section is usually recommended as the mode of birth in higher multiples, monoamniotic and other twin pregnancies, where the first twin has a presentation other than cephalic. However, where higher multiples have been born vaginally, adverse neonatal outcomes are not increased (Crowther 1996). The options available for the birth should be discussed with the woman during the prenatal period (Moll 2003a).

## First stage of labour

Care of the woman during the first stage is little different from that in any other type of high-risk situation but will include specific aspects of care (Moll 2003a).

An ultrasound scan should be performed on admission to confirm the cephalic presentation of the first twin and two separate fetal hearts. There should be continuous CTG monitoring using two external transducers. When the membranes rupture or elective amniotomy is performed in established labour, the first twin, if more than 34 weeks' gestation, should have scalp electrode monitoring and the second twin should continue with external monitoring. Fetal distress in either twin during the first stage will usually result in an emergency Caesarean section.

Uterine muscle dysfunction is more likely; therefore, the contractions should be carefully assessed to ensure progress. Any delay should be discussed with the obstetrician and augmentation using an oxytocin infusion may be an option.

Epidural anaesthesia is the method of choice for pain relief in labour for women with multiple pregnancy. One advantage is that it offers pain relief without the fetal respiratory depression associated with pethidine administration. However, there is also adequate pain relief *in situ* should alternative procedures be required, such as forceps or ventouse delivery, internal version or emergency Caesarean section.

Intravenous access is essential and must be maintained throughout labour and birth.

The woman should be encouraged to adopt whatever positions are most comfortable for her, excluding ambulation, if epidural anaesthesia is used. Aortocaval compression is more common and should be taken into account when positioning, perhaps using wedges for support.

Preparations for the birth will include a full blood count, having blood grouped and saved, and cross-matched blood available if the woman's haemoglobin is less than 10 g/dL.

Staff from the neonatal unit should attend when the birth is imminent. Two resuscitaires and one NNU team for each baby should be available.

## Second stage of labour

The vaginal birth of the first twin should be conducted in the usual way and any deviations managed as per the standard protocols. When born, the baby should be identified as the first twin, as should the baby's umbilical cord on the maternal side of the clamps before the cord is cut. If necessary, the baby can be given to the NNU staff for resuscitation and the parents kept appraised of his or her progress. Otherwise the baby can be given to the mother and preferably enabled to suckle at the breast to stimulate uterine contractions.

As the first twin is born, an experienced midwife or doctor should stabilize the second twin to help achieve a longitudinal lie. After the first twin is born, the lie and presentation of the second twin must be confirmed by palpation and vaginal examination, or preferably ultrasound scan. If the lie is oblique or transverse, external version to longitudinal lie should be attempted. If this is not achieved, emergency Caesarean section is usually performed. Longitudinal lie is more important than presentation as an assisted breech birth can be achieved for the second twin. Other manoeuvres are no longer recommended because of the associated high mortality. However, in specific situations, internal podalic version and breech extraction may be undertaken by an experienced operator (Moll 2003a).

When uterine contractions are re-established, cord presentation has been excluded and there is descent of the second twin's head into the pelvis, amniotomy and placement of a scalp electrode can be performed. If there is delay in descent of the fetal head into the pelvis despite adequate uterine contractions, a controlled amniotomy to facilitate descent can be considered. If uterine contractions do not re-establish, augmentation with intravenous oxytocin should be commenced (Moll 2003a).

The birth of the second twin should be conducted as for the first twin, with careful identification and labelling of the baby and the maternal side of the umbilical cord as the second twin.

If the condition of the mother and the second twin are within acceptable limits, the interval between the births of the babies is unimportant. However, the midwife and the obstetrician would usually discuss the management plan after 30 minutes. Inappropriate haste may result in avoidable complications. However, if the birth interval is prolonged owing to complications or there is any fetal distress, the birth must be expedited using instruments or Caesarean section as appropriate.

## Internal podalic version

A fetal foot is identified by recognizing a heel through intact membranes. The foot is grasped and pulled gently and continuously into the birth canal (Figure 9.3). The membranes are ruptured as late as possible. This procedure is easiest when the transverse lie is with the back superior or posterior. If the back is inferior or if the limbs are not immediately palpable, ultrasound may help to show the operator where they would be found. This will minimize the unwanted experience of bringing down a fetal hand in the mistaken belief that it is a foot.

## Non-vertex first twin

When the first twin presents as a breech, clinicians usually recommend delivery by elective Caesarean section. This is largely because of the increased risks associated with singleton breech vaginal delivery. Other factors include dwindling experience of breech delivery and the rarely seen phenomenon of 'locked twins'. In this latter case, the chin of the first (breech) baby locks against the chin of the second (cephalic) twin.

## Third stage of labour

Active management of the third stage is recommended with administration to the woman of either syntometrine or oxytocin with the birth of the second twin. Controlled cord traction is applied to both cords

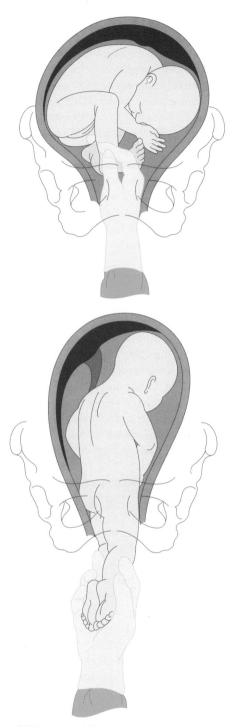

**Figure 9.3** Internal podalic version.

simultaneously. Following delivery of the placentae and membranes, adequate haemostasis is assured. There is an increased risk of postpartum haemorrhage owing to the large placental site and uterine overdistension; therefore, an oxytocin infusion should be available for immediate use should haemorrhage ensue or be used prophylactically to maintain haemostasis for some hours after the birth (Moll 2003a).

The placentae and membranes must be carefully examined for completeness, determination of the type of multiple pregnancy and identification of any deviations. The umbilical cords should also be examined and the vessels counted. Usually the placentae and membranes are sent for histological examination to confirm zygosity and chorionicity.

## Caesarean section

Caesarean section, whether elective or emergency, is conducted in the standard manner following the usual protocols. The principles of preparation that are followed for a vaginal birth of dizygotic twins should also be made for the Caesarean birth of multiples. This would include the availability of multiple NNU staff to receive and care for each of the babies, facilities to identify each baby and their respective umbilical cords, and prophylaxis for postpartum haemorrhage.

## Postnatal care

The needs of the woman in the postnatal period are likely to be similar to those of a woman following a singleton birth, so the same principles of care must be adhered to. However, some needs will be different and so specific midwifery care will be required (Moll 2003a).

Physically, involution can be slower and afterpains can be more painful. Puerperal haemorrhage is a possible complication; therefore, careful assessment of lochia, urine and faecal elimination and for signs of infection is required. Adequate analgesia must be prescribed.

The woman may need additional assistance to breast feed the babies, especially in relation to positioning. While feeding babies together may be beneficial, feeding each separately can enable the woman to get to know her babies as individuals. Being able to tell same-sex babies apart can be problematic for some women and techniques for doing so should be discussed and implemented.

A significant problem for many women is the tiredness or exhaustion they experience recovering from the pregnancy and trying to adjust to mothering more than one baby simultaneously. This problem may be complicated by anaemia. Apart from the practical assistance that the midwife can offer and appropriate treatment of any anaemia, strategies for help once the woman is at home should be planned.

The relationships with her partner and with her other children may be negatively affected by the amount of time and energy the woman spends with her new babies. Discussion, counselling and practical assistance may help, as might appropriate involvement of the family in the care of the babies.

If the babies are being cared for with the woman, their needs are similar to those of a singleton, with particular attention being paid to temperature regulation, nutrition, comfort, sleep and interaction.

If any of the babies requires care in the NNU, the parents should be able to see them before transfer and should be kept appraised of their condition and treatment. A photograph of the babies together may help confirm the reality of the multiple birth, with each baby clearly identified as to their birth order, gender and name, if available. Arrangements to visit the babies in the NNU or view them by video link should be made as soon as the mother's condition will allow. The father may visit the NNU before the mother and relay information to her. Frequent subsequent visiting should be encouraged.

The problems the babies encounter during the neonatal period and beyond are usually those related to being born preterm, and their management is no different to those of a singleton with the same problems.

The woman and her family may benefit from contact with appropriate support agencies. In the UK these include Home Start, The Twins and Multiple Births Association, and The Multiple Births Foundation.

## Conclusion

The incidence of multiple pregnancy is increasing mainly due to increased maternal age at the first pregnancy and assisted reproductive techniques. There are increased mortality and morbidity risks for the woman and the fetus/newborn, leading to problems for families, the health care system and society. The midwife has an important role as part of the team caring for the woman and her babies in trying to prevent, reduce or eliminate these risks.

## CASE HISTORY

### Miss A

Aged 32, single supported research scientist, high body
 mass index
Otherwise fit and well
Para = zero
Subfertility requiring clomiphene ovarian
 stimulation
Triplet pregnancy noted on transvaginal scan at 8 weeks
Now 12 weeks: trichorionic, triamniotic triplet pregnancy; all
 fetuses appear structurally normal and all have nuchal
 measurements that represent a considerable reduction in
 her age-related risk of Down's.

### What obstetric risks does Miss A face?

The risks of miscarriage and extremely preterm delivery are
far higher with a triplet pregnancy. The mean gestation at
delivery is approximately 34 weeks, and perinatal morbidity
and mortality are much increased over a singleton
pregnancy. Maternal complications, such as pre-eclampsia
and thromboembolism are slightly more frequent in multiple
pregnancy. She will suffer much more from the 'minor'
disorders of pregnancy: backache, varicose veins, heartburn
and anaemia, particularly.

### Is there any way of predicting her risk of preterm delivery?

Transvaginal ultrasound cervical length assessment at 20–24
weeks may be useful. However, there is no clear treatment that
reduces the chances of an early birth in those identified as
high risk. Nevertheless, a negative test may offer reassurance
and minimize the risk of inappropriate medical intervention.

### What aspects of prenatal care may identify/prevent complications?

More frequent prenatal visits for examination and discussions
with the midwife. She will be offered ultrasound scanning at
20 weeks' gestation to define any congenital abnormalities
and 2–4-weekly thereafter to evaluate fetal growth. She is
more likely to be prescribed iron supplements due to
increased requirements. As she is at high risk of very preterm
delivery, screening for group B streptococcus colonization, an
intrapartum care plan and a neonatal consultation may all be
helpful. Prophylactic steroids for fetal lung maturity will be
administered if preterm labour threatens.

Miss A is likely to give birth to her babies by Caesarean
section and, if born preterm, the babies will require care in
the NNU.

### What specific aspects of Miss A's midwifery care in the postnatal period would be addressed?

Prolonged involution and the risk of puerperal haemorrhage
would require careful assessment by the midwife. Miss A is
more likely to be anaemic, so should be screened and, if
diagnosed, appropriate treatment should be prescribed. Early
mobilization to prevent thromboembolic problems would be
essential given Miss A's obesity and post-Caesarean section
status. Interaction with and caring for the babies would
require particular attention, especially related to feeding and
identification of each baby. Ensuring that Miss A had
sufficient rest for her needs is important. She should be
given contact numbers for the local multiple birth support
groups.

### Key Points

- Twins account for approximately 1.5 per cent of all
 pregnancies
- Not all dichorionic pregnancies are dizygotic
- All monochorionic pregnancies are monozygotic
- Serious maternal and fetal complications can occur

## References

Crowther CA. Caesarean delivery for the second twin. *The
Cochrane Database of Systematic Reviews* 1996; Issue 1, Art.
no: CD000047. DOI: 10.1002/14651858. CD 000047. www.nelh.
uk/cochrane.asp (accessed November 2004).

Moll E. Multiple pregnancy; general. In: James DK, Mahomed K,
Stone P et al. (eds). *Evidence-based obstetrics,* 2nd edition.
London: Saunders, 2003a: 324–8.

Moll E. Multiple pregnancy; specific problems. In: James DK, Mahomed K, Stone P et al. (eds). *Evidence-based obstetrics, 2nd edition.* London: Saunders, 2003b: 328–31.

Royal College of Obstetricians and Gynaecologists. *Prevention of early onset neonatal Group B Streptococcal disease.* Guideline 36. November 2003. www.rcog.org.uk/resources/Public/GroupB strep no36.pdf (accessed November 2004).

Royal College of Obstetricians and Gynaecologists. *Antenatal steroids to prevent respiratory distress syndrome.* Guideline 7. February 2004. www.rcog.org.uk/resources/Public/Antenatal corticosteroids no7.pdf (accessed November 2004).

## Annotated bibliography

Boyle M (ed.). *Emergencies around childbirth; a handbook for midwives.* Oxford: Radcliffe Medical Press, 2002.
The chapters related to the general complications of multiple pregnancy and their management include a good overview of midwifery care, including excellent line drawings of aspects of management.

Marsh MS, Rennie JM, Groves PA. *Clinical protocols in labour.* Boca Raton: The Parthenon Publishing Group, 2002: Chapter 22.
An excellent overview of the management of complications associated with multiple pregnancy.

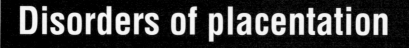

# Disorders of placentation

## OVERVIEW

Normal placental development is essential for successful pregnancy and depends on the proliferation, migration and invasion of trophoblast cells into the maternal decidua and myometrium in early gestation. The process of trophoblast invasion results in the transformation of the maternal spiral arteries. These small narrow arteries, which supply the placenta with blood, are gradually converted into large-capacity vessels, as the endothelium and the internal elastic lamina are replaced by trophoblast. The placental vascular supply becomes a low-pressure, high-flow system, allowing an adequate blood flow to the placenta and fetus.

The Confidential Enquiry into Maternal Deaths has repeatedly identified pre-eclampsia and eclampsia as leading causes of maternal mortality. Furthermore, pre-eclampsia is frequently accompanied by intrauterine growth restriction, which accounts for considerable perinatal mortality and morbidity. Although fetal growth is determined by a number of factors, including genetic predisposition, maternal nutritional status and ability of the placenta to allow nutrient exchange, it is now apparent that the origins of both pre-eclampsia and much of the fetal growth restriction seen in clinical practice lie in defective placental development. A further condition frequently related to impaired trophoblast invasion is abruptio placentae or premature separation of a normally sited placenta, which is usually of sudden onset and associated with a high fetal mortality, and substantial maternal mortality and morbidity. Knowledge of the early events in the invasion of the maternal uterine wall by placental trophoblast cells is, therefore, helpful in understanding the aetiology of these important clinical conditions.

## The placenta

The placenta is usually regarded as a fetal organ, although it contains adjacent maternal and fetal vascular beds. It receives the highest blood flow of any fetal organ (40 per cent of fetal cardiac output) and towards the end of pregnancy competes with the fetus for maternal nutrients, consuming the major fraction of glucose and oxygen taken up by the pregnant uterus.

The mature human placenta has about 10–40 cotyledons, lobes or lobules, each containing at least one primary villus stem arising from the chorionic plate and supplied by primary branches of fetal vessels. The primary stems divide to form secondary and tertiary stems from which arise the terminal villi, where maternal–fetal exchange takes place. The fetal cotyledons appear to develop around the entries of the maternal spiral arteries from the decidual plate and the centre of each cotyledon is hollow, where the pulsatile jet of blood from the spiral artery enters the intralobular space (Figure 10.1). Blood from the spiral arteries rises high to the chorionic plate, then disperses laterally between and over the surface of the terminal villi, becoming increasingly desaturated of oxygen and nutrients, and picking up carbon dioxide and waste products. The blood then filters into narrow venous channels between the cotyledons before falling back to the maternal decidual plate, where the maternal veins return the desaturated blood to the maternal circulation (Figure 10.2).

Three microscopic tissue layers separate maternal and fetal blood: trophoblastic tissue, connective tissue and the endothelium of the fetal capillaries. However, microscopic examination of the terminal villi, surrounding the intralobular space, shows numerous vasculosyncytial membranes where the fetal capillaries and trophoblast fuse to form a very thin membrane, where most of the transfer of nutrients and blood gases takes place (Figure 10.3).

## Normal placentation

Maternal blood flow to the placenta increases throughout pregnancy from 50 mL/minute in the first trimester to 600 mL/minute at term. This 12-fold increase in perfusion is accommodated by a series of adaptations, which convert the maternal spiral arteries from narrow muscular to wide-bored flaccid vessels. In the first 12 weeks, the decidual segments of the spiral arteries are invaded and replaced by trophoblast and fibrinoid. At the end of this period, the trophoblast plugs, which occupy the lumen of the spiral arteries, are released and this is associated with a sudden increase in blood flow to the intervillous space. Following this, the trophoblast invasion of the myometrial segment of the spiral arteries occurs, which further reduces resistance

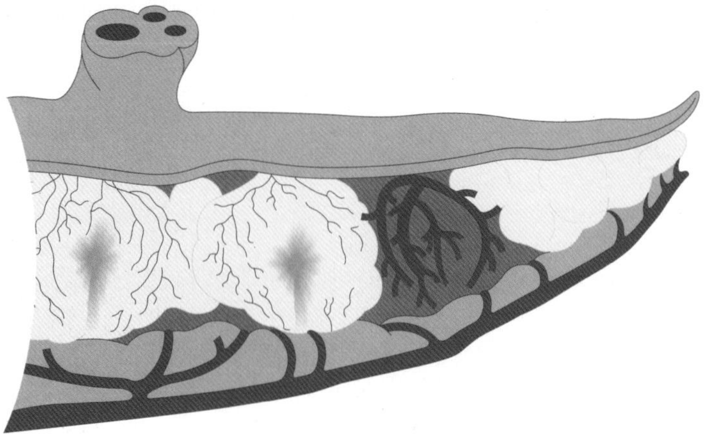

**Figure 10.1** Diagram of placenta showing the arrangement of fetal cotyledons, and the maternal and fetal vascular systems.

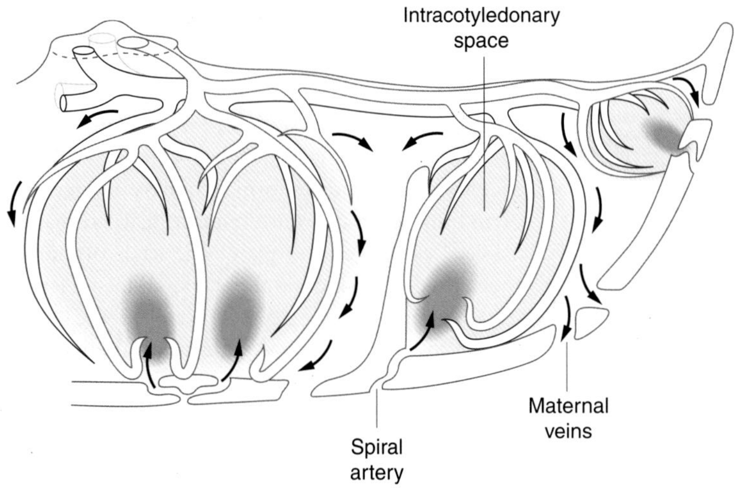

Intracotyledonary space

Maternal veins

Spiral artery

**Figure 10.2** Diagram showing the direction of maternal blood flow through the fetal cotelydons.

to blood flow to the placenta and is associated with a mid-trimester fall in the maternal blood pressure. This process should be complete by 20 weeks. The transformed spiral arteries permit increased perfusion because they lack smooth muscle and are less likely to respond to vasoactive substances (Figure 10.4).

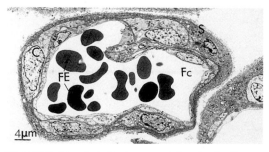

**Figure 10.3** A terminal villus in cross-section showing the vasculo-syncytial membrane. FE, fetal erythrocyte; Fc, fetal capillary; C, cytotrophoblast; S, syncytiotrophoblast.

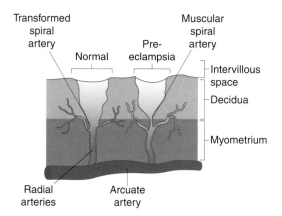
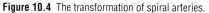

**Figure 10.4** The transformation of spiral arteries.

## Abnormal placentation

Pre-eclampsia, intrauterine growth restriction (IUGR) and abruptio placentae are clinical manifestations of total or patchy failure of trophoblast invasion of the myometrial segments of the spiral arteries. It is still not clear why trophoblast invasion fails and why this pathological maladaption can produce a pregnancy with either pre-eclampsia, IUGR or abruptio placentae, or all three. It is likely that the more complete the failure of trophoblast invasion, the more likely that pre-eclampsia will develop. There are other general conditions associated with impaired perfusion of the placenta, such as collagen vascular disease, antiphospholipid syndrome, severe diabetes mellitus and chronic hypertension (see Chapters 8 and 12). All of these may result in a small placenta with gross morphological changes. The most serious of these changes are infarcts and basal haematomas.

An infarct is an area of ischaemic necrosis of a cotyledon resulting from spiral artery occlusion, usually by thrombosis (Figure 10.5). Multiple placental infarcts are significantly associated with intrauterine fetal death and growth restriction. Placental haematomas, which consist of a mass of blood in the centre of the fetal cotyledon due to rupture of a damaged spiral artery, are closely associated with infarcts (Figure 10.6). They are also associated with maternal hypertension and increased perinatal mortality. These pathological

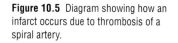

**Figure 10.5** Diagram showing how an infarct occurs due to thrombosis of a spiral artery.

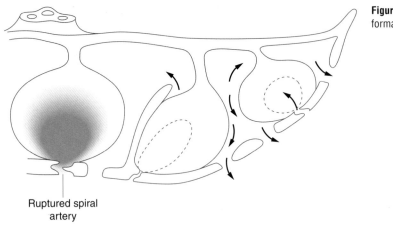

**Figure 10.6** Diagram showing the formation of a massive haematoma.

Ruptured spiral
artery

lesions should not be confused with calcification or fibrin deposits, which give the placenta an 'unhealthy' appearance but are benign.

## Pre-eclampsia

### Definition

In the past, the diagnostic criterion for pre-eclampsia has varied. This has led to difficulty in comparing studies on treatments, or outcomes, in different populations. The following definition provided by the International Society for the Study of Hypertension in Pregnancy (ISSHP) for pre-eclampsia is now widely accepted.

*Hypertension of at least 140/90 mmHg, recorded on two separate occasions at least four hours apart and in the presence of at least 300 mg of protein in a 24 hour collection of urine, arising after the 20th week of pregnancy in a previously normotensive woman and resolving completely by the 6th post partum week (Davey and MacGillivray 1988).*

### S Symptoms of pre-eclampsia

- May be asymptomatic
- Headache
- Visual disturbances
- Epigastric and right upper abdominal pain
- Oedema

### ☞ Signs of pre-eclampsia

- Elevation of blood pressure
- Fluid retention (non-dependent oedema)
- Brisk reflexes
- Ankle clonus (more than three beats)
- Uterus and fetus may feel small for gestational age

*Chronic hypertension* with or without renal disease, and existing prior to pregnancy, is of a different aetiology to pre-eclampsia (see Chapter 12), although it can predispose to the later development of superimposed pre-eclampsia.

*Gestational hypertension alone* (i.e. hypertension arising for the first time in the second half of pregnancy and in the absence of proteinuria) is not associated with adverse pregnancy outcome and, as such, should be clearly distinguished from pre-eclampsia.

*Eclampsia* is a serious and life-threatening complication of pre-eclampsia. It is defined as convulsions occurring in a woman with established pre-eclampsia in the absence of any other neurological or metabolic cause. It is an obstetric emergency and the management of this condition is discussed further in Chapter 16.

### Incidence

Pre-eclampsia complicates approximately 3 per cent of pregnancies, but the incidence varies according to the definition used and the population studied. Eclampsia is relatively rare in the UK, occurring in approximately 1:2000 pregnancies. The Confidential

Enquiry into Maternal and Child Health (CEMACH) 2000–2002 (Lewis and Drife 2004) recorded 14 maternal deaths due to pre-eclampsia or eclampsia, making this the second commonest cause of death in late pregnancy and puerperium. Worldwide it is a far greater problem with an estimated 72 000 deaths annually.

## Epidemiology

Pre-eclampsia is more common in primigravid women. The normal fetal–maternal transfusion occurring during pregnancy and delivery is thought to expose the mother to fetal (and hence paternal) genetic material, protecting her in subsequent pregnancies. In keeping with this concept, prolonged exposure to paternal antigens (e.g. through unprotected sex) prior to conceiving appear to reduce the risk of pre-eclampsia and conversely the protective effect of first pregnancy is partially lost if a women has a child with a new partner. There also appears to be a maternal genetic predisposition to pre-eclampsia, as there is 3–4-fold increase in the incidence of pre-eclampsia in first-degree relatives of affected women. Finally, there are a number of general medical conditions and pregnancy-specific factors that predispose to the development of pre-eclampsia (see box).

> ### Risk factors predisposing to the development of pre-eclampsia
>
> - Conditions where the placenta is enlarged (multiple gestation, diabetes, hydrops)
> - Pre-existing hypertension or renal disease
> - Pre-existing vascular disease (including diabetes or autoimmune vasculitis)

## Aetiology

Pre-eclampsia only occurs in pregnancy, but has been described in pregnancies lacking a fetus (molar pregnancies) and in the absence of a uterus (abdominal pregnancies), suggesting that it is the placenta that provides the stimulus for the disorder. Placental bed biopsies have demonstrated that, in pre-eclampsia, trophoblast invasion is patchy and the spiral arteries retain their muscular walls. This is thought to prevent the development of a high-flow, low-impedance utero-placental circulation. The reason why trophoblast

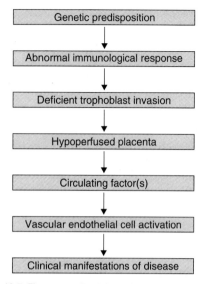

**Figure 10.7** The proposed aetiology of pre-eclampsia.

cells invade less effectively in these pregnancies is not known. It is thought that defective trophoblast invasion results in relative underperfusion of the placenta and that this releases a factor(s) into the maternal circulation, which targets the vascular endothelium (Figure 10.7). The nature of this factor has not yet been identified, although numerous candidates have been proposed, including a variety of growth factors, cytokines (small secreted proteins that mediate and regulate immunity, inflammation, and haematopoiesis) and products of abnormal lipid metabolism.

## Pathophysiology

There is abundant evidence that the clinical syndrome of pre-eclampsia is due to dysfunction of the vascular endothelial cells, which line the inside surfaces of blood vessels. The concentration of substances released when endothelial cell damage occurs (including fibronectin, adhesion molecules and von Willebrand factor) is increased in the plasma of women with pre-eclampsia.

Normal pregnancy is characterized by marked peripheral vasodilatation, resulting in a fall in total peripheral resistance despite an increase in cardiac output and circulating volume. This peripheral vasodilatation occurs because maternal blood vessels are less sensitive to vasoconstrictors, such as angiotensin, and possibly as a result of increased production of certain vasodilators by vascular endothelial cells. In pre-eclampsia, vessels do not develop reduced sensitivity to vasoconstrictors observed in normal pregnancy; experimental studies have shown that vessels are also less sensitive to vasodilators and more sensitive to vasoconstrictors.

Altered responses to vasoconstrictors and vasodilators in pre-eclampsia may result in vasospasm, a sudden decrease in the internal diameter of the blood vessels that increases peripheral vascular resistance. Endothelial cell dysfunction causes changes in shape, adhesiveness and clumping of platelets termed *platelet activation*. These processes account for many of the pathological features of pre-eclampsia seen in almost every major organ system (see box). Endothelial cell damage also results in increased vascular permeability and contributes to the formation of generalized oedema, which is often found in women with pre-eclampsia. Dependent oedema of the feet is very common in healthy pregnant women; however, rapidly progressing oedema of the face and hands is suggestive of pre-eclampsia.

---

### Organ-specific changes associated with pre-eclampsia

**Cardiovascular**
- Generalized vasospasm
- Increased peripheral resistance
- Reduced central venous/pulmonary wedge pressures

**Haematological**
- Platelet activation and depletion
- Coagulopathy
- Decreased plasma volume
- Increased blood viscosity

**Renal**
- Proteinuria
- Decreased glomerular filtration rate
- Decreased urate excretion

**Hepatic**
- Periportal necrosis
- Subcapsular haematoma

**Central nervous**
- Cerebral oedema
- Cerebral haemorrhages

---

In the kidney, a highly characteristic lesion (called glomeruloendotheliosis) is seen. This consists of endothelial and mesangial cell swelling, basement membrane inclusions but little disruption of renal epithelial podocytes. This is relatively specific for pre-eclampsia and is associated with the development of proteinuria, reduced renal clearance of uric acid and oliguria. It is not seen with hypertension due to other causes.

In the liver, subendothelial fibrin deposition is associated with elevation of liver enzymes. This can be associated with haemolysis and a low platelet count due to platelet consumption (and subsequent widespread activation of the coagulation system). The presence of these findings is called the HELLP syndrome (**H**aemolysis, **E**levation of **L**iver enzymes and **L**ow **P**latelets). The HELLP syndrome is a particularly severe form of pre-eclampsia. It occurs in approximately 2–4 per cent of women with pre-eclampsia and is associated with a fetal loss rate of up to 60 per cent if occurring antenatally and a maternal mortality of up to 24%. (The management of HELLP syndrome is discussed further in Chapter 16.)

Vasospasm and cerebral oedema have both been implicated in the cerebral complications of pre-eclampsia and the progression to eclampsia. Retinal haemorrhage, exudates and papilloedema (oedema of the optic disc) are characteristic of hypertensive encephalopathy and are rare in pre-eclampsia, suggesting that hypertension alone is not responsible for the cerebral pathology.

## Screening tests

Over 160 substances have been shown to be increased in the circulation of women with pre-eclampsia. Unfortunately, this has not yet led to the development of a sensitive and specific screening blood test.

The ability of Doppler ultrasound uterine artery waveform analysis to identify women at risk of pre-eclampsia and other adverse pregnancy outcome has been investigated with varying success. In pregnancies with inadequate or incomplete trophoblast invasion of the spiral arteries, a characteristic 'notch' can be seen in the waveform pattern (see Chapter 6). Such screening may have a place in women already identified as being at risk of pre-eclampsia because of their medical or past obstetric history. However, it has limited diagnostic potential for adverse pregnancy-related complications in a low-risk population.

Screening has been criticized on the basis that it will cause unnecessary alarm in pregnant women at a time when prevention of pre-eclampsia has not yet been proven. The most commonly used preventive therapy is low-dose aspirin (at 75 mg daily), on the basis that this dose will inhibit platelet activation and the release of vasoconstrictors, particularly thromboxanes, without impairing the synthesis of vasodilatory prostaglandins produced by the vascular endothelium. Large placebo-controlled studies have failed to show any significant benefit of aspirin therapy in preventing pre-eclampsia (CLASP 1994). However, there is some evidence that aspirin may be effective if given to a more targeted group at very high risk of developing the disease, if given at night and if given in doses that affect bleeding times (e.g. 150 mg daily). Recently, there has been increasing interest in a possible therapeutic role for antioxidants in the prevention and treatment of pre-eclampsia, based on evidence that oxidative stress, an imbalance between reactive oxygen species and antioxidant defences is a key factor in the disease process. A study of 283 women at high risk of pre-eclampsia demonstrated that supplementation with vitamins C and E (major antioxidants) reduced the incidence and severity of hypertensive disease (Chappell et al. 1999) however, the large *Vitamins in Pregnancy* (VIP) study failed to show any beneficial effect.

The development of early and effective screening tests for pre-eclampsia is important to allow initiation of preventative treatment. Accurate identification of women at risk of developing pre-eclampsia will facilitate targeting of increased antenatal surveillance, allowing women at low risk of the condition to participate in community-based antenatal care.

## Care and treatment

The mainstay of treatment for pre-eclampsia remains ending the pregnancy by delivery of the fetus and placenta. This can cause significant neonatal problems if pre-eclampsia occurs at 24–28 weeks' gestation, thus many strategies have been proposed to delay the need for delivery.

The principles of care of woman with pre-eclampsia are as follows:
- early recognition of the symptomless syndrome;
- awareness of the serious nature of the condition in its severest form;
- adherence to agreed guidelines for admission to hospital, investigation and the use of antihypertensive and anticonvulsant therapy;
- well timed delivery to pre-empt serious maternal or fetal complications;
- postnatal follow-up and counselling for future pregnancies.

A diagnosis of pre-eclampsia usually entails the woman being admitted to hospital for more intensive investigations and monitoring. When the blood pressure (BP) is only mildly elevated (i.e. a diastolic BP of 90–95mmHg) and there is minimal proteinuria with normal haematological and biochemical parameters, it may be possible to monitor her condition as an outpatient, attending a day-unit regular fetal and maternal assessment. In the presence of higher blood pressure values, greater proteinuria or abnormal haematological and biochemical parameters, admission to hospital is strongly advised. Investigations indicated in the further management of this condition are listed (see box). The aim of antihypertensive therapy is to lower the blood pressure and reduce the risk of maternal cerebrovascular accident without reducing uterine blood flow and compromising the fetus.

### Investigations for pre-eclampsia

These investigations will be repeated at intervals depending on the overall clinical picture
- Urinalysis by dipstick (quantitatively inaccurate)
- 24-hour urine collection (total protein and creatinine clearance)
- Full blood count (platelets and haematocrit)
- Blood chemistry (renal function, protein concentration)
- Plasma urate concentration
- Liver function
- Coagulation profile
- Ultrasound assessment:
  – fetal size
  – amniotic fluid volume
  – maternal and fetal
  – Dopplers

There are a variety of antihypertensives used in the management of pre-eclampsia in the UK. Labetalol is an alpha- and beta-blocking agent. It can be given orally or intravenously, and has a good safety record in pregnancy. Methyldopa is a centrally acting antihypertensive agent. It too has a long established safety record in pregnancy, but can only be given orally and takes upwards of 24 hours to take effect. Nifedipine is a calcium-channel blocker with a rapid onset of action. It can, however, cause severe headache that may mimic worsening disease. In severe pre-eclampsia, an intravenous infusion of hydralazine or labetalol can be titrated rapidly against changes in the blood pressure.

The drug of choice for the treatment of eclampsia is magnesium sulphate (Duley and Henderson-Smart 2003a,b). This is given intravenously and has been shown to reduce the incidence of further convulsions in women with eclampsia. Magnesium sulphate has also been shown to be useful in prevention of eclampsia in cases of severe pre-eclampsia (MAGPIE 2002).

Most of the maternal deaths related to pre-eclampsia occur due to a failure to recognize a deteriorating condition after delivery and result from multiple organ failure including disseminated intravascular coagulation (DIC), adult respiratory distress syndrome and renal failure. Obstetricians should involve clinicians from other specialities (intensive care, haematology) promptly where indicated.

## Additional points in care

Premature delivery of the fetus is often required in severe pre-eclampsia. This necessitates optimizing the fetal condition prior to delivery. Antenatal steroids (e.g. two doses of betamethasone 12 mg intramuscularly 24 hours apart; Royal College of Obstetricians and Gynaecologists 1999), should be given to the woman to reduce the chance of neonatal pulmonary insufficiency between 24 and 34 weeks' gestation. If the woman's condition permits, she should be transferred to a tertiary centre prior to delivery, to improve both her own management and the facilities for her baby. Delivery before term is usually by Caesarean section. Women with pre-eclampsia are at particularly high risk for thromboembolism and should be given prophylactic subcutaneous heparin and issued with antithromboembolic stockings. In the case of spontaneous or induced labour, and if clotting studies are normal, epidural anaesthesia is indicated, as it helps control blood pressure. Ergometrine is avoided in the management of the third stage, as it can significantly increase blood pressure.

## CASE HISTORY

Mrs AA
41-year-old non-smoker, weight 90 kg
Gravida 1
No past history of note
Booked for antenatal care at 11 weeks: BP 120/75 mmHg.
Ultrasound screening, confirmed dates, no fetal abnormality
  detected. Normal antenatal course to 30 weeks' gestation.
  Seen by community midwife in clinic. BP found to be
  150/95 mmHg and urinalysis revealed + + proteinuria.

### How should AA be cared for and treated?

AA has a positive screen for pre-eclampsia. She should have her blood pressure taken again several times to ensure it is not simply related to attending the clinic. She should also be screened for a urinary tract infection, a common cause of proteinuria. Assuming her blood pressure is elevated, she should be referred to hospital for obstetric assessment. Investigations should include 24-hour urine collection (to quantify protein and creatinine clearance), and blood for baseline platelet count, renal and hepatic function. An ultrasound scan should be performed to assess fetal growth and liquor volume. Doppler studies may also be performed.

### Should she be commenced on medication?

At this blood pressure, there is no proven advantage to commencing antihypertensives; the only aim of treatment is the prevention of an acute episode such as cerebrovascular accident (CVA). As she is overweight and has been admitted for rest, she should be commenced on heparin prophylaxis against thromboembolism. As she may require delivery in the near future, she should be given a course of steroids to promote fetal lung maturation.

### If delivery is the main treatment for pre-eclampsia, when should this be carried out?

The decision to deliver must balance the beneficial effect on the mother's health against detrimental effects on the baby's prognosis. Many women with pre-eclampsia run a chronic course and prolonging gestation will improve fetal maturity. There is no correct answer to this question. The decision to deliver will be based on frequent repetition of investigations into maternal and fetal health, and will occur at a time when it is felt that either maternal health is becoming compromised by further delay to delivery, or that the fetus can be better looked after *ex utero* than *in utero*.

## Intrauterine growth restriction

There are a variety of reasons why a fetus may be small, including congenital anomaly, fetal infections and chromosomal abnormality. However, the majority of fetuses that appear to be small are either constitutionally small (i.e. born to small parents and are fulfilling their genetic potential) or are small secondary to abnormal placental function.

## Significance of intrauterine growth restriction

Intrauterine growth restriction is a major cause of neonatal morbidity and mortality. It results in significant costs of special and intensive care of affected infants. In addition, there is a growing appreciation that individuals who were small or thin at birth may have an increased risk of developing certain adult diseases such as hypertension and diabetes (Barker 1992).

## Definitions and incidence

Intrauterine growth restriction is defined as failure of the fetus to achieve its genetic growth potential. This usually results in a fetus that is small for gestational age (SGA) and babies born below a particular centile weight for gestation (e.g. below the third or fifth centile) are frequently classified as IUGR. While this is convenient and makes it simple to calculate the incidence of IUGR (3 per cent if the third or 5 per cent if the fifth centile is chosen), the terms SGA and IUGR are not synonymous. The term SGA implies that the fetus or neonate is below a certain defined centile of weight or size for a particular gestational age, and some SGA fetuses are constitutionally small due to normal genetic influences. IUGR indicates that a particular pathological process is operating to modify the intrinsic growth potential of the fetus by reducing its growth rate. Some IUGR fetuses may not fall into any definition of SGA, but will have failed to achieve their full growth potential.

## Aetiology

There are many causes of IUGR (Table 10.1). They are best grouped into two main categories: factors that directly affect the intrinsic growth potential of the fetus and external influences that reduce the support for fetal growth. Postnatal 'catch up' growth is more likely to occur in fetuses in the latter category than in the former (Figure 10.8), as chromosome abnormalities, genetic

**Table 10.1** – Causes of intrauterine growth restriction

| Investigations | Cause |
| --- | --- |
| Reduced fetal growth potential | Chromosome defects (e.g. trisomy 18, triploidy) <br> Single gene defects (e.g. Seckel's syndrome) <br> Structural abnormalities (e.g. renal agenesis) <br> Infections (e.g. cytomegalovirus, toxoplasmosis) |
| Reduced fetal growth support | *Maternal factors* <br> Undernutrition (e.g. poverty, eating disorders) <br> Maternal hypoxia (e.g. altitude, cyanotic heart disease) <br> Drugs (e.g. cigarette smoke, alcohol, cocaine) <br><br> *Placental factors* <br> Reduced uteroplacental perfusion (e.g. inadequate trophoblast invasion, antiphospholipid syndrome, diabetes mellitus, sickle cell disease, multiple gestation) <br> Reduced fetoplacental perfusion (e.g. single umbilical artery, twin–twin transfusion syndrome) |

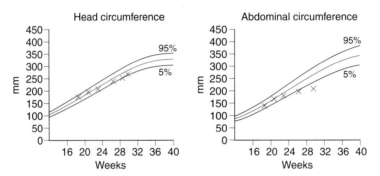

**Doppler:**

| | | | |
|---|---|---|---|
| L. uterine artery | RI | 0.71 | |
| | **Notch** | | |
| R. uterine artery | RI | 0.86 | |
| | **Notch** | | |
| Umbilical artery | PI | 1.34 | |
| | RI | 0.78 | |
| | End-diastolic flow: positive | | |
| Fetal aorta | PI | 2.29 | |
| | End-diastolic flow: positive | | |
| Middle cerebral artery | PI | 1.15 | |
| | RI | 0.07 | |
| | End-diastolic flow: positive | | |
| Ductus venosus | PIV | 0.880 | |

Diagnosis: Stable moderate redistribution. Increased DV PI.

**Figure 10.8** The growth pattern of a fetus with intrauterine growth restriction. Note the relative brain-sparing effect, with head circumference less affected than abdominal circumference. The Doppler chart demonstrates high resistance and notches in the uterine artery. There is fetal hypoxia, as demonstrated by low-resistance waveforms in the fetal brain (low pulsatility index) and probable acidaemia owing to the high pulsatility in the ductus venosus. DV, ductus venosus; PI, pulsatility index; PIV, pulsatility index for veins; RI, resistance index.

syndromes, infections and drugs can alter intrinsic fetal growth potential. Many chromosome abnormalities, such as trisomy 18 and triploidy, and single-gene defects such as Seckel's syndrome, will alter the genetic potential of the fetus, as will some multifactorial structural abnormalities, such as anencephaly and renal agenesis. Viral infections, such as cytomegalovirus and rubella, and protozoal infections, such as toxoplasmosis, can also affect fetal growth potential.

External influences that affect fetal growth can be subdivided into maternal systemic factors and placental insufficiency. Maternal undernutrition is globally the major cause of IUGR and, even in developed countries, it is now recognized that maternal eating disorders, such as anorexia or bulimia, can significantly affect fetal growth. Low maternal oxygen saturation, which can occur with cyanotic heart disease, chronic respiratory disease or at high altitude, will reduce fetal oxygen saturation and metabolism. Smoking increases the amount of carboxyhaemoglobin

in the maternal circulation and effectively reduces the amount of available oxygen to the fetus, thus causing growth restriction. A wide variety of drugs other than tobacco can affect fetal growth: alcohol, cannabis, heroin and cocaine are all associated with fetal growth restriction, probably through multiple mechanisms affecting fetal enzyme systems, placental blood flow and maternal nutrient levels.

In developed countries, the most common cause of IUGR is poor placental function, secondary to inadequate trophoblast invasion of the uterine decidua and myometrial spiral arteries. This results in reduced perfusion of the placental intravillous space, which leads to abnormal development of the terminal villi, and impaired transfer of oxygen and nutrients to the fetus. Less frequently, reduced perfusion can occur from other conditions, such as a severe diabetes mellitus, the antiphospholipid syndrome and sickle cell disease. Multiple gestation usually results in a sharing of the uterine vascularity, which causes a relative reduction in the blood flow to each placenta. On the fetal side of the placental circulation, abnormalities of the umbilical cord, such as a single umbilical artery, is associated with IUGR as are the intraplacental vascular connections found in monochorionic twins.

## Pathophysiology

Fetuses with IUGR are frequently described as symmetric or asymmetric in terms of their body proportions. Symmetrically small fetuses are usually associated with factors that directly impair the intrauterine growth potential of the fetus (i.e. chromosome abnormalities, viral infections, etc.), while asymmetric growth restriction is classically associated with uteroplacental insufficiency. The cause of fetal asymmetry follows upon the reduced oxygen transfer to the fetus and impaired excretion of $CO_2$ by the placenta. The resulting fall in $PO_2$ and rise in $PCO_2$ in the fetal blood will induce a chemoreceptor response in the fetal carotid bodies with resulting vasodilatation in the fetal brain, myocardium and adrenal glands, and vasoconstriction in the kidneys, limbs and subcutaneous tissues. The liver circulation is also severely reduced; normally 50 per cent of the well-oxygenated blood in the umbilical vein passes to the right atrium through the ductus venosus eventually to reach the fetal brain, with the remainder going to the portal circulation in the liver. When there is fetal hypoxia, more of the well-oxygenated blood from the umbilical vein is diverted through the ductus venosus, which means that the liver receives less.

The result of all these circulatory changes is an asymmetric fetus with relative brain sparing, reduced abdominal girth and skin thickness. The vasoconstriction in the fetal kidneys results in impaired urine production and oligohydramnios. The fetal hypoxaemia also leads to severe metabolic changes in the fetus, reflecting intrauterine starvation. Antenatal fetal blood sampling has shown reduced levels of nutrients such as glucose and amino acids (especially essential amino acids), and hormones such as thyroxine and insulin. There are increased levels of corticosteroids and catecholamines, which reflect the increased perfusion of the adrenal gland. Haematological changes also reflect the chronic hypoxia with increased levels of erythropoietin and nucleated red blood cells.

The fetal hypoxia eventually leads to fetal acidaemia, both respiratory and metabolic, which, if prolonged, can lead to intrauterine death, if the fetus is not removed from its hostile environment. IUGR fetuses are especially at risk from profound asphyxia in labour owing to the further compromise of the uteroplacental circulation caused by the uterine contractions.

## Investigation

Detecting fetal growth restriction is an important aim of antenatal care and, the earlier the diagnosis is made, the better the chance of improving the outlook for the fetus. On the premise that most IUGR fetuses are SGA, most antenatal screening programmes for IUGR judge their efficacy on the ability to predict the birth weight of an infant below the tenth centile birth weight for gestation. The detection of an SGA infant contains two elements: first, the accurate assessment of gestational age and, second, the recognition of fetal smallness. As described in Chapter 6, early measurement of the fetal crown–rump length before 12 weeks or the biparietal diameter between 12 and 20 weeks is routinely carried out in most centres and provides the most accurate assessment of gestational age. If there is any discrepancy between the assessments made at 12 weeks and 20 weeks, then the prediction from the earlier measurement should be accepted. Abdominal palpation and symphyseal–fundal height, which are measured at every antenatal visit, have only limited ability to predict SGA (Neilson 2000). Therefore, ultrasound biometry, particularly measurement of the abdominal circumference (AC) and estimation of birth weight (EFW), are used to predict SGA pregnancies where the fundal height measurement is more than 3 cm below the expected size for the gestational age. Serial ultrasound biometry may also be indicated in the following circumstances.

- Women who have had a previous SGA baby, who are of low body mass index (BMI), who are heavy smokers, drug abusers, have a medical condition such as hypertension, antiphospholipid syndrome or diabetes, or who give a history of eating disorders or persistent hyperemesis.
- Pregnancies where twins have been diagnosed at the first or second trimester scan.
- Pregnancies where there are abnormal uterine artery waveforms at the mid-pregnancy scan (this is only performed in a few hospitals).

When a diagnosis of SGA has been made, the next step is to establish whether this represents IUGR or whether the fetus is 'small normal'. A detailed ultrasound scan of the fetal anatomy should be offered to detect any fetal abnormalities to explain fetal smallness that may have been missed on the second trimester scan. Up to 19 per cent of fetuses with AC and EFW below the fifth centile may have chromosomal abnormalities. The risk is higher when IUGR is associated with structural abnormalities and normal Doppler waveforms; in these circumstances, an amniocentesis and fetal karyotype should be offered. Features suspicious of uteroplacental insufficiency would be an asymmetric fetus with a relatively small abdominal circumference, oligohydramnios and a high umbilical artery resistance.

## Care and treatment

At present, there are no specific treatments available for growth restriction related to placental dysfunction. Women should be encouraged and offered support to stop or reduce smoking, alcohol and drug abuse where possible. Management of coexisting disease (diabetes, thyroid dysfunction, etc.) should be optimized. When growth restriction is severe, and the fetus is considered too immature to be delivered, rest in hospital is often advised in an effort to maximize placental blood flow and allow monitoring. The aim of these interventions is to gain as much maturity as possible before delivering the fetus, thereby reducing the morbidity associated with prematurity. A growth-restricted baby weighing 1 kg and delivered at 32 weeks' gestation usually has a less stormy neonatal course than does a normally grown baby delivered at 28 weeks' gestation with the same birth weight.

Timing delivery to maximize gestation without the baby dying *in utero* involves intensive fetal surveillance. The most widely accepted methods of monitoring the fetus are discussed in Chapter 6. In brief, serial ultrasound scans are performed to establish that some fetal growth is maintained; cessation of fetal growth may be an indication in itself for delivery. However, fetal biometry cannot give meaningful estimates of growth rate at intervals less than 2 weeks so dynamic tests of fetal well-being, such as Doppler ultrasound and fetal cardiotocography, are now the principal means of determining fetal well-being. Absence of blood flow in the umbilical artery during fetal cardiac diastole or reversed flow (i.e. back towards the heart) requires delivery in the near future, as it reflects high placental resistance and is usually a pre-terminal

event. When this situation is seen at early gestation (24–28 weeks), more complicated fetal arterial and venous Doppler studies are used in some tertiary centres in an attempt to delay delivery. Unlike the umbilical artery Doppler, the role of other fetal Doppler studies has not yet been proven by large prospective trials.

No effective drug therapy for IUGR has yet been found. Small studies have suggested that aspirin, nitric oxide donors or antioxidants may be helpful in some cases. These drugs may act by reducing platelet activation in the uteroplacental circulation, or may be acting directly as vasodilators. Larger, prospective, placebo-controlled studies are awaited to assess the use of these agents in either prevention, or treatment, of IUGR.

## Prognosis

The main danger to the baby is intrauterine death, owing either to failure in making the diagnosis, or excessive delay prior to delivery. Some babies will suffer morbidity, or die, as a result of premature delivery. The long-term prognosis for survivors is good, with low incidences of mental or physical handicap. Whilst height and weight curves for these infants remain slightly below the 50th centile, most infants with IUGR secondary to placental insufficiency show 'catch up' growth after delivery, when feeding can be optimized. Where IUGR is related to a congenital infection, or chromosomal anomaly, subsequent development of the child will be determined by the precise abnormality present.

## Placental abruption

### Definition

This is uterine bleeding following premature separation of a normally sited placenta. It is concealed in approximately one-third of cases (i.e. no blood loss is seen per vaginam) and revealed in two-thirds of cases.

### Incidence

This has been documented as between 0.5 and 2.0 per cent of pregnancies, but varies depending on the diagnostic criteria. Where diagnosis is based on histological examination of the placenta, the incidence has been reported to be as high as 4 per cent.

## Aetiology

This is unknown in the majority of cases, although there is evidence of an association with defective trophoblastic invasion. Other associations include direct abdominal trauma (e.g. road traffic accidents, assault, external cephalic version), high parity, uterine overdistension (polyhydramnios and multiple gestation), sudden decompression of the uterus (e.g. after delivery of the first twin or release of polyhydramnios) and smoking. The association with hypertension may reflect a direct cause or may be a manifestation of poor trophoblastic invasion.

---

### Risk factors for placental abruption

- Hypertension
- Smoking
- Trauma to abdomen
- Crack cocaine usage
- Anticoagulant therapy
- Polyhydramnios
- Intrauterine growth restriction

---

## Clinical presentation

The classical presentation is that of abdominal pain, vaginal bleeding and uterine contractions. The vaginal bleeding is usually dark and non-clotting; however, as the bleeding may be concealed, its absence does not preclude the diagnosis. Placental abruption often occurs close to term and frequently during labour. Although abdominal pain is a common feature, and is probably due to extravasation of blood into the myometrium, 'silent' abruptions have also been described. Some women also present with nausea, restlessness and faintness.

---

### Clinical features of placental abruption

- Tender, tense uterus
- Tachycardia and hypotension out of proportion to vaginal bleeding
- Renal compromise
- Coagulation disorders: possibly disseminated intravascular coagulation

---

If blood loss is significant, there may be signs of hypovolaemic shock, with increased pulse rate, hypotension and signs of peripheral vasoconstriction. Abdominal palpation reveals a tender uterus that is often described as being 'woody hard'. The uterus may be larger than gestation suggests and the fetus is often difficult to palpate. Depending on the size of the abruption, and the area of placental separation, the fetus may be dead, in distress or be unaffected. Vaginal examination may reveal blood or cervical dilatation, if the abruption has precipitated labour.

## Diagnosis

This is usually made on clinical examination. Where abruption has not been severe, the diagnosis may only be made by inspection of the placenta after the third stage of labour is complete. Ultrasound can be helpful in some cases, demonstrating retroplacental clot and excluding placenta praevia. Ultrasound examination is also important where abruption is managed conservatively (see 'Effects on the fetus' later). The differential diagnosis of placental abruption can be broadly divided into two groups: other causes of vaginal bleeding and other causes of abdominal pain in pregnancy.

## Effects on the mother

### *Hypovolaemic shock*

There is a tendency to underestimate the amount of blood loss. This is due to some haemorrhage being concealed behind the placenta and within the uterine wall. In addition some patients will have been hypertensive prior to the abruption, masking the hypotensive effect of blood loss. Central venous pressure measurement is extremely helpful both in assessing the degree of blood loss and in accurate fluid replacement.

### *Disseminated intravascular coagulation*

Disseminated intravascular coagulation (DIC) is a secondary event following a trigger to generalized activation of coagulation systems. Consumption of fibrin, clotting factors and platelets occurs, resulting in continued bleeding and further depletion of these factors. The triggers known to precipitate DIC include tissue thromboplastin release, endothelial damage to small vessels and procoagulant phospholipid production secondary to intravascular coagulation. The incidence is very variable but serious DIC probably affects about 0.1 per cent of pregnancies. Laboratory investigations include measuring the thrombin time, fibrin degradation products (FDPs) and platelet count. These tests should be repeated at regular intervals as resuscitation takes place. In cases of significant DIC, it is vital to involve a haematologist in the early care of the woman.

### Acute renal failure

This is a consequence of poor renal perfusion, secondary to hypovolaemia, hypotension and DIC (microthrombi in the kidneys). The patient initially becomes oliguric and may develop acute tubular necrosis, if the reduced renal perfusion is prolonged. After adequate fluid replacement and treatment of the DIC the patient may become polyuric, during which phase the plasma urea and creatinine concentrations may continue to rise. Fluid, acid–base and electrolyte balance must be carefully monitored. Dialysis may be required. In general, the prognosis for acute renal failure after placental abruption, in women who are adequately resuscitated, is excellent.

### Fetomaternal haemorrhage

This can lead to sensitization of the mother to fetal blood group antigens. This is particularly important for the rhesus D blood group, and all mothers who are D negative should have a Kleihauer test to quantify the size of the fetomaternal haemorrhage and an appropriate dose of anti-D immunoglobulin.

### Maternal mortality

Successive Confidential Enquiries into Maternal Mortality continue to record placental abruption as a significant cause of death, usually as a consequence of the complications listed above.

### Recurrence

After a single episode of abruption, the recurrence rate is approximately 10 per cent, increasing to 25 per cent after two episodes.

## Effects on the fetus

### Perinatal mortality

Abruption is a significant cause of fetal and neonatal loss. Perinatal mortality rates are influenced by the size of abruption, interval to delivery, gestational age at which the abruption and delivery have occurred, and other associated factors, such as growth retardation related to poor placentation.

### Intrauterine growth restriction

This probably has two main components. The first cause is probably inadequate trophoblast invasion of the maternal decidua and spiral arteries, as with the increased risk of pre-eclampsia. Where abruption is chronic or recurrent, the area of placenta available for nutrient and waste exchange between the fetus and the mother is reduced. This may also contribute to fetal growth restriction.

## Care and treatment following placental abruption

A large placental abruption is an obstetric emergency as it is life-threatening for both mother and fetus. The immediate management of a patient with a large antepartum haemorrhage due to placental abruption is discussed in detail in Chapter 16.

Where smaller degrees of abruption have occurred and there is no evidence of fetal distress, particularly where gestational age favours delaying the delivery to allow greater fetal maturity, conservative management may be instituted. This will require close monitoring of fetal well-being, using ultrasound scans of fetal growth, amniotic fluid volume, umbilical artery Doppler and cardiotocography. As with many complicated obstetric problems, timing of delivery will be when the perceived risks of leaving the fetus undelivered outweigh the risk of premature delivery, and the decision is best taken in conjunction with either local paediatricians or with the regional neonatal unit.

### Key Points

- Abnormal trophoblast invasion in the first trimester of pregnancy prevents a low-resistance, high-flow uteroplacental circulation from developing.
- Failed transformation of maternal spiral arteries can be detected by uterine artery Doppler ultrasound in the second trimester: 'notched' uterine artery waveforms indicate high resistance to blood flow before any problem is manifest.
- The consequences of abnormal placentation are pre-eclampsia, intrauterine growth restriction, placental abruption and intrauterine death.
- The search for effective prevention and treatment of these conditions has been only partially successful to date, and remains a major aim of perinatal research for the future.

# References and further reading

Barker DJ. Fetal growth and adult disease. *British Journal of Obstetrics and Gynaecology* 1992; **99**(4):275–6.

Chappell LC, Seed PT, et al. Effect of antioxidants on the occurrence of pre-eclampsia in women at increased risk: a randomised trial. *Lancet* 1999; **354**(9181):810–16.

CLASP: a randomised trial of low-dose aspirin for the prevention and treatment of pre-eclampsia among 9364 pregnant women. Collaborative Low-dose Aspirin Study in Pregnancy Collaborative Group. *Lancet* 1994; **343**(8898): 619–29.

Davey DA, MacGillivray I. The classification and definition of the hypertensive disorders of pregnancy. *American Journal of Obstetrics and Gynecology* 1988; **158**(4):892–8.

Duley L, Henderson-Smart D. Magnesium sulphate versus diazepam for eclampsia. *Cochrane Database of Systematic Reviews* 2003a; (4):CD000127.

Duley L, Henderson-Smart D. Magnesium sulphate versus phenytoin for eclampsia. *Cochrane Database of Systematic Reviews* 2003b; (4):CD000128.

Lewis G, Drife J (eds). *Confidential Enquiry into Maternal and Child Health; why mothers die 2000–2002.* Sixth report of the confidential enquiries into maternal deaths in the UK. London: RCOG Press, 2004.

MAGPIE. Do women with pre-eclampsia, and their babies, benefit from magnesium sulphate? The Magpie Trial: a randomised placebo-controlled trial. *Lancet* 2002; **359**(9321):1877–90.

Neilson JP. Symphysis–fundal height measurement in pregnancy. Cochrane Database of Systematic Reviews 2000: (2) CD000944.

Royal College of Obstetricians and Gynaecologists. *Antenatal corticosteroids to prevent respiratory distress syndrome.* London: RCOG, 1999.

# Preterm labour

## OVERVIEW

Spontaneous preterm labour and preterm rupture of membranes account for approximately two-thirds of preterm births. They usually proceed to preterm deliveries in up to 80 per cent of the cases. They are the predominant causes of perinatal mortality and morbidity particularly in those before 32 weeks' gestation. The care and management of preterm labours must be individualized to the needs of the mother, the fetus and the family, with an aim to reduce perinatal mortality and morbidity. The midwife has a unique role in the care and management of the mother and her family in this critical period.

## Definition

Preterm birth refers generally to the delivery of the baby occurring between 24 + 0 and 36 + 6 weeks of pregnancy. Preterm labour with intact membranes accounts for over 50 per cent of cases presented at maternity units and will be the focus of discussion in this chapter. Preterm prelabour rupture of membranes with subsequent preterm labour is thought to have a different pathophysiology and is also discussed in Chapter 8.

## Prevalence

The UK has the highest rate of preterm births in Europe, currently up to 7 per cent of all births. This figure is higher in socioeconomically deprived inner-city areas and lower in more affluent areas. In the USA, the rate of preterm births are reported to be higher at up to 11 per cent compared to the Nordic countries, with very reliable statistical data, which quote significantly lower rates of below 5 per cent. Factors such as socioeconomic and cultural differences between the countries may have some bearing on the figures. Alarmingly, the incidence of preterm births appears to be rising, in part due to an increase in the numbers of multiple births, and other social and cultural changes in society. The incidence of all low birth weight babies of less than 2500 g is greater at up to 7.7 per cent; this includes all preterm births as well as term babies with intrauterine growth restriction and marcosomic preterm babies.

Spontaneous preterm labour and preterm rupture of the membranes proceed to preterm deliveries in up to 80 per cent of cases.

## Classifications and categories of preterm births

Preterm births are divided into three gestational periods:
- *moderately preterm births* occur between 35 and 37 weeks (incidence 5.5 per cent);
- *very preterm births* occur between 29 and 34 weeks (incidence 0.7 per cent);
- *extremely preterm births* occur between 24 and 28 weeks (incidence 0.4 per cent).

Earlier deliveries are usually referred to as miscarriages, as the current age of viability is 24 weeks' gestation, unless the baby has shown signs of life at delivery.

*Indicated preterm deliveries* are preterm births that occur because the delivery is felt to be in the best interest of either the mother or the baby.

Spontaneous preterm births are preterm births that occurring due to:
- *spontaneous preterm labour*; and
- *spontaneous preterm prelabour rupture of membranes* (PPROM).

Each of these groups accounts for one-third of early births (Figure 11.1).

## Classification of the preterm baby

The birth weight as well as the gestational age is an important consideration in the management of a preterm baby after its delivery:
- *low birth weight babies* weigh less than 2500 g (5.5 lb);
- *very low birth weight babies* weigh less than 1500 g (3.0 lb);

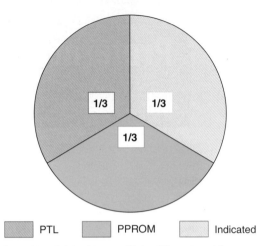

**Figure 11.1** Origin of preterm births. PTL, preterm labour; PPROM, preterm prelabour rupture of membranes.

- *extremely low birth weight babies* weigh less than 1000 g (2.2 lb).

Some babies may be both small for gestational age and premature, as a result of intrauterine growth restriction.

Birth weight is the major determinant of neonatal mortality. Very low birth weight (i.e. 500–1499 g) accounts for nearly half of all infant deaths.

## Survival rates

The survival rate of preterm babies is dependent on the aetiology, outcome and recurrence risk:
- babies born at 23 weeks have a 17 per cent chance of survival;
- babies born at 24 weeks have a 39 per cent chance of survival;
- babies born at 25 weeks have a 50 per cent chance of survival.

From 32 weeks onwards babies have a >50 per cent chance of survival, but may require medical and technological help. Preterm delivery is associated with massive expenditure of financial resources to sustain the preterm baby. The estimated costs for a providing care for a neonatal intensive care cot in the UK averages £1000 per day in terms of staffing, drugs, equipment and other running costs. There is much debate regarding the health economics and the ethics of this area of health care owing to the poor outcomes that are found in surviving children.

Preterm delivery accounts for 65 per cent of neo-natal deaths and up to 50 per cent of neurological disabilities in childhood. Longitudinal studies of preterm infants have found that one in ten will develop permanent disability, such as lung disease, cerebral palsy, blindness or deafness, irrespective of their gestational age.

A total of 50 per cent of preterm babies born before 26 weeks' gestation are disabled, a quarter with severe disabilities. Eighty per cent of these infants will have physical, psychomotor and intellectual impairment with boys having more profound disabilities than girls.

## Aetiology

There are many theories and much debate as to the causes of preterm labour. Its prediction is difficult owing to the diversity of risk factors that individually may be the key cause or a combination of several risks may be present. Extensive research has been undertaken in this area of obstetric medicine but the condition remains an enigma. The underlying physiology and molecular biology of preterm labour is still not fully understood, particularly regarding the activation of the maternal or fetal hypothalamic–pituitary–adrenal axis that initiates labour.

The causes can be divided into two main groups: physiological and non-physiological.

## Physiological causes

### Infections

Some mothers may experience illnesses, such as urinary tract infections, pyelonephritis, appendicitis or pneumonia, and these are associated with preterm labour. In these cases, preterm labour is probably due to direct blood-borne spread of infection to the uterine cavity, or indirectly through chemical by-products either from micro-organisms or from inflammatory responses by the body.

Subclinical infection of the choriodecidual space and amniotic fluid is the most widely studied aetiological factor underlying spontaneous preterm births. Inflammatory responses in the placenta, fetal membranes and maternal decidua lead to the production of endotoxins, cytokines, such as interleukin 1-beta

and interleukin 6 from endothelial cells, and tumour necrosis factor-alpha from macrophages. This activates the production of prostaglandin, which will stimulate cervical ripening and uterine contractions. Early onset of neonatal sepsis, maternal postpartum endometritis and histological chorioamnionitis are significantly common after the delivery. The midwife must be vigilant in assessing the mother for possible signs and symptoms of infection during the pregnancy, and routine antenatal infection screening programmes must be offered to all mothers.

### Overdistension

In pregnancy, there are two main causes of overdistension: multiple pregnancy and polyhydramnios. The incidence of multiple births has statistically shown an increase owing to the advancement of assisted conception techniques and treatments. Polyhydramnios is strongly associated with gestational diabetes and fetal congenital abnormalities. There is a significant rise in clinical obesity and diabetes mellitus in the general population, and some mothers may have these underlying conditions.

Overdistension may cause premature prelabour rupture of the membranes and also stretches receptors in the myometrium, which may perceive that the pregnancy is at term and ready for delivery. The midwife in her antenatal abdominal palpation of the mother should observe for any sign of overdistension of the uterus, and observe for signs of uterine irritability during the pregnancy.

### Vascular problems

Antepartum haemorrhage and abruption are commonly reported prior to spontaneous preterm deliveries. Blood is an irritant to the myometrium, weakens the membranes and will cause uterine contractions. Emergency contact numbers should be available for the mother to contact for midwifery advice if there are signs of bleeding.

### Cervical weakness

Cervical weakness, previously know as cervical incompetence, may cause both late miscarriage and preterm labour. There may be dilatation of the cervix with or without uterine contractions or spontaneous rupture of membranes. Previous cervical surgery, such as cone biopsy, will increase the risk of preterm delivery, low birth weight and Caesarean section. Large loop excision of the transformation zone for cervical dyskaryosis will increase the risk of prelabour rupture of membranes. Surgical termination of pregnancy with resulting cervical trauma and damage has been associated with the inability of the cervical os to remain tightly closed during the pregnancy.

## Iatrogenic causes

Up to 30 per cent of preterm births may be due to medical indications for induction of labour or surgical deliveries. The most common indication is for fulminating pre-eclampsia in the mother (see Chapter 16), or signs of serious intrauterine growth restriction to the singleton fetus or to one of the fetuses in a multiple pregnancy. The midwife is responsible for the full antenatal assessment of the mother in order to monitor for normal progress and to detect any abnormal conditions.

## Idiopathic causes

In up to 75 per cent of preterm labours and deliveries, the cause is unknown and is categorized as idiopathic preterm labour. However, there are other well-known causative risk factors that will precipitate a preterm delivery. These are the socioeconomic, racial and cultural factors, namely the non-physiological reasons.

## Other physiological predictors of preterm labour

### Cervical length

Current research into transvaginal ultrasonogragphy to assess the cervical length and the shortening of the cervix in pregnancy has generated much debate regarding which length is discriminatory, the accuracy of the scanning routes and the gestation at which the predictive scanning test should be performed on the mother. The normal cervical length is approximately 35 mm (Figure 11.2a). Significant cervical shortening is often accompanied by dilatation and funnelling of the membranes down the cervical canal (Figure 11.2b). Recent research has found that a cervical length of less than 15 mm has a risk of nearly 50 per cent of early spontaneous preterm delivery before 32 weeks' gestation.

### Fibronectin

Fetal fibronectin (fFN) is a glue-like glycoprotein produced by the chorionic cells that binds the choriodecidual membranes layers. It is present in vaginal secretions in early pregnancy up to 22 weeks' gestation. Swabs can be taken from the ectocervix or from the posterior vaginal fornix. An enzyme-linked immunosorbent assay (ELISA) containing FDC-6 monoclonal antibody can be used to detect fetal fibronectin. The levels are negligible between 24 and 34 weeks followed by a rise in levels before the onset of labour. If there is any disruption at the choriodecidual interface as a result of damage, infection or bleeding, then fFN may appear in the vaginal secretions earlier. This may be a useful predictor of impending preterm labour and delivery; several studies have found the majority of mothers who tested positive

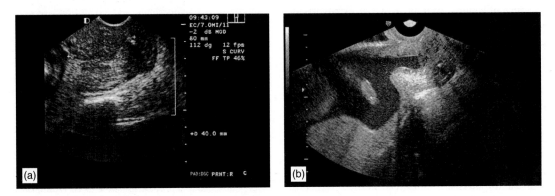

**Figure 11.2** (a) Normal cervix. (b) Cervical length and funnelling on ultrasound.

have delivered within 7 days. While the cervico-vaginal fetal fibronectin test has been proposed as a predictive test, critics have stated that its accuracy is variable and should, therefore, be part of an overall framework for decision-making and management for preterm labour.

### Salivary oestriol

Current research by the PREMET study is comparing and investigating levels of salivary oestriol, fetal fibronectin, bacterial vaginosis infection, interleukin (IL)-6 and IL-8 as predictive and effective tests for preterm labour.

---

**Physiological causes of preterm labour**

- Infections
- Overdistension
- Vascular
- Cervical weakness
- Iatrogenic
- Idiopathic
- Cervical length
- Fibronectin
- Salivary oestriol

---

**Non-physiological risk factors**

### Maternal age

The age of the mother has a significant influence on the possibility of a preterm labour and delivery, the very young (i.e. under 18 years of age) or those over 35 years have been shown statistically to have a higher incidence of preterm labours. Second births among women between 15 and 19 years were associated with three-fold risk of extremely preterm birth and still-birth compared to women between 20 and 29 years. Death rates for babies and young children born to teenage mothers are 60 per cent higher than older women. As women are delaying having their first babies in favour of establishing a career, the national age of the primigravida has now risen to 29 years. Preterm labour is also associated with older women as they may have some underlying medical or gynae-cological problems, or have conceived through *in-vitro* fertilization (IVF) treatment, which is also likely to precipitate a multiple pregnancy as well as other potential associated problems of infertility treatment.

### Lower social class or socio-economic factors

Many socioeconomic factors have been cited as pre-disposing risks to preterm births. Research from both the UK and USA has found that low-income women, or women who have little or poor financial support from partners, have a higher risk of preterm labour and of having babies who are small for gestational age, and have greater gestational complications. The midwife may be able to make such an assessment of the mother by undertaking the first booking history interview in the mother's own home environment. In the UK, government initiatives such as Sure Start pro-grammes are available for mothers from poor socioeconomic groups. Sure Start provides financial incentives for women to attend antenatal appointments and parent education classes, which may help them to prepare for their role and responsibilities as a poten-tial parent, and the additional monies may help to reduce their financial burden.

### Unmarried or unsupported women

An extensive study by Zeitlin et al. (2002) of 16 European countries has found that there is a signifi-cant risk of preterm birth associated with co-habitation and single motherhood.

Research studies have also found that the lack of a relationship with a husband or partner was related to greater risk of having a low birth weight baby. There was also a strong correlation between single mothers and the increased incidence of lowered gestational age of their babies. The midwife may be able to establish the presence or absence of a supportive partner during the initial booking interview. If the mother is unsup-ported, the midwife should monitor the mother closely and, if necessary, refer the mother to the medical social workers after discussion with the mother.

### Maternal weight – underweight and overweight

Women who are underweight as a result of previous anorexia nervosa are more susceptible to preterm labour and low birth weight babies. At the other end of the weight spectrum, women who are clinically obese are also at risk of preterm labour and delivery, as they have a tendency to develop gestational diabetes during the pregnancy. Moreover, they are also at higher risk of developing pre-eclampsia, which is strongly associated with preterm delivery. The midwife must make an assessment of the maternal weight and body mass index (BMI) as part of the initial first 'top-to-toe' booking check, and monitor the mother's weight at subsequent antenatal checks.

## Maternal diet

A mother's poor diet around the time of conception is linked to possible preterm births and low birth weight babies. Recent work in the USA found that mothers who ate less frequently than average delivered their babies earlier. Comparative studies of Indian women in rural India found that they delivered a week earlier when compared with Indian women in Southampton, UK. The most likely explanation is that the mothers in India were undernourished. Researchers estimated that up to 40 per cent of women of a childbearing age in the UK do not consume the recommended daily intake of vitamins and other important nutrients to allow for optimum health. The demands of a pregnancy will quickly exhaust the mother's own stores and, if the maternal diet is poor, then the fetus will be compromised and a possible preterm delivery may result. It is the midwife's responsibility to provide information and advice on nutrition in preparation for childbirth (Article 4 of the EU Second Midwifery Directive 80/155/EEC) to help ensure an adequate diet for health during the pregnancy for both mother and baby.

## Smoking, alcohol and drugs misuse

The Tommy's national pregnancy week survey in 2004 found that one in five mothers smoked through their pregnancy, with 24 per cent continuing to smoke throughout the pregnancy and only one-third giving up before the birth. (Tommy's is a UK charity dedicated to maximizing maternal and fetal health through research; www.tommys.org) Smoking is associated with adverse outcomes, notably an increased risk of up to 26 per cent with preterm labours, reduced birth weight of up to 200 g lighter and perinatal deaths.

With alcohol consumption, the survey found two out of five mothers drank alcohol during their pregnancy, with one in four (28 per cent) drinking up to 5 units of alcohol a week, which is double the recommended weekly limit. High volumes of alcohol consumption by the mother may result in higher risk of preterm labour as well as fetal alcohol syndrome of the baby.

Drugs and substance misuse has also been found to be a major causative factor in preterm labours and deliveries. This may be due to the self-neglect of the mother resulting in nutritional deficiencies and also the adverse effects of the smoking, alcohol and drugs misuse. There may have been fetal compromise from possible fetal hypoxia, systematic infections, placental abruptions, and poor placental perfusions of blood, nutrients and oxygen. As the intrauterine environment becomes more hostile and unfavourable, there is strong likelihood of a preterm delivery. The midwife must actively encourage and support the mother to reduce her smoking, alcohol or drug consumption in pregnancy, as well as possible lifestyle modification. Referral to specialist practitioners, such as a smoking cessation midwife, or an alcohol and drugs rehabilitation practitioner for entering a withdrawal programme, can help the mother for long-term support.

## Previous premature labour

When there has been a previous history or histories of preterm labour and delivery of unknown cause, the risk of preterm delivery will be greatly increased.

## Race

Racial and ethnic origins of the mother have been found to be a significant factors in the length of the gestational age and birth weight of the baby. Studies in the USA by Mackey et al. (2000) have found a significant difference between black and white women in relationship to their birth outcomes from preterm labours. Black women had consistently higher fatigue, work stress and future security concerns correlating with many also having a higher incidence of low birth weight and low gestational age babies. There were twice as many black preterm and low birth weight babies born when compared to white mothers' births. Researchers have attributed this phenomenon to the possibility that black women have higher rates of heavy drugs and alcohol use, poor antenatal attendance, late antenatal registration, poorer educational status, unwanted pregnancies, poorer nutrition and high stress factors, which may lead to preterm labour and delivery. However, researchers have also found that even healthy middle class black women have a higher rate of preterm deliveries compared to matched white control groups of mothers.

In a recent observational study by Field et al. (2002), population characteristics or demographics of the local population of a particular area were found to influence the outcomes of the preterm delivery rates and mortality rates. Despite more available intensive care delivered by the neonatal services or by a more specialized neonatal service, the outcomes may still be worse.

## Work

Preterm labours and deliveries have been found in women whose jobs require prolonged standing, long working hours and heavy manual labour. Research has also found that mothers who are unemployed have higher incidence of preterm labour and delivery. Of the women who worked, those who were in jobs where they had little control over the pace and structure, as well as being psychological demanding were more at risk of preterm labour. In the UK, women are entitled to attend antenatal appointments during work time and the Health and Safety at Work Act 1974 stipulates that the employer must ensure the health and safety of their employees at all times.

## Stress and birth outcomes

As no interventions have been shown to decrease the rate of preterm birth significantly, researchers have now called for the research emphasis to be towards the social and biological factors, such as stress, social deprivation and poverty, along with infections and inflammations of the urogenital tract. Researchers believe that maternal stress may be a major factor in inducing preterm labours via one or both of two physiological pathways.

First, they postulate that maternal stress may affect the neuroendocrine pathway, which will activate the maternal–placental–fetal endocrine systems that promote parturition. Lockwood and Kuczynski

1999) theorize that activation of the hypothalamic–pituitary–adrenal axis (HPA), as a result of stress, can induce preterm labour and birth.

Second, the immune–inflammatory pathway may be involved. Maternal stress may affect systematic and local (placental–decidual) immunity to increase susceptibility to intrauterine and fetal infectious–inflammatory processes, and cause parturition through the pro-inflammatory mechanisms identified previously (Wadhwa et al. 2001).

Midwives are in a unique position to assess risk during the first booking visit, for the mothers who are especially susceptible to stress and/or infections, as well as to identify the socioeconomic factors that may contribute to the woman going into preterm labour. Social and psychological support from midwives and other health professionals has been shown to be an important factor in the management and possible prevention of preterm births. The Sighthill project in Scotland and the UK Newcastle antenatal care project in the 1980s initiated by midwives have been successful in reducing low birth rate babies and prevention of preterm labours. Many countries and many different models of care have been implemented for women who may be at risk of preterm labours, with many of these women being from socially deprived backgrounds. These programmes offer advice and support on nutrition, rest, stress management, alcohol and recreational drug use. Many also provided financial and practical assistance, such as transportation to antenatal clinics, and home help and support workers have also been made available. Moreover, emotional support, such as counselling, reassurance, sympathetic listening, as well as professional psychiatric help, was made available for mothers who required it. Such programmes may help to predict the potential birth outcomes and birth weights of the babies.

## Birth spacing

Research has found that the closer the interpregnancy spacing, the greater the risk of preterm labour and birth. The World Health Organisation (WHO) recommends a minimum 24-month interval in order for the body to recover from the childbirth process. Mothers should be given appropriate advice by midwives for conceptual care and pregnancy planning as required by the Nursing and Midwifery Council (NMC; 2004) *Midwives rules and standards*. Moreover, in accordance to Article 4 of the European Union *Second midwifery directive* 80/155/EEC (1980), midwives must provide sound family planning information and advice.

## Risk factors for preterm labour

- Maternal age
- Lower social class or socioeconomic factors
- Unmarried or unsupported women
- Maternal weight – underweight and overweight
- Maternal diet
- Smoking, alcohol and drug misuse
- Previous premature labour
- Race
- Work
- Stress and birth outcomes
- Birth spacing

## Clinical features of preterm labour

The preterm labour may present, as would normal labour at term, by spontaneous onset of regular painful uterine contractions, with or without spontaneous rupture of membranes. Some cases may have preterm prelabour spontaneous rupture of membranes followed by the onset of regular painful contractions. Some women may present with a history of vague backache and low-grade abdominal discomfort.

This may or may not be the onset of preterm labour and a differential diagnosis needs to be made to eliminate the possibility of urinary incontinence as opposed to preterm rupture of membranes. The likelihood of a urinary tract infection causing the abdominal and backache rather than the onset of labour must be investigated.

## Diagnosis of preterm labour

Diagnosis of preterm labour is made when there is evidence of regular uterine contractions with accompanying effacement and dilatation of the cervix before 37 weeks' gestation.

## Investigations

### Nitrazine testing

As amniotic fluid is alkaline, it will turn a nitrazine stick black, indicating the possible presence of amniotic fluid in the vaginal canal. However, there are occasional false positives owing to the contamination from blood, semen and even sometimes urine. So it is not a definitive test for determining preterm rupture of membranes and, in particular, the forewaters, as there may be a hindwater rupture.

### Genital tract swabs

A high vaginal swab should always be taken for microbiology, culture and sensitivity to help guide antibiotic therapy, if there is an infection present. Screening for group B streptococcus (GBS) can also be performed, especially if labour is likely to occur in the next 24–48 hours.

### Maternal well-being

Maternal vital signs should be monitored regularly, and bloods taken for full blood count, group and cross-matching, as the preterm labour may be due to antepartum haemorrhage and the mother's condition may deteriorate rapidly owing to haemorrhage. Serial high white-cell counts and C-reactive proteins may be indication of an infection.

### Fetal well-being

Full assessment of the fetal condition is crucial in establishing baseline observations. Either intermittent or continuous cardiotocography (CTG) may be required to monitor the fetus. Fetal tachycardia is suggestive of intrauterine infection.

### Ultrasound

An ultrasound scan may help to establish the volume of liquor, and there is a direct correlation between the amount of amniotic fluid remaining and the latency period. This may help the obstetric and midwifery staff in the planning of care and management of the mother and baby for both the delivery and subsequent postnatal period.

## Treatment

### Maternal steroids

Current evidence shows that a single course of maternal steroids (two injections 12–24 hours apart) given between 28 and 34 weeks' gestation, and received within 7 days of delivery results in markedly improved neonatal outcomes. This is due to a reduction in neonatal respiratory distress syndrome. The greatest benefit is seen after 48 hours postinjection. Courses received less than 48 hours or more than 7 days before delivery may still lead to benefit, as may courses given to labours before 28 weeks' gestation. Although long-term follow-up of preterm infants has not found any adverse consequences from intramuscular steroids, there have been concerns raised regarding the adverse outcomes of repeated dosing, as there is the potential for harm with repeated continued steroid use.

### Tocolytics

There are several types of drug used to reduce uterine contractility: most are smooth muscle relaxants and are useful for ensuring the administration of maternal steroids prior to delivery, when transferring mothers to a specialist unit and for acute episodes of uterine contractions of less than 48 hours. Tocolytics should not be use when there is rupture of membranes, any signs of chorioamnionitis, fetal anomaly and antepartum haemorrhage. The midwife must adhere to the NMC (2004) Guidelines on the safe administration of medicines when caring for mother who are prescribed tocolytics.

Beta-agonists, such as ritodrine, salbutamol and terbutaline, may be given orally or intravenously. They act on the beta-2 adrenergic receptors, which relax the muscle. The side effects of beta-agonists include tachycardia, sweating and headaches. The most serious adverse side effect for the mother is cardiovascular compromise with pulmonary oedema, which can cause maternal deaths.

The use of tocolytics such as ritodrine was found by the Canadian Preterm Labour Trial to have no significant benefit on the perinatal mortality or the prolongation of pregnancy to term, although it did reduce the number of mothers delivering within 48 hours by 40 per cent (Canadian Preterm Labour Investigators Group 1992). For many obstetricians, this window of opportunity is the sole reason for its continued usage. Tocolytics are probably inappropriate once steroids have been given and special neonatal intensive care cots are available.

Other smooth muscle relaxants used are:
- *Calcium-channel blockers* (e.g. oral nifedipine). The side effects are mild headaches and flushing in the mother. Glyceryl trinitrate, a nitric oxide donor and magnesium sulphate have been used to cause smooth muscle relaxation, but there is no strong evidence that any one drug is more effective in arresting labour or improves the birth outcomes.
- Non-steroidal anti-inflammatory drugs, such as indomethacin, given orally or rectally will block the release of prostaglandin and reduce uterine contractions. Indomethacin has been shown to be effective in postponing delivery with fewer maternal side effects and is being adopted for use in many National Health Service Trusts. However, if the drug is used for >24 hours, the side effects on the fetus include oligohydraminos, intraventricular haemorrhage and a risk of patent ductus arteriosus in the neonate that may require corrective surgery.

### Antibiotics

The Medical Research Council Oracle study concluded that the routine use of antibiotics in uncomplicated preterm labour has no significant benefits for the mother, but a slight benefit for the baby after prelabour preterm rupture of the membranes (Kenyon et al. 2001a,b). However, most Trusts continue in prescribing routine prophylactic antibiotic treatment. The midwife must ensure that the mother does not have any allergies to an antibiotic prior to its administration.

### Cervical cerclage

The surgical intervention of cercival cerclage, involving the insertion of a cervical suture using either the Shirodkar or McDonald techniques, has been found to have only a marginal benefit in preventing preterm labour. However, greater success was found when used on women who had been diagnosed with a short cervix, and better outcomes with the transabdominal cerclage in comparison to the transvaginal route.

## Fetal assessment

The baby must be monitored to assess the fetal heart rate as maternal steroid therapy can affect the fetal heart rate and its variability. Doppler studies are not influenced by the steroid therapy. The presentation of the fetus should be confirmed by ultrasound scan, as clinical abdominal palpation may be unreliable before the age of 28 weeks. The estimation of fetal weight by ultrasound scan may be useful to give a predictive birth weight in order to assess the survival rate of the preterm baby. Continuous CTG monitoring of the fetal heart is required for assessment of the fetus' reaction to uterine contractions. It is thought that there may be considerable difficulties in interpreting the fetal heart rate pattern in extremely preterm infants; nonetheless, continuous CTG monitoring may help to provide useful information on the fetal heart for base rate, variability and reaction to any uterine activity or rise in intrauterine pressures.

## Management of the high-risk asymptomatic woman

The mother who has been assessed by the midwife as being at high risk of having a preterm labour or delivery will require close antenatal monitoring and assessment for any signs of labour. It will be essential to establish the expected day of delivery of the baby and an early dating scan may be useful in confirming the baby's gestational age. Routine antenatal infection screening tests must be performed to ascertain any possible presence of asymptomatic urinary tract infection or other infections. The fetal fibronectin levels should be tested, if there are any signs of infection. The measurement of cervical length is not universally offered as a routine but may be useful for mothers who have had previous preterm deliveries, and cervical cerclage could be offered as a possible intervention to sustain the pregnancy where there is a diagnosis of cervical weakness.

There are currently research trials examining the use of progesterone given intramuscularly or by vaginal pessary, and the use of supplements of fish oils in the antenatal period for mothers who are at high risk of preterm labour. Preliminary results have been promising in showing some benefit in reducing preterm deliveries for high-risk mothers. The most effective and conclusive antenatal intervention in preventing preterm labour is to stop mothers smoking. Women must be educated and information given to them to help them modify their smoking, and their use of alcohol and other drugs and substances. The mother will require support and advice from the midwife to help her change her lifestyle and dietary regime.

## Delivery management

### Communication

Effective communication is vital to the care and management of the mother in preterm labour. The midwife must ensure that the two vital areas of communication regarding the management of the preterm labour and possible preterm delivery are fully explained to the mother and her family. In accordance with the NMC (2004) Code of Professional Conduct, they must be fully informed of the risks involved in the different possible care pathways (i.e. to attempt to arrest the labour or to allow the delivery to take place) and the subsequent management of the preterm baby. Communication with the neonatal unit staff and paediatrician is vital to ensure that adequate and appropriate resources are made available for the delivery. If there is no neonatal cot available, then alternative care provision in neighbouring or nearest hospitals Trusts must be found to ensure the preterm baby has access to neonatal intensive care.

### In-utero transfer

Many of the Confidential Enquiries into Maternal Deaths and Child Health (CEMACH) recommend that mothers and their babies should be managed by specialist expert teams. If the maternity unit does not have a specialist team to manage preterm labours or does not have specialist neonatal care services for the newborn, an 'in-utero' transfer to a unit with specialist midwifery and specialist neonatal facilities is strongly recommended in order that the birth outcome may be improved.

## Analgesia

The use of epidural analgesia is useful in the management of preterm labour as it may help to prevent and avoid expulsive maternal efforts before full dilatation or a precipitous delivery that may cause fetal damage. It will also aid a relaxed pelvic floor and perineum, and the ability to proceed quickly to abdominal delivery if so required. Although the more traditional analgesics such as Entonox and pethidine may be administered, their usage must be with reference to the fetal condition.

## Fetal and maternal vital signs

Close monitoring of the maternal and fetal vital signs is critical in ensuring the safety of the mother and baby, especially with mothers who may have an underlying physiological problem, such as bleeding or an infection, as the condition may deteriorate and adversely affect the mother and baby. A partogram may be commenced to assess the progress of the labour and continuous CTG of the fetal heart should also be applied.

## Management of the membranes

The membranes should be kept intact for as long as possible in the labour so that the liquor can act as a buffer against the intrauterine pressures of the contracting uterus. It may help to protect the fragile fetal body and especially the fetal head from birth trauma. It may help to minimize fetal head compression to prevent cerebral intraventricular haemorrhages postdelivery.

## Mode of delivery

An experienced and skilled midwifery, obstetric and paediatric team must be available to care for the mother and baby. The mode of delivery is dependent on the presentation of the fetus or fetuses. If the presentation is breech, or there are twins or multiple births, then a Caesarean section is the most likely option. Caesarean section is also indicated if there is fetal or maternal compromise, such as severe eclampsia with convulsions. Most preterm labours have a tendency to be rapid and of short duration with the likelihood of a vaginal

birth. Forceps may be used to protect the fetal head with an aim to reduce intracranial trauma. Ventouse should not be used on babies less than 34 weeks, as it can cause intracranial trauma and haemorrhages.

Preterm labours and deliveries should ideally be conducted in a consultant hospital unit; however, the midwife may be called to a mother in the community in advanced labour and unsuitable for *in-utero* transfer. The midwife must call for additional midwifery support and the services of the paramedic, if there is no obstetric 'flying squad' available. The midwife may have to resuscitate and intubate the preterm baby after delivery and rearrange for immediate transfer to the neonatal intensive care unit.

---

### Delivery management

- Communication
- *In-utero* transfer
- Analgesia
- Fetal and maternal vital signs
- Management of the membranes
- Mode of delivery

---

### New developments

The new focus of preventing preterm labours and births is to target high-risk mothers and provide psychosocial and financial support interventions that may help to reduce the rates of preterm labours and births, as well as low birth weight babies. The implementation of Sure Start programmes nationally may help to provide social and financial support for women. The government recommendations for tackling inequalities in health may help to target high-risk populations and reduce their risk levels. Women's and children's mental health and well-being are being addressed though the National Service Framework directives as well as the recommendations from CEMACH to assess the mental well-being of women in early pregnancy, so that early interventions can be put into place.

The detection of fetal fibronectin levels and the use of ultrasound scanning to measure cervical length in order to predict the likelihood of preterm labour in women has been very useful in managing asymptomatic high-risk mothers and also in helping to plan for the delivery.

## Conclusion

The prediction, prevention and management of preterm labour and preterm births remain a challenge to health professionals. It is widely considered that there is still a current lack of in-depth knowledge regarding the causes of preterm labours and a lack of effective preventative interventions. The aim of care is:

- first, to assess and recognize risk factors that may lead to preterm labours;
- second, to achieve a safe and timely delivery for the mother and baby by skilled and experienced health professionals;
- finally to provide appropriate and specialist neonatal care, which will improve neonatal outcomes for the preterm baby.

The role and responsibilities of the midwife are to provide support and advice for the mother and her family during the pregnancy to help the mother minimize her own risk factors by adopting healthy lifestyle changes.

## Key Points

- Preterm deliveries complicate up to 7 per cent of UK pregnancies.
- Major risk factors are physiological (e.g. previous preterm labour, infections) or socioecomonic (e.g. maternal diet, smoking and alcohol use).
- Predicting and managing preterm labours is difficult until advanced cervical dilatation has occurred.
- The use of transcervical ultrasound scanning of cervical length and testing for levels of fetal fibronectin are useful in the assessment of preterm labours.
- Midwives have a key role in the education and support of mothers to help them reduce their risk of preterm labour.
- Preterm labour and deliveries should be managed by a specialist team of midwives, obstetricians and paediatricians.
- The use of maternal steroid therapy is essential for improving neonatal outcome.
- Effective communication is vital between the mother, her family and the health care professionals.

## CASE HISTORY

Angela, a 24-year-old single mother, is pregnant for the third time with a new partner. Her first child a girl weighing 1.8 kg was born at 32 weeks' gestation when she was 17. Angela had a spontaneous vaginal delivery 48 hours after preterm rupture of membranes. Two years later, her second child, a boy weighing 1.9 kg was born at 34 weeks' gestation, and the pregnancy was prolonged for 1 week until she went into spontaneous labour and delivery. Angela smokes up to ten cigarettes a day and is reluctant to give up, as she says she needs it to help her through the stresses and strains of the day. Angela's children are at school full time and she works part time in a shop to coincide with the school hours. She has little family support apart from her new partner, who does not live with her full time.

Angela's care and management will automatically be put into the high-risk category in accordance with the National Institute for Clinical Excellence guidelines as she has had two previous preterm deliveries. Therefore, she will require close and regular monitoring by the midwifery and obstetric team. Full antenatal screening and infection screening must be performed to assess for possible infections. Early ultrasound scanning to determine gestational age of the fetus is crucial in the planning and management of the pregnancy and delivery for Angela. The use of predictive

assessment tests, such as ultrasound scanning of the cervical length and assessment of fetal fibronectin levels in vaginal secretions, may help to provide a more rounded assessment of the mother's potential for going into preterm labour.

The midwife must give help and advice to Angela regarding her smoking habits and referral to the smoking cessation midwife, who may help Angela to reduce the number of cigarettes she smokes. The midwife will need to assess and discuss the level of support that Angela may need postdelivery, as she has had minimal contact with her family and her partner does not live with her full time. The midwife may request social support for Angela, but only if Angela is receptive and happy to allow social worker support. The help may just be a temporary domestic 'home help' scheme for mothers with newborn babies for the first few months of life when the mother has two or more young children.

Full discussion of the possibility of a third preterm labour and delivery should be conducted between Angela and the midwifery and obstetric teams, so that Angela is given full and objective information regarding the possible interventions that may be required. This is necessary in order for her to have informed choice about her care, and fully participate and be proactive in planning her own care with the health care professionals.

# References

Canadian Preterm Labour Investigators Group. Treatment of preterm labour with the beta-adrenergic agonist ritodrine. *New England Journal of Medicine* 1992; **327**:308–12.

European Union. *Second midwifery directive* (80/155/EEC). Brussels: European Union, 1980.

Field D, Petersen S, Clarke M, Draper ES. Extreme prematurity in the UK and Denmark: population differences in viability. *Archives of Diseases in Childhood, Fetal and Neonatal Edition* 2002; **87**(3):F172–5.

Kenyon SL, Taylor DJ, Tarnow-Mordi W, ORACLE Collaborative Group. Broad-spectrum antibiotics for preterm, prelabour rupture of fetal membranes: the ORACLE I randomised trial. *Lancet* 2001a; **357**:979–88.

Kenyon SL, Taylor DJ, Tarnow-Mordi W, ORACLE Collaborative Group. Broad-spectrum antibiotics for spontaneous preterm labour: the ORACLE II randomised trial. *Lancet* 2001b; **357**:989–94.

Lockwood CJ, Kuczynski E. Markers of risk for preterm delivery. *Journal of Perinatal Medicine* 1999; **27**:5–20.

Mackey MC, Williams CA, Tiller CM. Stress, preterm labour and birth outcomes. *Journal of Advanced Nursing* 2000; **32**(3):666–74.

Nursing and Midwifery Council. *Midwives rules and standards*. London: NMC, 2004.

Wadha PD, Culhane JF, Rauh V, et al. Stress, infection and preterm birth: a biobehavioural perspective. *Paediatric and Perinatal Epidemiology* Supplement 2001: **15**(Suppl 2): 17–29.

Zeitlin JA, Saurel-Cubizolles M-J, Ancel, P-Y, EUROPOP Group. Marital status, cohabitation, and the risk of preterm birth in Europe: where births outside marriage are common and uncommon. *Paediatric and Perinatal Epidemiology* 2002; **16**(2):124–30.

# Additional reading

Fowlie PW, McGuire W. *ABC of preterm birth*. London: BMJ Publishing, 2002.

Hodnett ED, Fredericks S. Support during pregnancy for women at increased risk of low birth weight babies. *The Cochrane Database of Systematic Reviews* 2003; Issue 3, Art. no CD000198.

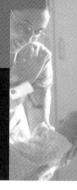

# Chapter 12

# Medical conditions associated with pregnancy

## OVERVIEW

Pregnancy is a normal physiological event and most women remain healthy throughout the duration of their pregnancy. However, pregnancy may be complicated by a variety of disorders and conditions that can affect the well-being of the woman and her fetus. Furthermore, it is not uncommon to encounter pregnant women with pre-existing medical conditions. Both pregnancy-specific and pre-existing medical conditions may in some circumstances be associated with significant maternal and fetal morbidity and, more rarely, mortality. It is, therefore, important for the midwife to not only understand how pregnancy may affect pre-existing medical conditions, but also how the condition and/or treatment may affect the pregnancy.

Assessment of medical conditions and discussion regarding the implications for pregnancy should be available and offered to the woman and a plan of care documented before pregnancy. Counselling prior to conception allows women who have a pre-existing medical condition to understand the possible risks in pregnancy and the level of antenatal care they will require. Although such preconception counselling does occur, it is not universal, and often takes place following a pregnancy where the outcome has not been a positive one.

Such pregnancies are often considered to be high risk, and a multidisciplinary collaborative approach is recommended to ensure that the health of the woman and her fetus is carefully monitored. It is also vital that the woman and her family be involved in decision-making in order to promote feelings of autonomy and control over a condition that has the potential to result in the medicalization of childbirth. This chapter discusses the most common medical disorders that may complicate pregnancy and the important role that the midwife plays in supporting the woman and her family. This should involve ensuring not only the physical needs, but also psychological and sociological needs, and that the pregnancy is treated as normal as far as is possible.

## Cardiac disease

### Prevalence and aetiology

Although cardiac disease in pregnancy is rare, complicating approximately 1 per cent of all pregnancies, it is potentially serious and continues to contribute significantly to maternal morbidity and mortality. Maternal death from cardiac disease in the UK increased in the last triennial report from 35 (1997–99) to 44 (2000–2002) (Lewis and Drife 2004). However, this prevalence varies from one community to another, principally because the incidence of rheumatic heart disease and undiagnosed or uncorrected congenital heart disease is higher in developing countries and immigrants from such countries. In the UK 50 years ago, rheumatic heart disease accounted for 90 per cent of all cardiac disease in pregnancy but, since the widespread use of antibiotics in streptococcal infection, this figure has fallen dramatically. Rheumatic heart disease nonetheless remains an important cause of cardiac disease in ethnic minority groups.

In contrast, advances in paediatric cardiac surgery since the mid-1960s have resulted in an increase in the number of women with congenital heart disease surviving to reach childbearing age. Congenital heart disease now accounts for approximately 50 per cent of pregnant women with heart disease in the UK. Furthermore, acquired ischaemic heart disease is becoming more common in pregnancy, as it is related to a delay in the average age of women experiencing childbirth as well as to smoking.

## Physiology

Irrespective of the underlying condition, pregnancy imposes a significant burden on the heart owing to the normal physiological changes that occur. Both blood volume and cardiac output increase by 40 per cent. The increase in cardiac output is achieved by an increase in stroke volume and a rise in heart rate of 12–15 beats per minute. These changes are discussed in more detail in Chapter 4.

## Maternal risks

The majority of pregnancies complicated with cardiac disease can be expected to have a favourable outcome for both the mother and fetus. However, maternal mortality is most likely to be seen in conditions that restrict an increase in pulmonary blood flow, typically pulmonary hypertension and mitral stenosis. In these circumstances, an obstruction exists either within the pulmonary vessels or at the mitral valve. The maternal mortality in pulmonary hypertension and Eisenmenger's syndrome is 40–50 per cent. In other complex cardiac conditions, such as Fallot's tetralogy, the risk of maternal mortality is much lower (i.e. 5 per cent), as there is no pulmonary

hypertension. Other common cardiac causes of maternal death are cardiomyopathy, rupture or dissection of the aorta or its branches, and ischaemic heart disease. Infective endocarditis is rare since the routine use of antibiotics but fatal cases do occur when the underlying heart defect (often a bicuspid aortic valve) is not recognized. Prior episodes of arrhythmia, cardiac failure, severe impairment of left ventricular function, left heart obstruction from aortic stenosis or hypertrophic cardiomyopathy may also have some effect on maternal morbidity during pregnancy.

## Fetal risks

The incidence of congenital heart disease in the general population is 8:1000 live births. If a parent is affected, the risk to the fetus is increased to 5 per cent. Therefore, all pregnant women with congenital heart disease should be referred for expert fetal cardiology scanning during the antenatal period. It is known that the fetus is at increased risk of intrauterine growth restriction (IUGR) and preterm birth in pregnancies complicated by cyanotic congenital heart disease. In some instances, the perinatal mortality rate may be as high as 40 per cent. Uncorrected coarctation of the aorta is also associated with IUGR in over 10 per cent of fetuses owing to reduced placental perfusion.

## Preconception management

Most women with cardiac disease will be aware of their condition prior to becoming pregnant. Ideally these women should be fully assessed before embarking on a pregnancy and the maternal and fetal risks carefully explained to them and their partners. A cardiologist should be involved in this assessment, which usually includes maternal echocardiography and electrocardiography (ECG). Any concurrent medical problems are promptly treated to optimize medical therapy. If there is a possibility that the cardiac disease will require surgical correction, it is recommended that this should be undertaken before conception if at all possible. Key points for discussion in preconception counselling of women with cardiac disease are shown (see box on p. 165).

## Antenatal management

The management of pregnant women with significant cardiac disease should take place in a joint obstetric cardiac clinic by experienced physicians and obstetricians. Continuity of care makes the detection of subtle changes in maternal well-being more likely. This is important because many of the symptoms and signs of cardiac failure, such as breathlessness, tachycardia, ankle swelling, a third heart sound and an ejection systolic heart murmur, are also common in low-risk pregnancies. In trying to distinguish between these normal symptoms and impending cardiac failure it is important that the woman is asked about any experiences of breathlessness at night when at rest, changes in her heart rate or rhythm, and increased tiredness or reduction in exercise tolerance. The physical examination of pregnant women with cardiac disease should include assessment of those aspects identified in the box below.

**Essential elements of the physical examination of pregnant women with cardiac disease**

- Pulse rate and rhythm
- Blood pressure
- Jugular venous pressure
- Presence of basal crepitations
- Ankle and sacral oedema
- Symphysis–fundal height measurement

In the majority of cases, women with cardiac disease will remain well during the antenatal period and outpatient management is usually possible. Midwives have a vital role to play in health promotion in order to optimize the health of the woman with cardiac disease and reduce the risk of her developing heart failure as a result of the pregnancy. This should include advice about reducing her normal physical activities, eating a well-balanced diet to avoid excessive weight gain and anaemia, and how to recognize respiratory, urinary and vaginal infections. It is important that any infection is treated promptly. Furthermore, midwives should also advise these women to seek an early dental appointment to detect and treat any caries and gum disease that may precipitate endocarditis. It is, therefore, important that the midwife recognizes the risk factors that may contribute to the development of cardiac failure.

**Risk factors contributing to cardiac failure**

- Respiratory or urinary infections
- Anaemia
- Obesity
- Multiple pregnancy
- Hypertension
- Arrhythmias
- Pain-related stress
- Fluid overload

Any signs of deteriorating cardiac status should be carefully investigated and treated. The condition of each woman should be assessed on an individual basis regarding the need for hospital admission for bed rest in order to reduce the workload of the heart. Psychological support from the midwife is important for those women who are admitted to hospital with complications, particularly in relation to the emotional effects of being separated from their families. Wherever possible, and providing the woman can get adequate rest at home, antenatal care provision within the community setting is preferred.

The hypercoagulable state in pregnancy increases the risk of thromboembolic disease in women who have arrhythmias, mitral valve stenosis or who have had mitral valve replacements. The use of anticoagulant therapy during pregnancy is both a complicated and controversial issue and will depend on the perceived degree of thrombotic risk and the woman's choice once the risks and benefits have been carefully explained.

In the non-pregnant state, warfarin is commonly used, but is teratogenic if used in the first trimester and is also associated with a high fetal loss rate. It also increases the risk of haemorrhage in the woman and fetus when used in the third trimester. Should labour commence whilst the woman is receiving warfarin, fresh-frozen plasma (FFP) and vitamin K should be given to reduce the risk of bleeding. Consequently, the use of unfractionated heparin may be used in early and late pregnancy, as it does not cross the placenta. However, prolonged use can result in heparin-induced complications, such as thrombocytopenia and osteoporosis. More recently, low-molecular-weight heparin in the form of enoxaparin given subcutaneously to women throughout pregnancy has been found to provide effective thromboprophylaxis with very few side effects. If the woman is admitted to hospital during pregnancy for rest and assessment, full-length thromboembolic (TED) support stockings should be worn. The woman should also continue to wear them during labour and in the immediate postnatal period.

## Treatment of cardiac failure in pregnancy

The development of cardiac failure in pregnancy may potentially have serious consequences for the woman and her fetus. The principles of treatment are the same as in the non-pregnant individual. The woman should be admitted to hospital and the diagnosis confirmed by clinical examination and echocardiogram. Drug therapy may include diuretics, vasodilators and digoxin. Oxygen and morphine may also be required. Dysrhythmias also require urgent correction and drug therapy, including selective beta-adrenergic blockade, may be required. In all cases, assessment of fetal well-being is essential and should include ultrasound to assess fetal growth and regular cardiotocography (CTG). If there is evidence of fetal compromise, premature birth may have to be considered. Similarly, in cases of intractable cardiac failure, the risks to the woman of continuing the pregnancy and the risks to the fetus of prematurity must be carefully balanced.

## Management of labour and birth

The least stressful labour for a woman with cardiac disease will be spontaneous in onset as this will minimize the risk of intervention and maximize the chances of a normal birth. It is, therefore, important that labour is planned and managed carefully with a coordinated team approach and good communication between midwife, obstetrician, cardiologist, neonatologist, anaesthetist and the woman and her family. Women with cardiac disease often have quite rapid, uncomplicated labours. Vaginal birth is preferred unless there is an obstetric indication for Caesarean section owing to the latter being associated with an increased risk of haemorrhage, thrombosis and infection: conditions that are less likely to be tolerated in women with cardiac disease. Induction of labour should be avoided if possible and only considered in very high-risk pregnancies to ensure that the birth occurs at a reasonably predictable time when all the relevant personnel are present or available. Prostaglandins should be used with particular caution, as they can cause a marked increase in cardiac output owing to their vasodilatory properties. Similarly, intravenous infusions of oxytocin cause a degree of fluid retention and may necessitate the use of a central venous pressure (CVP) line to monitor the woman's fluid balance closely and prevent fluid overload.

### The midwife's intrapartum management of a woman with cardiac disease

- Frequent measurement of temperature, pulse, blood pressure and urine output
- Pulse oximetry: administering oxygen therapy if oxygen saturation levels are <92 per cent
- Accurately monitoring and recording fluid balance
- Advising the woman on appropriate pain relief (e.g. epidural to reduce cardiac output and heart rate)
- Advising the woman on optimal position during labour: upright/left lateral to avoid supine hypotension
- Administering prophylactic antibiotics to those women with a structural heart defect to reduce bacterial endocarditis
- Encouraging the woman to push according to her own natural instinct giving several short pushes during each contraction
- Ensuring the second stage of labour is short: if the woman's condition deteriorates, a ventouse or forceps delivery should be undertaken
- Slowly administering intravenously no more than 5 IU syntocinon to deliver the placenta and membranes, and assist in controlling postpartum bleeding

## Specific congenital heart conditions affecting pregnancy

### Mitral stenosis

Mitral stenosis is the commonest acquired cardiac lesion accounting for 90 per cent of rheumatic valvular problems. The stenosis produces a left atrial obstruction with a consequent elevated left atrial and pulmonary wedge pressure (Figure 12.1). Eventually pulmonary oedema and atrial fibrillation may occur. There is a fixed cardiac output with limited ability to adapt to the increased demands placed on the heart during pregnancy by a raised intravascular volume and heart rate. The woman is at particular risk as the cardiac output increases in early pregnancy and also around the time of the baby's birth as the third stage of labour leads to

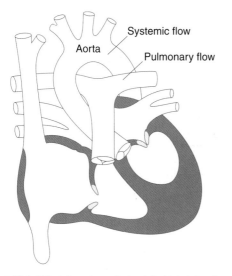

**Figure 12.1** Mitral stenosis producing left atrial obstruction.

autotransfusion of blood from the uterus into the venous circulation. Surgical valvotomy in suitable cases should ideally be undertaken before pregnancy, although it may be safely performed during pregnancy.

### Eisenmenger's syndrome

Eisenmenger's syndrome is associated with a very high maternal mortality rate: between 40 and 50 per cent. It is a condition that is caused by a left to right shunt of blood through a ventricular septal defect, atrial septal defect or a patent ductus arteriosus, resulting in an increase in pulmonary blood flow. In time, this leads to fibrosis and the development of pulmonary hypertension. Eventually the shunt reverses and cyanosis occurs (Figure 12.2). The major risk in pregnancy is during labour and birth when there may be sudden changes in systemic vascular resistance leading to increased right to left shunting and reduction in oxygen saturation. Women with this condition are advised against pregnancy because of the very high maternal mortality rate. Where the woman decides to continue with the pregnancy, miscarriage, prematurity and IUGR are common because of the relative hypoxia and cyanosis to the fetus.

### Coarctation of the aorta

Although coarctation of the aorta may be detected in childhood, and has consequently usually been repaired, in less severe cases it may not present until the second and third decades when hypertension develops. The principal risk is of dissection of the aorta associated with the increased cardiac output of pregnancy and a possible increase in medial vessel degeneration. In addition, endocarditis, intracranial haemorrhage and death have been reported. There is

**Figure 12.2** Eisenmenger's syndrome: initial left-to-right shunting is reversed, with consequent cyanosis.

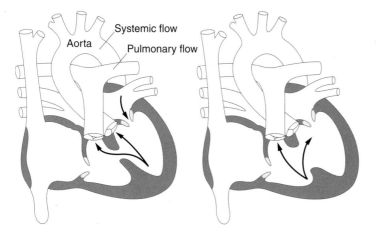

a 2 per cent risk that the fetus will also develop coarctation of the aorta. Furthermore, where coarctation of the aorta has not been repaired, the risk of maternal death is approximately 15 per cent and so the option of termination should be discussed with the woman and her family. During the antenatal period, the development of hypertension is the most serious sign and should be promptly treated so as to reduce the consequential effects on maternal morbidity and mortality.

## Marfan's syndrome

Marfan's syndrome is caused by an autosomal dominant defect on chromosome 15. It is a connective tissue abnormality that affects the musculoskeletal system, the cardiovascular system and the eyes. The cardiovascular abnormalities are the most life-threatening, as the elastic fibres in the media of the blood vessels weaken. This may lead to mitral valve prolapse and aortic regurgitation, as well as aortic root dilatation, which may be followed by aortic dissection or rupture, or both. The mean age at which these events occur is 32 years, often resulting in premature death. Pregnancy increases the risk of aortic rupture or dissection and has been associated with maternal mortality of up to 50 per cent where there is very marked aortic root dilatation. Echocardiography is the principal investigation, as it is able to determine the size of the aortic root and the degree of regurgitation. Serial echocardiography should be performed throughout pregnancy, especially in women who enter pregnancy with an aortic root that is already dilated.

## Hypertensive disorders

## Prevalence

Hypertensive disease complicates 5–7 per cent of all pregnancies and is a significant cause of maternal and fetal/neonatal morbidity and mortality. It is considered that the placenta is the main contributory cause, as the disease regresses following the birth of the baby. The aetiology and pathophysiology are detailed in Chapter 10. The National High Blood Pressure Education Program – Working Group on High Blood Pressure in Pregnancy (2000) defines five major categories of hypertension during pregnancy as follows.

- *Chronic hypertension/pre-existing hypertension.*
  This is hypertension diagnosed before pregnancy

or assumed when a woman is diagnosed with a rise in blood pressure >140/90 mmHg before 20 weeks of pregnancy that persists 6 weeks after the baby is born.
- *Gestational hypertension/pregnancy-induced hypertension.* This occurs when hypertension first develops in a woman who is known to be normotensive after 20 weeks of pregnancy without any significant proteinuria or any other features of pre-eclampsia. It is diagnosed when, after resting, the woman's blood pressure rises above 140/90 mmHg on at least two occasions no more than 1 week apart. However, it is also recommended that pregnant women should be closely observed where there is a rise in diastolic blood pressure of at least 15 mmHg, or a rise in systolic blood pressure of at least 30 mmHg (compared to the blood pressure at the initial antenatal visit), especially if there is also proteinuria.
- *Pre-eclampsia and eclampsia* These are considered in Chapters 10 and 16.
- *Pre-eclampsia superimposed by chronic hypertension.* This may occur in women with pre-existing hypertension before 20 weeks of pregnancy who consequently develop proteinuria, a sudden increase in pre-existing hypertension, thrombocytopenia and abnormal liver enzymes.

## Physiology

As the blood pressure falls in the first trimester, pregnancy may mask pre-existing hypertension. Blood pressure rises again in the third trimester and, therefore, if hypertension is noted for the first time in the third trimester, this may be due to unrecognized chronic hypertension, pregnancy-induced hypertension or pre-eclampsia. Often a clear diagnosis is only possible several months after birth when the blood pressure either reverts to normal or remains elevated.

Significant proteinuria is defined as 0.3 g/L or more in a 24-hour urine sample. Although reagent strips give an indication as to the degree of proteinuria, accurate quantification relies on a 24-hour collection. Other causes of proteinuria include renal disease, vaginal discharge or contamination, and urinary tract infection. Oedema is a non-specific generalized accumulation of fluid, which affects more than 50 per cent of pregnant women and, therefore, is not a useful indicator to diagnose pre-eclampsia.

## Chronic hypertension/pre-existing hypertension

Essential hypertension is the underlying cause in 90 per cent of cases presenting with hypertension in pregnancy. The causes are listed separately (see box below). Before a diagnosis of essential hypertension is made, these other possible causes need to be excluded. Irrespective of the underlying cause, the principal concern for health professionals caring for the woman is the possibility she may develop pre-eclampsia. This may occur in up to one-third of women with pre-existing hypertension and is more likely in women with severe hypertension, defined as a diastolic blood pressure of 110 mmHg or higher before 20 weeks' gestation, and in those with renal disease. Risk factors for women developing pre-eclampsia superimposed by chronic hypertension with the consequential risk of placental abruption, heart failure and intracerebral haemorrhage are listed separately (see box). Abruption is rare but, in severe hypertensive disease, the risk is approximately 10 per cent. Fetal risks include IUGR from placental insufficiency. Maternal and neonatal morbidity and mortality are closely related to the degree of severity of maternal hypertension and the gestational age of the fetus at the time of birth.

---

**Causes of chronic hypertension**

- Essential hypertension
- Renal disease
  - Glomerulonephritis
  - Polycystic disease
  - Diabetic nephropathy
- Renal artery stenosis
- Collagen vascular disease
  - Systemic lupus erythematosus
  - Scleroderma
- Coarctation of the aorta
- Endocrine disease
  - Phaeochromocytoma
  - Conn's syndrome

---

**Risk factors for women developing pre-eclampsia superimposed by chronic hypertension**

- Blood pressure >160/100 mmHg in early pregnancy
- Renal disease
- Maternal age >40 years
- Diabetes mellitus
- Connective tissue disease (e.g. systemic lupus erythematosus and antiphospholipid syndrome)
- Coarctation of the aorta

---

## Management of hypertension in pregnancy

The midwife is in a unique position to identify women who are at risk of developing hypertensive disorders in pregnancy by undertaking a comprehensive history at the first antenatal visit. This should include identifying any social factors, underlying medical conditions and aspects of the woman's family history that may increase her risk of developing hypertension. Blood pressure should never be assessed immediately after a woman has experienced anxiety, pain, undertaken a period of exercise or has smoked. An interval of at least 10 minutes is recommended before measuring the blood pressure in these circumstances.

Whenever the midwife discovers a woman's blood pressure is elevated for the first time in pregnancy, she should refer the management to the obstetrician. Consequently, appropriate investigations should be performed to exclude renal, cardiac and autoimmune disease. These may include assessment of creatinine, electrolytes and urate levels, liver function tests, 24-hour urinary protein/creatinine clearance, renal scan and cardiac investigations, such as ECG and echocardiography. In mild cases (blood pressure <150/100 mmHg), there is no immediate indication to treat. The pregnancy, however, should be monitored carefully by the community midwife to detect any rise in blood pressure or features of pre-eclampsia, such as proteinuria, or IUGR. If the latter is detected, serial ultrasound examination may be necessary in such pregnancies.

If the blood pressure is consistently noted to be >150/100 mmHg, antihypertensive therapy will need to be introduced or recommended. This is to reduce the risk of severe hypertension and the consequential risks of maternal intracerebral haemorrhage and heart failure. However, women who are receiving antihypertensive therapy before pregnancy are often able to discontinue this for the first part of pregnancy because of the physiological fall in blood pressure during this time. Some antihypertensives, such as the angiotensin-converting enzyme (ACE) inhibitors, should be discontinued because of the teratogenic effect on the developing fetus. Care should be taken not to lower the blood pressure excessively, as this may adversely affect the fetus by reducing placental blood flow. Preferred antihypertensive agents include methyldopa (centrally acting agent), labetalol (alpha- and beta-blocker) and nifedipine (calcium-channel blocker). The aim of antihypertensive medication is to maintain the blood pressure below 160 mmHg systolic and 100–110 mmHg diastolic. The optimum target blood pressure to reduce the risk to the woman, without compromising the fetus, however, is disputed and is currently the subject of clinical studies.

## Management of labour and birth

When caring for a woman with hypertensive disease during labour, the midwife should remain with her at all times should her condition suddenly worsen. It is essential to monitor the maternal and fetal condition carefully, noting any marked deviations and seeking prompt medical assistance. The woman with mild hypertensive disease will require less intensive care than a woman with severe pre-eclampsia. However, continuous fetal monitoring is advocated in labour, especially if the fetus is IUGR. An epidural may provide the best pain relief, reduce the blood pressure and facilitate a prompt Caesarean section should the need arise. Depending on the maternal and fetal condition, a short second stage of labour may be advocated and, if the woman is unable to birth her baby, a ventouse or forceps delivery may be indicated. Oxytocin is the preferred agent for the management of the third stage of labour, as ergometrine and syntometrine will cause vasoconstriction and increase hypertension.

## Renal disease

Having a good understanding of the changes that occur in renal physiology and function in low-risk pregnancies (Chapter 4) will assist the midwife in understanding the effects that pregnancy may have on existing renal disease, and the predisposition that

many women have to develop urinary tract infections in pregnancy.

## Asymptomatic bacteriuria

Asymptomatic bacteriuria occurs in 2–10 per cent of pregnant women and the most common causative organism is *Escherichia coli* (*E. coli*) and less commonly streptococci, *Proteus*, *Pseudomonas* and *Klebsiella* are implicated. It is, therefore, important that all women should be screened for bacteriuria at their first antenatal visit with the midwife. Diagnosis is made if there are more than 100 000 bacteria/mL of urine. If the infection is not treated, 20–30 per cent of these women will develop symptomatic urinary tract infections, such as cystitis and pyelonephritis. Such infections may pose a risk to maternal and fetal well-being and precipitate the onset of preterm labour. Consequently, it is considered beneficial to treat all women diagnosed with asymptomatic bacteriuria with antibiotics. Furthermore, women who develop recurrent urinary tract infections may require prophylactic antibiotics throughout pregnancy.

## Cystitis

This is an infection of the urinary bladder and occurs in approximately 1.5 per cent of pregnancies. Women usually experience dysuria, haematuria, frequency/urgency of micturition accompanied by suprapubic pain. Diagnosis is made by culture from a midstream specimen of urine (MSSU) and treatment is by antibiotics, usually ampicillin or oral cephalosporins. Further testing of the urine should be undertaken, as the condition may recur. Midwives should encourage women to drink plenty of fluids, to avoid acidic and carbonated drinks, and advise them regarding perineal hygiene and emptying the bladder immediately following sexual intercourse. If women are able to tolerate acidic drinks, midwives can also advise them to drink cranberry juice. The tannin in cranberries is thought to prevent p-fimbriated *E. coli* from attaching themselves to uroepithelial cells, thereby inhibiting infection. Should signs and symptoms of further infection occur, the woman should be advised to notify her midwife or general practitioner (GP) as ascending infection could lead to the more serious condition of pyelonephritis.

## Pyelonephritis

Pyelonephritis occurs in 1–2 per cent of all pregnancies. It is a condition in which the renal tubules become inflamed and their ability to reabsorb sodium is greatly affected. Consequently, this leads to oedema and increased pressure on the cardiovascular system with decreased urine output. The woman feels extremely unwell and shows signs and symptoms consisting of pyrexia (which may reach 40°C), rigors, tachycardia, nausea and vomiting, leading to dehydration. In addition, there is usually pain and tenderness over the loin area, which may be accompanied by muscle guarding. Anaemia may be present and the woman may also complain of dysuria and frequency of micturition. It is important that the woman is referred to a doctor immediately. Diagnosis is confirmed by microscopic examination of a MSSU. This will reveal pus cells and 100 000 bacteria/mL of urine, the causative organism often being *E. coli*. The urine is usually cloudy, acidic and has an offensive smell.

Pyelonephritis also poses a marked risk to the fetus in that the incidence of miscarriage and preterm labour is increased. In addition, maternal pyrexia may result in intrauterine fetal death. IUGR and fetal hypoxia may also result owing to reduced maternal plasma volume leading to poor placental perfusion. Furthermore, the diagnosis of preterm labour may not always be easily recognized as the severe pain the woman experiences may mask the pain of uterine contractions. Consequently diagnosis can be made by CTG.

### Subsequent management

Once pyelonephritis has been diagnosed, the woman is usually admitted to hospital for rest, observation and treatment as, in the acute stages, significant complications such as preterm labour, transient renal failure, acute respiratory distress syndrome, sepsis and shock may develop. Intravenous antibiotics (e.g. cephalosporins or gentamicin) are usually administered initially and, once the pyrexia and any vomiting settles, oral antibiotics may be taken. Although the woman is encouraged to drink plenty of fluids to avoid urinary stasis, if there is severe nausea and vomiting, intravenous fluids may be required to prevent dehydration. It is important that the midwife maintains an accurate record of fluid balance in order to assess renal function.

The midwife should undertake 4-hourly observation of temperature, pulse and respiration and, if the woman is pyrexial, tepid sponging, a fan and antipyretics may be used. Lying on the unaffected side may help to reduce the woman's pain and assist urinary drainage. Analgesics are prescribed and administered as and when required. Bearing in mind the risks of immobility, the midwife should ensure the woman is wearing TED stockings, and is encouraged to perform circulatory leg and deep breathing exercises, as she feels able. The doctor may prescribe low-dose heparin therapy to women who are considered at high risk of developing deep vein thrombosis. In addition, the haemoglobin is assessed and any anaemia treated.

Antibiotic therapy usually continues for 10 days and then a further MSSU is obtained for bacteriological examination 2 weeks after the completion of the treatment and monthly until the baby is born to ensure there is no recurrence. If the woman has a urinary tract infection at the time of birth, the baby is at substantial risk of congenital infection and will need antibiotic therapy in the neonatal period. Three months following the baby's birth, an intravenous pyelogram and other renal investigations, such as a cystoscopy, may be carried out to ensure there is no abnormality of the renal tract giving rise to the persistent or recurrent infection that is with or without symptoms.

## Chronic renal disease

The underlying pathophysiology associated with pyelonephritis leads to the same maternal and fetal sequelae in chronic renal disease. This condition is further complicated by impaired blood supply to the kidneys as a result of renal tissue damage. When this occurs, renin is produced to increase the blood supply resulting in a rise in blood pressure. A number of conditions may give rise to chronic renal disease, such as chronic pyelonephritis, glomerulonephritis, diabetic nephropathy and systemic lupus erythematosus (SLE), which the midwife needs to be aware of when taking a medical history from the woman during the antenatal period.

The outcome of pregnancy is dependent on the nature and severity of the renal disease, and the degree of loss of renal function. Where renal function is mildly affected (serum creatinine <125 μmol/L) and there is no hypertension, the outcome is usually good. However, renal disease combined with hypertension is associated with miscarriage, superimposed pre-eclampsia, IUGR, preterm birth and increased perinatal mortality.

Ideally, assessment of renal function prior to conception should take place in order to advise the woman and her partner about the dangers of embarking on a pregnancy.

*Subsequent management*

The overall aim of antenatal care is to prevent further deterioration in renal function. This may necessitate more frequent antenatal visits to assess maternal and fetal well-being with close liaison between the midwife, obstetrician and nephrologist. Renal function tests that involve serum urate, electrolyte, urea and creatinine levels, 24-hour creatinine clearance and urinalysis to screen for glycosuria, proteinuria and haematuria should be undertaken on a regular basis along with monitoring the woman's blood pressure. Urine cultures should also be undertaken frequently in order to detect urinary tract infections. The midwife can advise the woman about recognizing the signs and symptoms of such infections so that treatment can be promptly commenced. In chronic renal disease, the production of erythropoietin is suppressed resulting in anaemia. Fetal well-being is assessed by the use of serial ultrasound scans and Doppler flow studies from 24 weeks of pregnancy. If renal function deteriorates, proteinuria increases and blood pressure rises and, if there is any evidence of fetal compromise, the woman should be advised that hospital admission is necessary.

The course of the pregnancy will determine the mode and time of labour and birth: labour consequently may be spontaneous or induced. If the maternal condition becomes life threatening at any stage of the pregnancy, the risks and benefits of continuing with the pregnancy should be discussed with the woman and her partner/family; for some, this may indicate a Caesarean section.

## Acute renal failure

The first sign of acute renal failure is a fall in urinary output of $<500$ mL in 24 hours. However, in pregnancy, such a condition is rare being $<0.005$ per cent, but mild to moderate renal impairment may occur in 1:8000 pregnancies. The kidneys are unable to excrete creatinine and urea leading to acidosis. Acute renal failure is associated with severe haemorrhage, preeclampsia and eclampsia, and infection, including septic abortion. However, it is rarely attributed to pyelonephritis. Despite this condition being rare, it is serious and unpredictable and, as a result, all women with renal failure should be transferred to a unit where renal dialysis is available. The management of acute renal failure will depend on the cause: either renal or prerenal (e.g. hypovolaemia).

*Subsequent management*

Midwives need to be aware that management of acute renal failure involves the avoidance/treatment of uraemia, acidosis, hyperkalaemia and fluid overload, and renal dialysis may be required in some cases. It is essential that, whilst the woman is extremely ill, the multidisciplinary team (including the midwife) provide psychological support to her and her family during such a stressful period. It is also important that, during the postnatal period, the woman is made fully aware of the nature of her illness and its effects on subsequent pregnancies.

## Renal transplant

Pregnancies occur in 1:20 women following a successful renal transplant. Preconception advice is important, however, to ensure that the woman is in optimal health before embarking on a pregnancy, This will include ensuring that the woman is normotensive, that her serum creatinine levels are within the normal range and that there is an absence of urinary tract infections/asymptomatic bacteriuria. It is also recommended that the woman avoids pregnancy for at least 2 years after transplantation to ensure success of the graft.

*Subsequent management*

Throughout pregnancy, the woman's health is closely monitored by the midwife, obstetrician and nephrologist with frequent assessment of renal function including urinalysis, blood pressure, haemoglobin levels and the status of the graft being undertaken. Close monitoring of the fetus is also required to detect any IUGR. Immunosuppressive drug therapy, such as prednisolone and azathioprine, is usually continued throughout pregnancy with the dose at the lowest possible maintenance level. Although the effect of such drugs on the pregnancy and fetus are unknown, they are likely to make the woman more susceptible to infection, especially urinary tract infections. The woman may also develop hypertension and anaemia.

Labour may be spontaneous unless there are obstetric reasons to intervene earlier. During labour, steroid therapy is increased and antibiotics given prophylactically for any surgical intervention, including episiotomy. The newborn baby will be more vulnerable to infection as immunosuppressive therapy reduces the transmission of maternal antibodies to the fetus. Whilst breast feeding should be possible, it is usually not advised owing to the uncertainties surrounding the effects of some of the drugs.

## Endocrine disorders

## Diabetes mellitus

### Definition
The World Health Organization has defined diabetes mellitus as either a raised fasting blood glucose level of >7.8 mmol/L or a level of >11.1 mmol/L 2 hours following a 75 g oral glucose load (WHO 1999). The significance of impaired glucose tolerance (2-hour value 7.8–11.1 mmol/L) in pregnancy has been much debated, but many now feel that it is unlikely to have any untoward effect on pregnancy outcome unless the WHO criteria for diabetes are reached.

### Physiology
Significant hormonal changes affect carbohydrate metabolism during pregnancy. In particular, there is an increase in human placental lactogen and cortisol, both of which are insulin antagonists and, therefore, the woman develops relative insulin resistance. These changes are most marked during the third trimester. To balance these changes during normal pregnancy, the maternal pancreas secretes increased amounts of insulin to maintain carbohydrate metabolism. Typically, in pregnancy, this will result in a fall in the fasting level of glucose. In contrast, following a carbohydrate challenge, the levels of glucose are higher than in the non-pregnant state. Glucose crosses the placenta by means of a facilitated diffusion process and the fetal blood glucose level closely follows the maternal level. Fetal glucose levels are, therefore, normally maintained within narrow limits, if the maternal levels are also well controlled.

Diabetes may complicate a pregnancy either because a woman has pre-existing insulin-dependent diabetes mellitus (IDDM) or non-insulin dependent diabetes mellitus (NIDDM) before pregnancy, or she may develop an impaired glucose tolerance or diabetes during the course of her pregnancy (gestational diabetes).

Approximately 1–2 per cent of pregnant women will develop gestational diabetes. Certain groups of women are more likely to develop diabetes at some time during their life and are recognized as potential diabetics. There are a number of important risk factors of which the midwife should be aware (see box below).

---

**Risk factors for the development of diabetes mellitus in pregnancy**

- Obesity (body mass index >30)
- Family history of diabetes
- Previous baby >4.5 kg
- Previous unexplained stillbirth
- Previous congenital abnormality

---

### Maternal mortality and morbidity
Maternal mortality as a consequence of diabetic pregnancies has become a very rare event. Those at most risk are women with pre-existing coronary artery disease. In general, the maternal morbidity is related to the severity of diabetic-related disease preceding the pregnancy. The complications associated with diabetic pregnancies that may affect the health of the woman are identified (see box).

---

**Maternal complications of diabetic pregnancies**

- Nephropathy (temporary worsening: improves after the birth of the baby)
- Retinopathy (progression)
- Coronary artery disease
- Hyperglycaemia/hypoglycaemia/ketoacidosis
- Pre-eclampsia (increased 2–4-fold)
- Infection
- Thromboembolic disease (as a result of increased incidence of operative births)

---

The importance of good glycaemic control during pregnancy is reinforced by the direct relationship between blood glucose levels and the incidence of fetal and maternal complications. For this reason, women who plan to become pregnant should be advised to aim for optimal control of their diabetes prior to conception and throughout pregnancy. This may necessitate a change to insulin therapy prior to conception in women with NIDDM. Midwives can play a part in advising women of the risks of pregnancy and diabetes, and the importance of diet, exercise and the careful self-monitoring of their glucose levels: a critical aspect of care. This helps to highlight excessive swings in blood glucose levels. Women who have IDDM are likely to require increased insulin doses during pregnancy and, if they are using insulin twice daily, they may often have to change to a four times daily insulin regime.

### Fetal and neonatal complications

As there is an increased risk of miscarriage and congenital fetal abnormality associated with diabetes, it is important that there is good diabetic control, particularly prior to conception, in order to reduce these risks substantially. Measurement of glycosylated haemoglobin (HbA1c) gives a retrospective assessment of diabetic control: high levels in early pregnancy are associated with neural tube defects, congenital heart disease, cleft palate and other spinal anomalies, including the rare caudal regression syndrome. Congenital abnormalities are the most common cause of morbidity and mortality in diabetic pregnancies, and are 2–4 times more common than in low-risk pregnancies. Currently, malformations contribute to 40 per cent of the perinatal mortality associated with diabetic pregnancies. The mechanism that gives rise to these abnormalities is not fully understood, but it is thought that hyperglycaemia in the critical stages of organogenesis may be the underlying cause.

Apart from structural malformations, fetal macrosomia as shown in Figure 12.3, is a major problem associated with traumatic birth and shoulder dystocia (Chapter 16) and, therefore, possible hypoxic damage. Accelerated growth patterns are typically seen in the late second and third trimesters, and are associated

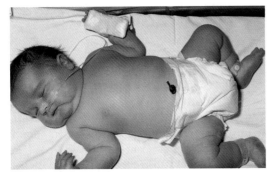

**Figure 12.3** The 5.1-kg macrosomic infant of a diabetic mother.

with poorly controlled diabetes. Sudden, unexplained, late stillbirths occur in 10–30 per cent of diabetic pregnancies but have become much less common since the importance of good diabetic control and appropriate time of birth has been appreciated. However, there still remains a risk of late stillbirths in women whose diabetes is poorly controlled or who have vascular disease, and in pregnancies complicated by macrosomia or polyhydramnios. The reasons for such an event are not fully understood, although several possible mechanisms may contribute to chronic hypoxia and fetal acidosis.

### Neonatal complications

Neonatal morbidity in diabetic pregnancies has fallen dramatically over the last three decades, as a consequence of the improvement of glucose control during the antenatal period. However, morbidity still remains significantly higher in this group of babies compared to those babies born to non-diabetic women. Babies born to women with diabetes should be closely monitored in the early neonatal period for possible complications, especially hypoglycaemia and respiratory distress syndrome.

---

**Causes of neonatal morbidity associated with diabetic pregnancies**

- Congenital abnormalities
  - cardiac
  - neural tube defects
- Macrosomia
  - birth asphyxia
  - traumatic birth injury (e.g. brachial plexus injury)
- Respiratory distress syndrome
- Hypoglycaemia
- Hypomagnesaemia
- Polycythaemia
- Hyperbilirubinaemia

---

Neonatal hypoglycaemia following the birth of the baby is anticipated, particularly in the first 24 hours, because the infant continues to produce large amounts of insulin in the immediate neonatal period due to recent fetal hyperglycaemia. However, once the umbilical cord is clamped, the baby is no longer exposed to high levels of glucose from the mother. Midwives should encourage women to breast feed their baby straight after the birth and at frequent intervals

(3–4 hourly) to prevent hypoglycaemia. The baby's blood glucose levels should be assessed 1–2 hours following birth and then every 4–6 hours for the first 24–48 hours with the aim to maintain the blood glucose of at least 2 mmol/L. Less common complications include hypocalcaemia and magnesium deficiency that can lead to apnoeic episodes and convulsions in extreme cases. Fetal hyperinsulinaemia during pregnancy also leads to an increase in red cell production resulting in polycythaemia, which may need correction by a partial exchange blood transfusion. The rapid breakdown of the excess red blood cells and the relative immaturity of the newborn liver predisposes these babies to jaundice. This may also be exacerbated if there is bruising as a result of any birth trauma.

## Screening for diabetes in pregnancy

This is an extremely controversial area since there is no agreed definition for gestational diabetes in terms of specific blood glucose levels and it is disputed whether treatment of gestational diabetes, however defined, improves fetal and neonatal outcome. Many confounding variables, especially maternal weight, increase both the risk of diabetes and of macrosomia, thus making causality hard to prove. Screening for diabetes in pregnancy can be justified to diagnose previously unrecognized cases of pre-existing diabetes and to identify a group of women who are at risk of developing NIDDM later in life. No single screening test has been shown to be perfect in terms of high sensitivity and specificity for gestational diabetes. Urinary glucose is unreliable and most screening tests now rely on blood glucose estimation. Many maternity units use an oral glucose tolerance test, but this is expensive, time-consuming and does not have good reproducibility in pregnancy. Other units use a random blood glucose test (interpreted according to the time since the last meal) or a blood glucose test undertaken 1 hour following a 50-g glucose meal (sometimes called a mini glucose tolerance test).

## Antenatal management

Pregnant women with diabetes and their partners should be seen in a combined clinic by a multidisciplinary team that includes a physician, an obstetrician with a specialist interest in diabetes in pregnancy, a specialist diabetic nurse, a specialist midwife and dietician. The aim of treatment is to maintain the blood glucose level as near normal as possible, with a combination of diet and insulin (i.e. the pre-meal blood glucose level between 5.0 and 6.0 mmol/L and post-meal levels of <7.8 mmol/L). In women with IDDM, this will usually require three or four daily doses of insulin or the newer rapidly acting insulin analogues. All women with diabetes should be encouraged and supported by the team to monitor their condition at home using their own glucose meters. Long-term control may be assessed using glycosylated haemoglobin measurements, which should be ≤7 per cent, and the dose of insulin adjusted accordingly.

Women with diabetes also have a predisposition to urinary and vaginal infections in pregnancy. These should be discussed with the midwife so that the women are more able to recognize the signs and symptoms, and seek treatment as soon as possible. Furthermore, in view of the potential risks to fetal development of maternal diabetes, it is important that these women and their partners are advised regarding appropriate screening tests in order to make an informed choice. This may include nuchal translucency scanning, detailed ultrasound assessment for fetal anomalies and fetal echocardiography. Serial growth scans may also be recommended to detect fetal macrosomia, although this is rarely a problem before the third trimester, and developing polyhydramnios. In addition, increased surveillance may include Doppler ultrasound and CTG. Any concern that the midwife may have regarding maternal and fetal well-being should be promptly relayed to the obstetrician and other members of the multidisciplinary team. In principle, if the pregnancy has remained uneventful, the management attempts to achieve a vaginal birth between 38 and 40 weeks' gestation. However, the development of macrosomia, reduced fetal movements at or near term, with a non-reassuring CTG, or maternal complications, such as pre-eclampsia, should lead to the birth of the baby being expedited as a priority. The rate of failed induction is such that the Caesarean section rate amongst pregnant women with diabetes can be as high as 50 per cent.

The management of preterm labour or polyhydramnios is particularly difficult in diabetic pregnancies. Tocolytics, such as ritodrine or salbutamol, are also diabetogenic and will tend to elevate blood glucose levels. In addition, the administration of intramuscular steroids to improve fetal lung maturity will also destabilize diabetic control. Under these circumstances, increasing doses of insulin are required and an intravenous infusion of insulin and glucose may be appropriate to ensure normoglycaemia.

## Management of labour and birth

During either spontaneous or induced labour, the midwife should ensure that normoglycaemia is maintained using a sliding scale of insulin (i.e. <7.0 mmol/L) and testing the blood glucose levels at hourly intervals. As women with diabetes are susceptible to infection, the midwife should ensure that vaginal examinations are kept to a minimum. Continuous fetal monitoring is advised and fetal scalp blood sampling should be undertaken in the presence of an abnormal CTG. Pain relief, such as epidural analgesia, assists in regulating the blood sugar levels and preventing the development of metabolic acidosis in women with diabetes. An epidural is also useful if difficulties arise with the birth of the shoulders or an operative birth is required.

## Postnatal and neonatal care

Following the birth of the baby, the insulin requirements of women with IDDM will rapidly fall and return to pre-pregnancy levels. The intravenous insulin infusion should be reduced by at least 50 per cent and, once carbohydrate metabolism returns to normal, the woman can resume her pre-pregnancy insulin regimen with the infusion discontinued. The diabetic team should review those women who have NIDDM or gestational diabetes to ascertain the best management to maintain normoglycaemia (e.g. oral hypoglycaemics or dietary control). If the woman chooses to breast feed her baby, midwives should be aware that an additional carbohydrate intake of 40–50 g/day is recommended to sustain lactation and the woman's insulin therapy may also need adjusting. In addition, midwives should be aware that women with diabetes are susceptible to infection and delayed healing. It is important that the midwife ensures the baby is correctly positioned at the breast to avoid trauma to the nipples and carefully observes that any perineal/abdominal wound is healing satisfactorily. The administration of antibiotics as a preventative measure may be considered in such instances.

Throughout pregnancy and during the postnatal period, midwives are in an ideal position to offer contraceptive advice to diabetic women to ensure they achieve optimum metabolic control prior to planning the next pregnancy. As the combined oral contraceptive pill may alter carbohydrate metabolism, some women may need increased doses of insulin. Furthermore, the risk of thromboembolism is higher in diabetic women who take the combined contraceptive pill. However, intrauterine contraceptive devices can be an alternative method for diabetic women to choose as they are not only effective, but also the risk of infection is no different than in women who do not have diabetes. In those cases where diabetes is generally well controlled and the effects of a further pregnancy would not result in diabetic complications, the midwife could suggest barrier methods of contraception as a suitable method of contraception. The midwife should provide full details of each method to women with diabetes and their partners so that they are able to make an informed choice suitable to their individual lifestyles.

A full glucose tolerance test is usually performed in the puerperium at 6 weeks to ensure that the diabetes has subsequently resolved in those women who experienced gestational diabetes. However, it is recommended that women with IDDM, gestational diabetes or impaired glucose tolerance are reviewed at a combined diabetic clinic at 6 weeks, especially as gestational diabetes has a high recurrence rate in subsequent pregnancies.

# Thyroid disorders

Pregnancy has a significant impact on the normal maternal thyroid physiology. During pregnancy, the production of thyroid-binding globulin by the liver doubles as a result of oestrogenic stimulation. As a consequence there is an increased amount of total thyroxine (T4) and tri-iodothyronine (T3). However, there is no significant change in the amount of circulating free thyroid hormone (FT4 and FT3) (Chapter 4). The renal clearance of iodine increases in pregnancy. The physiological changes in metabolism during pregnancy make the diagnosis of thyroid conditions difficult, as the hormonal changes and metabolic demands result in complex alterations in the biochemical parameters of thyroid function.

## Maternal hyperthyroidism (thyrotoxicosis)

The incidence of maternal hyperthyroidism is approximately 1:500 pregnancies. In the majority of cases, the condition has been diagnosed before pregnancy and 90 per cent of cases are secondary to Graves' disease. This autoimmune disorder is associated with the presence of circulating thyroid-stimulating antibodies and an enlarged thyroid gland (goitre). Less common causes of hyperthyroidism include:

- toxic nodules;
- Hashimoto's thyroiditis;

- multinodular goitre;
- trophoblastic disease (extremely rare).

The condition should be suspected in any woman who fails to gain weight satisfactorily despite a good appetite. Other symptoms include goitre, exophthalmos, eyelid lag and persistent tachycardia. Clinical diagnosis is difficult as the physiological signs and symptoms pregnant women normally experience, such as heat intolerance, palpitations and mood lability, may mask this condition.

Antenatal management

If there is a past history, or clinical suspicion of thyroid disease, the midwife should refer the woman to the medical team, consisting of obstetrician and endocrinologist, to be reviewed on a monthly basis throughout pregnancy. Thyroid function tests (including a free T4) should be performed. Hyperthyroidism is confirmed by high levels of FT4 and FT3, with reduced levels of thyroid-stimulating hormone (TSH). Uncontrolled maternal hyperthyroidism is associated with maternal cardiac arrhythmias, including atrial fibrillation, diarrhoea, vomiting, abdominal pains and psychosis. If the underlying aetiology is autoimmune disease, the thyroid-stimulating antibodies may cross the placenta and cause fetal thyrotoxicosis and goitre. If untreated, there is an increased risk of pre-eclampsia, miscarriage, low birth weight, pre-term labour and perinatal mortality. In women who are poorly controlled, there is a risk of a thyroid crisis, or storm, precipitated by infection or stress. The woman presents with hyperpyrexia, palpitations and tachycardia that may lead to heart failure, especially in labour. It is a medical emergency requiring oxygen, cooling, hydrating, antibiotics and drug therapy to halt the production and reduce the effects of thyroid hormone.

Following the diagnosis of hyperthyroidism, the treatment during pregnancy should be drug therapy with carbimazole or propylthiouracil (PTU), aiming to maintain maternal FT3 and FT4 levels in the high/normal range. Radioactive iodine is contraindicated because it completely obliterates the fetal thyroid gland. The lowest dose of carbimazole or PTU must be used as high doses cross the placenta and may cause fetal hypothyroidism. However, in severe hyperthyroidism, it is important to control the disease as quickly as possible, if necessary with high doses of antithyroid drugs. Occasionally, beta-blockers and surgical treatment may also be indicated. Careful monitoring of maternal thyroid function is essential under these circumstances. The midwife has an important role in advising the woman about achieving a healthy diet, preventing infection and ensuring that, if nausea and vomiting become a problem, fluid loss is closely monitored and the woman is made aware of the signs of dehydration and how to prevent it.

Subsequent midwifery management

During labour, the midwife should carefully assess the woman's temperature, heart rate and rhythm in order to observe for signs of a thyroid crisis/storm developing and promptly summon medical assistance should it be necessary. Should a woman with hyperthyroidism wish to breast feed her baby, the midwife can advise her that this is possible. However, as PTU crosses into the breast milk to a lesser extent, this would be the drug of choice to use in the postnatal period. The dosage should not exceed 150 mg/day. It is debatable as to whether the thyroid function of a baby who is breast feeding should be monitored while the woman is taking antithyroid drugs. Furthermore, it is important that the woman's thyroid function should be assessed following the birth of her baby, as the condition may develop again in the postnatal period.

## Maternal hypothyroidism

Worldwide, the commonest cause of hypothyroidism is decreased activity of the thyroid gland as a result of iodine deficiency. However, in the UK this is rarely seen and the main factors contributing to maternal hypothyroidism are autoimmune thyroiditis (Hashimoto's disease) or induced following surgery, radioactive iodine or drug therapy for hyperthyroidism. Consequently, the body's metabolic processes can slow down resulting in mental and physical lethargy, excessive weight gain, cold intolerance, constipation, fluid retention, hair loss and dry skin. If left untreated, hypothyroidism may lead to infertility, increased risk of miscarriage and fetal loss. Thyroid hormone is essential for human brain development and the fetus receives this hormone almost entirely from its mother. Hypothyroidism in pregnancy consequently can result in poor neurological development in the fetus and congenital hypothyroidism – cretinism in the newborn.

Antenatal and subsequent management

As the symptoms may be non-specific, hypothyroidism in pregnancy can be difficult for midwives to recognize. Women who are diagnosed with hypothyroidism should continue full thyroid replacement during pregnancy. However, those treated with radioactive iodine frequently require thyroxine supplements. Provided a woman is receiving an adequate dose of thyroxine prior to pregnancy, there is rarely a need to increase this dose in pregnancy. Thyroid function tests should be undertaken in early pregnancy and subsequently at regular intervals, in order to ensure that appropriate levels of FT4 and FT3 are maintained with the dose of thyroxine adjusted accordingly. Following birth, the thyroid status of the baby should be assessed to identify whether neonatal hypothyroidism is present. There is no contraindication to breast feeding but thyroxine levels may need adjusting as a result of maternal weight loss following childbirth.

## Postpartum thyroiditis

This presents in around 5 per cent of women during the first year following childbirth. It is a transient thyroid disorder that presents with mild hyperthyroidism a few months after the birth of the baby followed by a period of hypothyroidism. In both phases, the woman experiences fatigue and a painless goitre and may also present with postnatal depression. Although treatment is not usually required, as recovery tends to be spontaneous, many women will suffer recurrence after a subsequent pregnancy and are at risk of permanent hypothyroidism.

## Pituitary disorders

Hyperprolactinaemia is an important cause of infertility and amenorrhoea. It is most often due to a benign pituitary microadenoma. It may also be due to drugs that act as dopamine antagonists, such as methyldopa and the phenothiazines. The diagnosis is confirmed with a combination of measurement of the prolactin level and computerized tomography (CT) scanning or magnetic resonance imaging (MRI) of the pituitary fossa. In 80 per cent of cases it may be treated with dopamine agonists, bromocriptine or cabergoline, which cause the tumour to diminish in size. Larger tumours may require surgery or radiotherapy, ideally undertaken before pregnancy. Once pregnancy has been confirmed, bromocriptine and cabergoline are discontinued. Although the pituitary gland enlarges during pregnancy, it is rare for microadenomas to cause any problem. It is important that the midwife

recognizes any deterioration in the woman's vision during pregnancy and ensures a referral is made for visual fields monitoring. If there is evidence of tumour growth during pregnancy, bromocriptine or cabergoline should be recommenced. In women with macroadenomas ($>1$ cm), it is recommended that dopamine agonists are recommenced because of the risk of the tumour enlarging under oestrogenic stimulation. There is no evidence that bromocriptine or cabergoline are teratogenic.

## Adrenal disorders

### Cushing's syndrome

All adrenal disease is rare in pregnancy. Cushing's syndrome is characterized by increased glucocorticoid production usually due to hypersecretion of adrenocorticotrophic hormone (ACTH) from a pituitary tumour. Most women with Cushing's syndrome are infertile and in the few reported cases of pregnancy, a high incidence of preterm birth and stillbirth is described. Diagnosis may be difficult because many of the symptoms mimic normal pregnancy changes, such as weight gain, striae gravidarum, glucose intolerance and hypertension. If suspected, plasma cortisol levels should be assessed and adrenal imaging with ultrasound, CT or MRI should be undertaken. However, when making a diagnosis, it must be acknowledged that, as cortisol levels are known to rise in pregnancy, this should not be the only feature considered.

### Addison's disease

Addisons's disease arises as a result of an autoimmune process and is insufficient production of the adrenal glands. The signs and symptoms of Addison's disease are exhaustion, nausea, hypotension, hypoglycaemia and weight loss. The diagnosis is difficult to make in pregnancy because the cortisol levels, instead of being characteristically decreased, may be in the low-normal range owing to the physiological increase in cortisol-binding globulin in pregnancy. Occasionally, the disease may present as a crisis, and treatment consists of glucocorticoid and fluid replacement. In adequately treated women, the pregnancy usually continues normally. It is important for the midwife to remember that replacement steroids should be continued in pregnancy and increased at times of stress should the woman experience hyperemesis gravidarum or during labour and birth.

## Phaeochromocytoma

Phaeochromocytoma is a rare catecholamine-producing tumour. The tumours arise from the adrenal medulla in 90 per cent of cases. In pregnancy, it may present as a hypertensive crisis and the symptoms may be similar to pre-eclampsia. A characteristic feature is paroxysmal hypertension, while the other symptoms of headaches, palpitations, blurred vision, anxiety and convulsions may occur in pre-eclampsia. The diagnosis is confirmed by measurement of catecholamines and their metabolites in a 24-hour urine collection. Treatment is by alpha-blockade with phentolamine. Caesarean section is the preferred mode of birth as it minimizes the likelihood of sudden increases in catecholamines associated with vaginal births.

## Respiratory conditions

## Asthma

Asthma is reversible bronchial airway obstruction and may complicate up to 5 per cent of pregnancies. In most cases, the condition can be controlled with inhaled beta-2 agonists (salbutamol = relievers) and corticosteroids (betamethasone = preventers). Pregnancy itself does not necessarily affect the maternal asthmatic status: some women may experience no change in symptoms, whereas others may have a distinct worsening of the condition. Women with severe asthma and those whose asthma is poorly controlled are at risk of adverse maternal and neonatal outcomes, including preterm labour and birth, hypertensive disorders of pregnancy, IUGR, abruptio placentae, chorioamnionitis and Caesarean birth. However, there appears to be improved perinatal outcomes in those cases where asthma is well controlled.

### Antenatal management

At the initial visit with the midwife, information about the frequency and severity of the asthma, family history, any known asthma triggers and current treatment should be discussed with the woman. Management of asthma during pregnancy should be through multidisciplinary collaboration between midwife, GP, chest physician and obstetrician. Care should be aimed at optimizing medical treatment to prevent exacerbations of asthma and the aggressive treatment of acute attacks. Inhalation techniques should be carefully reviewed. Regular respiratory peak expiratory flow rate

(PEFR) assessment, performed by the woman at home to monitor the level of resistance in the airways caused by the inflammation and/or bronchospasm, is the best way of monitoring the severity of the condition. In severe exacerbations where the woman is too breathless to complete sentences, and where the PEFR is <50 per cent of the normal range, hospital admission for nebulized treatment with bronchodilators, oxygen and steroids is indicated. The British asthma management guidelines (British Thoracic Society 1997) provide comprehensive multidisciplinary advice for best practice in asthma care.

### Management of labour and birth

During labour, the increase in cortisone and adrenaline (epinephrine) from the adrenal glands is thought to prevent asthma attacks. If an attack does occur, it should be treated with the same urgency as one outside of pregnancy and labour. Drugs that cause bronchospasm should be avoided in pregnancy and labour, especially intravenous, intra-amniotic and transcervical prostaglandins and ergometrine. In addition, general anaesthesia should be avoided, if possible, as it increases the risk of bronchospasm and chest infection. If a woman has received corticosteroids in pregnancy, the dose should be increased during labour to counterbalance the stress of labour: 100 mg hydrocortisone intramuscularly every 6 hours and up to 24 hours following the baby's birth.

### Postnatal and neonatal care

In the postnatal period, non-steroidal anti-inflammatory drugs (NSAIDs), often used for pain relief, should be avoided. The midwife should encourage breast feeding as this may protect babies from developing certain allergic conditions. Furthermore, none of the drugs used in the treatment of asthma is secreted in sufficient quantities in the breast milk to cause any detrimental effect to the baby.

## Cystic fibrosis

This is an autosomal recessive condition found in approximately 1:2000 live births. Cystic fibrosis affects the exocrine glands causing production of excessive secretions with abnormal electrolyte concentrations resulting in obstruction of the ducts and glands. This affects the pancreas, sweat glands and respiratory, digestive and reproductive systems. However, pulmonary disease is the primary cause of morbidity and mortality associated with cystic fibrosis, and accounts for up to 90 per cent of deaths. Traditional treatments have included chest physiotherapy, antibiotics and pancreatic enzyme supplements. More recent developments in treatment include improved nutrition, the use of the synthetic hormone Dornase alfa to break down mucus, and heart–lung transplantation. There is a possibility that, in future, gene therapy may be used to replace the cystic fibrosis gene with a normal healthy gene. As a result of the advances in treatment, the life expectancy of affected women has steadily increased and many more women are surviving to an age where pregnancy is possible, although fertility may be reduced because of the chemical alteration in the cervical mucus. Malabsorption due to pancreatic insufficiency is often a major problem and women are typically underweight. Many women with cystic fibrosis develop diabetes and this risk is increased during pregnancy. The main risks to the fetus include IUGR and preterm birth, the latter usually being iatrogenic, if there is evidence of deteriorating maternal respiratory function.

Prior to pregnancy, it is important that the woman with cystic fibrosis and her partner are offered genetic counselling as 1:25 of the population carry the defective gene. It is, therefore, important that the partner be tested for his cystic fibrosis carrier status to determine the risk of the fetus having the condition or only being a carrier. Women with mild pulmonary disease and good nutritional status generally do well in pregnancy. However, those women with severe complications associated with cystic fibrosis are likely to have a poor outcome and should be advised against becoming pregnant.

### Antenatal management
Once pregnancy is confirmed, a multidisciplinary approach that includes midwifery, obstetric, dietetic, medical and physiotherapy expertise is vitally important. Maternal well-being is assessed by pulmonary function tests, arterial blood gases, sputum culture, liver function tests, glucose tolerance tests, chest X-ray, ECG and echocardiogram. Most women will have a daily physiotherapy regime using postural drainage techniques; however, in late pregnancy, this may become more difficult due to the enlarging uterus. An important part of the midwife's role is to recognize acute exacerbations or pulmonary infections necessitating prolonged antibiotic therapy and

hospital admission, to assess the nutritional status of the woman and observe for signs of cystic fibrosis-related diabetes. Fetal growth and well-being are monitored by serial ultrasound scans.

### Management of labour and birth
If the birth is contemplated before 34 weeks' gestation, steroid therapy should be given to improve fetal lung maturation. During labour, the midwife should closely monitor cardiorespiratory function, and fluid and electrolyte balance, as women with cystic fibrosis can easily become hypovolaemic owing to the loss of large quantities of sodium in sweat. Epidural analgesia should be offered as pain relief. However, general anaesthesia should be avoided because of the potential risks from respiratory complications.

### Postnatal and neonatal care
Following birth, it is recommended that the woman with cystic fibrosis be carefully observed in a high-dependency unit as cardiorespiratory function often deteriorates in the postnatal period. Breast feeding is not contraindicated as the sodium content in the breast milk of women with cystic fibrosis has been found to be similar to women without the condition. The midwife, however, needs to encourage the woman to take a well-balanced diet and maintain an adequate calorie intake. It is recommended that, as cystic fibrosis is the UK's most common life-threatening inherited disorder, universal neonatal screening is undertaken; this is usually carried out by the midwife around 6 days of age with parental consent.

## Pulmonary tuberculosis

Tuberculosis (TB) is caused by the tubercle bacillus, *Mycobacterium tuberculosis*, and affects mainly the lungs, although other organs may also become affected. It is responsible for 6 per cent of all deaths worldwide. All forms of TB are notifiable under the Public Health (Control of Disease) Act 1984. TB is transmitted through the inhalation of infected airborne droplets from a person with active TB. Although the incidence of TB has been declining over the past number of decades, more recently the number of cases has begun to show signs of rising, particularly among people aged between 25 and 44 years of age. Consequently, TB has become more prevalent in women of childbearing age with some studies finding an incidence of 143.3 per

100000 births. Community nurses, midwives and specialist community public health nurses, therefore, have a vital role to play in the prevention, screening and treatment of TB.

Factors contributing to the increased incidence of TB involve those women who have immigrated to the UK from areas of South Asia and the Indian subcontinent, African countries such as Somalia, Russia, Eastern Europe and the Baltic states, where TB is endemic. In addition, the development of multidrug-resistant organisms, and the increase in adults and children infected with the human immunodeficiency virus (HIV) may also contribute to the rising incidence of TB in the UK. The greatest percentage increase has been seen in inner-city areas where additional social factors, such as poverty, poor nutrition, homelessness, overcrowding and substance misuse, contribute to the transmission of the disease.

The symptoms of primary TB are non-specific and include fatigue, malaise, loss of appetite, loss of weight, alteration in bowel habit and low-grade pyrexia, all of which can be considered as usual symptoms occurring in pregnancy. However, as the disease progresses, the classic symptoms of chronic cough, night sweats, haemoptysis, dyspnoea and chest pain occur quite late on and are often absent when TB is extrapulmonary. This may lead to a delay in diagnosis that includes microscopic examination and culture of sputum to confirm the presence of mycobacterial infection and identify drug sensitivity. If a chest X-ray is needed, a lead apron should be used to protect the woman's abdomen and the developing fetus.

### Antenatal management

All pregnant women with TB should be referred to a specialist physician with experience in the disease. It is vitally important there is collaboration with the midwife, GP and obstetrician to ensure continuity of care and advice. A social worker may also be involved where social and economic factors feature in the care of the woman with TB. Maternal morbidity and mortality rates are higher where women do not adhere to the prescribed treatment, where active TB is left untreated or when treatment is started late in pregnancy. The neonate is also at risk of prematurity, perinatal death and being of low birth weight.

The standard antituberculous therapy rifampicin, isoniazid and pyrazinamide is also recommended for the pregnant woman. These drugs are considered to be safe in pregnancy and do not have any teratogenic effect on the developing fetus. Within 2 weeks of treatment, TB is usually rendered non-infectious. Wherever possible, treatment is undertaken in the woman's home. However, admission to hospital would be necessary if the woman becomes severely ill, or when there are adverse reactions to the drug therapy, for obstetric reasons, such as preterm labour, for social reasons or for further investigations. Upon admission, the woman should be provided with a single room but strict barrier nursing is not required.

### Postnatal and neonatal care

Following birth, babies born to women with infectious TB should be protected from the disease by the prophylactic use of isoniazid syrup (5 mg/kg per day) for 6 weeks and then tested for tuberculosis. If negative, BCG (bacille Calmette–Guérin) vaccination should be given to the baby and drug therapy discontinued. If the tuberculin test is positive, the baby should be assessed for congenital or perinatal infection and drug therapy continued, if these are excluded. Antituberculous drugs are considered to be compatible with breast feeding, which is only contraindicated if the woman has active TB, as the disease is transmitted through the breast milk. These women will also need support to care for their babies and adequate rest and a good diet is vitally important to prevent the recurrence of the disease. Contraceptive advice is an important part of postnatal and preconception care, as it is advisable for a woman with TB to avoid pregnancies until there are no further signs of the disease for at least 2 years. When giving such advice, midwives should be aware that rifampicin reduces the effectiveness of the oral contraceptive pill.

## Haematological disorders

### Anaemia

Anaemia is a deficiency in the quality or quantity of red blood cells, resulting in reduced oxygen-carrying capacity of the blood. It is commonly found during pregnancy owing to a lack of haemoglobin (Hb) production because of low levels of essential precursors, such as iron and folate. Less commonly, it may be secondary to chronic haemorrhage or haemolysis. As a consequence, anaemia is a contributory factor of maternal mortality and morbidity particularly in developing countries. The WHO defines anaemia as a haemoglobin concentration of <11.0 g/dL. During pregnancy, although the red cell mass increases, the plasma volume expansion is relatively greater and, therefore, the haemoglobin concentration falls, leading to physiological anaemia.

## Microcytic anaemia/iron-deficiency anaemia

Iron demand in pregnancy increases from 2 to 4 mg daily. A healthy diet contains 10 mg. It is recommended that the woman's iron status should be assessed prior to pregnancy as iron deficiency in early pregnancy has the most significant effect on fetal growth. Signs and symptoms involve:

- pallor of the mucous membranes;
- tiredness, dizziness and fainting;
- dyspnoea on exertion;
- palpitations;
- oedema;
- loss of appetite, nausea and vomiting;
- chronic infections, such as pyelonephritis, may predispose to anaemia.

The diagnosis of iron deficiency is suspected if the mean corpuscular volume (MCV) is $<85\,\mu m^3$, assuming electrophoresis is normal. Low levels of serum iron and ferritin help to confirm the diagnosis, particularly as serum ferritin levels will show changes before the level of haemoglobin changes. Although iron supplementation is controversial, it is suggested that women with a serum ferritin of $<50\,\mu g/L$ will require oral iron supplementation of 120–160 mg daily. This can be in the form of ferrous sulphate tablets that contain 60 mg iron in every 200 mg tablet, or ferrous gluconate tablets containing 35 mg iron in 300 mg tablets. Those women who have a serum ferritin concentration of $>80\,\mu g/L$ are unlikely to require supplementation.

Not only can midwives give women dietary advice regarding improving their iron status, they can also advise them that vitamin C enhances iron absorption, tannin in tea can inhibit absorption and that, if supplementation is deemed necessary, taking iron after meals may reduce some of the side effects. Side effects may include blackness of stools, nausea, epigastric pain and constipation. However, if the woman is unable to tolerate iron because of these common side effects, different iron preparations are available including liquid formulae. Other means of increasing haemoglobin concentration have their drawbacks:

intramuscular iron (iron sorbitol) is painful, and intravenous iron (iron dextran) may cause allergic reactions and thus should be given slowly closely observing the woman for the first few minutes. Blood transfusions, although rarely used to treat anaemia in pregnancy, should be avoided if possible because of the small risk of antibody production and transfusion reactions. Those women who have iron-deficiency anaemia should continue with iron supplementation during the postnatal period, especially if they are breast feeding their baby. Blood tests should be undertaken at 6 weeks including any further investigations should anaemia persist.

## Macrocytic (megaloblastic) anaemia/folic acid deficiency

Folic acid is required for formation of the nuclei in all body cells and consequently the increased cell growth of both mother and fetus during pregnancy. The normal values of folate concentrations fall in pregnancy owing to the haemodilutional effect of plasma expansion. It is, therefore, more common for folic acid deficiency to manifest in late pregnancy when the growth of the fetus is more rapid. Although folate deficiency is less common in the UK, as many foods include folate supplements, it is usually diagnosed by an examination of the peripheral blood that would show large red blood cells (macrocytic), an increased MCV and serum folic acid levels $<4\,\mu g/mL$.

All women considering pregnancy should be encouraged to take folate supplementation (i.e. 0.4 mg daily), as it has been shown to reduce the incidence of neural tube defects. Folic acid deficiency is associated with a poor dietary intake, multiparous women and multiple pregnancies. Women who are taking anticonvulsant therapy, anticoagulants and long-term sulphonamides or who drink excessive amounts of alcohol, require an additional daily supplement of 5 g folic acid, as these substances interfere with folic acid metabolism.

*Vitamin $B_{12}$ deficiency (pernicious anaemia)* is another cause of macrocytic/megaloblastic anaemia, but is unlikely to present in pregnancy, as severe cases are associated with infertility. However, as vitamin $B_{12}$ is found exclusively in products of animal origin, including milk and cheese, women who are vegans are most likely to suffer from this deficiency. Diagnosed cases should, therefore, take vitamin $B_{12}$ supplements throughout pregnancy.

# Haemoglobinopathies

Haemoglobinopathies are inherited conditions in which one or more abnormal types wholly or partly replace the normal adult haemoglobin HbA. In the homozygous form, such conditions can be fatal. It is, therefore, important that those susceptible to such conditions are screened to detect different types of haemoglobin in their blood, and are offered genetic counselling before embarking on a pregnancy or prenatal diagnosis in order to make an informed decision (Chapter 7).

## Sickle cell disorders

These are autosomally inherited diseases commonly found in people of African or West Indian origin. Abnormal haemoglobin (HbS and/or HbC) contains beta-globin chains with an amino-acid substitution that results in it precipitating when in its reduced state. Both haemoglobins S and C are genetically inherited, and thus there are homozygous (HbSS/HbCC) and heterozygous (HbAS/HbAC) forms of the disease. Where HbS is present, the red blood cells have become sickle-shaped and occlude small blood vessels, resulting in sickling disease.

### Sickle cell anaemia

Sickle cell anaemia (HbSS) is a severe condition and, in pregnancy, women are at high risk of complications as the life span of erythrocytes is only 5–10 days as opposed to the normal life span of 120 days. The erythrocytes become sickle shaped under conditions of low oxygen tension, such as hypoxia, stress, infection, haemorrhage, acidosis and cold. They are easily haemolysed and cause extremely painful vaso-occlusive symptoms in joints, abdomen and chest, particularly in pregnancy, known as crises. Women are, therefore, at increased risk of chronic haemolytic anaemia, thromboembolic disorders, pre-eclampsia, retinopathy and infection owing to malfunction of the spleen. There is an increased risk of IUGR, miscarriage, premature labour and consequential perinatal mortality. Ideally, these potential risks associated with pregnancy should be discussed with the woman preconceptually.

### Homozygous CC disease

As there is no S haemoglobin in homozygous CC disease, women with this condition would not experience sickling crises as those with HbSS.

### Sickle cell trait

Women with sickle cell trait (HbAS/HbAC) are carriers of the disease, and are usually asymptomatic and fit and well. Although the sickle screening test is positive, the blood appears normal and there is no sign of anaemia. However, they are at increased risk of urinary tract infection and only very rarely may they suffer from a sickling crisis.

### Sickle cell haemoglobin C disease

In some instances, an individual may inherit two different abnormal haemoglobins, HbS from one parent and HbC from the other, and thus have sickle cell haemoglobin C disease (HbSC). Although HbSC may cause only mild degrees of anaemia, it can present with very severe crises that are more common throughout pregnancy. It is commonly found in Ghanaians. The danger of HbSC is that there is still a possibility of sickling, which doctors and midwives may not anticipate owing to the absence/mild degree of anaemia. Women with HbSC should be cared for during labour in the same way as women with HbSS.

### Antenatal management

Women who are at risk of sickle cell disorders are screened in early pregnancy and the midwife should also encourage their partner to be screened. If both parents are carriers (heterozygous), there is a 1:4 chance of the fetus being homozygous for the condition. This then creates an ethical dilemma for the parents in deciding whether the fetus should be screened and the pregnancy continued/terminated. No specific treatment exists to prevent sickle cell crises; however, hypoxia, dehydration and infection should be avoided by aggressive treatment with adequate analgesia, antibiotics, oxygen and rehydration. Ideally, a haemoglobin concentration of at least 10.0 g/dL with 60 per cent normal HbA will minimize the risk of crises. In some cases, blood transfusion or an exchange transfusion to remove HbS and replace it with HbA may be used to increase the percentage of circulating normal HbA; however, blood transfusions are not without risk and their role in pregnancies complicated with sickle cell disorders is controversial. Fetal well-being is monitored throughout pregnancy by serial ultrasound and Doppler assessment.

### Management of labour and birth

During labour, the midwife should ensure dehydration, cooling, infection or hypoxia is avoided to reduce the risk of a sickling crisis occurring in the woman. Continuous fetal monitoring is recommended with an epidural for pain relief in order to reduce the stress of labour. Intrapartum management should involve collaboration with haematologists who have expertise in the care and management of women with sickle cell disease. Unless there is an obstetric complication, a Caesarean section is not indicated and general anaesthesia should be avoided.

### Postnatal and neonatal care

Following the birth of the baby, women with sickle cell disease remain at increased risk of suffering a crisis as the postnatal period is also a stressful time. Antibiotics may be administered to prevent puerperal sepsis. Midwives should carefully discuss contraception with these women and the combined contraceptive or progesterone-only pill may both be safely used. Neonatal testing of all babies at risk undertaken at birth via a cord blood sample is debatable as the sickle cell test does not yield positive results until 3–4 months of age when HbF recedes. It is, therefore, important that all babies at risk should be followed-up in infancy in order to reduce the high infant mortality associated with sickle cell disease.

## Thalassaemia

The thalassaemia syndromes are the commonest genetic blood disorders and are found in people of Mediterranean and Asian origin. The condition arises from a defect in the alpha- or beta-globin chains, resulting in thin red blood cells that are often misshapen and deficient in haemoglobin and that have only a short life span. Consequently, the individual experiences profound anaemia. The syndromes are divided into the alpha- and beta-types depending on which globin chain is affected. The number of defective genes an individual inherits determines the severity of the condition.

### Alpha-thalassaemia major

In alpha-thalassaemia major, there are no functional alpha-chains, no normal haemoglobin is synthesized and the condition is incompatible with extrauterine life. The fetus develops marked hydrops and pregnancies are complicated by polyhydramnios and preterm birth. If affected, the baby will only survive a few hours following birth. These pregnancies may also be complicated by severe pre-eclampsia related to the enlarged and hydropic placenta. There is no treatment, but individuals can be offered the option of

genetic counselling and prenatal diagnosis in subsequent pregnancies.

### Beta-thalassaemia major

Beta-thalassaemia major usually presents between the ages of 3 and 18 months when the child becomes pale and fails to thrive. It occurs as a consequence of two defective beta-genes and has little significance in intrauterine life as the fetus produces HbF. However, once the baby is born, it is unable to produce normal HbA1 and severe anaemia develops requiring regular blood transfusions. Eventually this can lead to the problems of iron overload causing damage to the heart and liver. If left untreated, these children will die before the age of 8. However, with treatment, they may survive into adulthood.

### Thalassaemia minor/trait

In thalassaemia minor (sometimes referred to as thalassaemia trait), there is a deletion of one of the two normal alpha- or beta-genes required for haemoglobin production, resulting in alpha-thalassaemia minor (which is rare in the UK) or beta-thalassaemia minor. Although these conditions produce an anaemia that is similar to iron deficiency anaemia with low haemoglobin, mean cell volume and mean cell haemoglobin concentrations, they rarely produce obstetric complications except in cases of severe blood loss. Consequently, all pregnant women considered to be at risk should be offered electrophoresis as part of the antenatal screening process. It is also important to screen the woman's partner for thalassaemia and, should he also be a carrier, there is a 1:4 risk of the fetus inheriting alpha/beta-thalassaemia major. In pregnancy, the woman should take oral iron and folate supplements to maintain her iron stores. Parenteral iron should never be given. However, blood transfusions may be given if the haemoglobin level is thought inadequate for the stress of labour and blood loss at birth.

## Glucose-6-phosphate dehydrogenase deficiency

Glucose-6-phosphate dehydrogenase (G6PD) deficiency is inherited through an X-linked gene and, therefore, is predominant in males. The incidence is more common in Africa, Asia and Mediterranean countries. G6PD is an enzyme necessary for the survival of red blood cells. When it is deficient, the red blood cells are destroyed in the presence of substances such as broad (fava) beans, sulphonamides, vitamin K analogues, salicylates and camphor (found in products, such as Vicks Vaporub) and anaemia consequently develops.

Clinically, G6PD manifests in two forms. The first is prolonged jaundice in the neonatal period occurring on the second or third day of life, reaching a maximum by the sixth day and subsiding by the end of the first week. Alternatively, it may present as an acute self-limiting haemolysis as a result of contact with the substances listed above. This may be indirect contact via the placenta or breast milk. Death from haemolysis is, however, rare.

# Thrombocytopenia

Thrombocytopenia is a reduction in the number of platelets ($<150 \times 10^9$/L). There are many causes and these are classified below:
- incidental thrombocytopenia of pregnancy;
- autoimmune thrombocytopenia (e.g. systemic lupus erythmatosus, antiphospholipid syndrome);
- activated clotting mechanism (e.g. pre-eclampsia, HELLP syndrome, disseminated intravascular coagulation);
- thrombotic thrombocytopenic purpura;
- hypersplenism;
- decreased platelet production/bone marrow suppression (e.g. sepsis, HIV);
- malignant marrow infiltration.

## Incidental thrombocytopenia
Incidental thrombocytopenia is common and may be present in 7–8 per cent of pregnant women. Mild falls in platelet counts to between 100 and $150 \times 10^9$/L are only very rarely associated with poor maternal outcome. Bleeding is rarely a complication unless the count is $<50 \times 10^9$/L. The diagnosis of incidental thrombocytopenia is a diagnosis of exclusion and can only be made when autoimmune and other causes have been excluded.

## Autoimmune thrombocytopenia purpura
Acute autoimmune thrombocytopenia purpura (ITP) may present typically in children after a viral illness, whereas in adults, the presentation is more chronic.

The incidence in pregnancy is 1:5000. Autoantibodies are produced against platelet surface antigens leading to platelet destruction by the reticuloendothelial system. In pregnancy, the condition may present with bruising or be suspected for the first time following a routine blood test. The platelet count is typically $30–80 \times 10^9$/L and it is rare for it to fall to extremely low levels. Other associated autoimmune conditions should be considered including systemic lupus erythematosus and antiphospholipid syndrome (APS).

### Antenatal management
Management in pregnancy should include serial platelet counts, and providing the count remains $>80 \times 10^9$/L, no bleeding complications are likely and regional epidural/spinal anaesthesia and analgesia may be used. If the count falls $<80 \times 10^9$/L, other forms of pain relief for labour or general anaesthesia for Caesarean section may be indicated. If the platelet count falls to $<50 \times 10^9$/L approaching term, treatment with corticosteroids should be considered. These act by suppressing platelet autoantibodies. However, high doses are often required to improve the platelet count and long-term use is associated with weight gain, hypertension, diabetes and osteoporosis. Corticosteroids also take 2–3 weeks to have an effect.

Although much more expensive, the use of intravenous human immunoglobulin G (IgG) has been a major advance in the treatment of autoimmune thrombocytopenia. The precise mechanism of its action is not known, but it is thought that its administration prolongs the clearance time of IgG-coated platelets by the reticuloendothelial system. The platelet response is usually rapid. Because of the cost implications, this treatment is usually reserved for cases that do not respond to steroids, or when a rapid response is required prior to labour and birth, or if there is bleeding in the postpartum period. The resulting increase in platelets will normally provide the woman with adequate platelet cover for labour and birth to take place within the following 2–3 weeks and, therefore, the option of an epidural in labour can be considered. A final treatment is splenectomy, but this is very rarely undertaken in pregnancy, as it is associated with significant maternal and perinatal mortality.

In pregnancy, antiplatelet antibodies may cross the placenta and destroy the fetal platelets; however, severe fetal thrombocytopenia is unusual and is less than 5 per cent in maternal ITP.

## Neurological disease

# Epilepsy

Epilepsy is a condition of abnormal cerebral function in which characteristic convulsive seizures occur. The condition affects 1:200 of the general population and consequently the incidence in pregnancy is between 0.15 and 1 per cent. The seizures may be generalized (petit mal and grand mal), partial (temporal lobe epilepsy) or focal (Jacksonian seizure), and may frequently result in the loss of consciousness for periods of seconds to up to half an hour. In all cases, abnormal paroxysmal electrical discharges, recordable on an electroencephalogram (EEG), occur in the brain. In many cases, the cause is unknown (idiopathic) but epilepsy may be due to the following:

- cerebral trauma;
- congenital abnormality;
- eclampsia;
- infection: encephalitis/meningitis;
- space-occupying lesion;
- cerebral vascular accident;
- drug or alcohol withdrawal/toxic overdose;
- metabolic disturbance (hypoglycaemia).

In the event of a first seizure in pregnancy, it is important to exclude the other possible causes listed above, particularly eclampsia. In the last triennial report into maternal deaths (2000–2002), there were 13 deaths associated with epilepsy (Lewis and Drife 2004). The midwife should ensure that partners and families are fully aware of the first-aid measures necessary should a seizure occur, using the recovery position to maintain a clear airway and prevent aspiration. In addition, the dangers of the woman taking hot baths alone that may induce fainting and consequent drowning should also be emphasized.

### Preconception care

Although epilepsy can be controlled by the use of antiepileptic drugs (AEDs), such as sodium valproate (Epilim) or phenytoin sodium (Epanutin), it cannot be cured. Phenobarbitone or benzodiazepines may also be given. Many of the drugs have side effects, such as drowsiness, nausea and skin rashes. The majority of women will usually have commenced AEDs prior to pregnancy and should be encouraged to seek preconception counselling with their partner in order to receive full information about the risk of congenital abnormalities and the screening tests available to them. All AEDs are associated with an approximate doubling of the risk of fetal abnormality (6–7 per cent): the major fetal abnormalities being neural tube defects, facial clefts and cardiac defects. All women receiving AEDs should be advised to take a daily supplement of 5 mg folic acid prior to conception to reduce the risk of neural tube defects. However, midwives should also be aware that folic acid may reduce serum phenytoin levels in pregnancy, which may affect the control of seizures in some women.

### Antenatal management

Pregnancy has a variable effect on the pattern of seizures but, in general, the more severe the disorder, the greater the effect on the pregnancy. Successful pregnancy outcome relates to preconception assessment and counselling, the close monitoring of the epilepsy throughout pregnancy and cooperation of the woman in taking the prescribed medication. The care and management should, therefore, be shared between the neurologist, the obstetrician and the midwife at a combined clinic to maximize professional expertise and surveillance of the woman's condition.

The aim of antenatal management is to ensure there is a balance maintained between preventing seizures that could result in both maternal and fetal hypoxia and maternal injury, and maintenance of drug levels at the lowest maternal therapeutic doses possible. Physiological changes in pregnancy result in lower concentrations of AEDs, which may need to be increased, subject to assessment of plasma levels. Where women have been free of seizures for 2 years, consideration may be given prior to conception to discontinue AEDs. In general, the risk of recurrent seizures is about 25 per cent within 1 year of reducing the medication. The risk is higher in women with adolescent or adult-onset epilepsy, those requiring more than one AED to control their epilepsy, those who had seizures while on medication, and those with an abnormal EEG in the past year.

The principal concern related to epilepsy in pregnancy is the increased risk of congenital abnormality caused by AEDs. Many of these abnormalities are detectable by ultrasound and, therefore, all women should be offered detailed anomaly scanning. In addition, each AED has been associated with a specific syndrome that includes developmental delay, nail hypoplasia, IUGR and midface abnormalities. Such abnormalities occur more often in women taking combinations of AEDs and so, during pregnancy, treatment is recommended with one drug where possible. Counselling the woman is, therefore, vitally important with regard to the association between fetal abnormality and drug therapy, as some women may be fearful of the potential teratogenic effects of the drugs and consequently this may lead to their non-compliance. However, failure to take AEDs can lead to an increased frequency of uncontrolled epileptic seizures that can potentially be more harmful to the fetus than the potential risks of drug therapy.

Monitoring of drug levels in pregnancy, however, is difficult. Although the measured drug level falls, in the majority of cases, this is not associated with an increased frequency of seizures. An increase in dosage to combat the anticipated fall may lead to an increased fetal risk. Provided there is no increase in frequency of seizures, the prenatal drug dosage can be continued. However, an increase in frequency or a recurrence of seizures, especially in the context of subtherapeutic drug levels, should prompt an increase in dosage.

### Management of labour and birth

As tonic–clonic (grand mal) seizures only occur in 1–2 per cent of women during labour, the care and management of the woman with epilepsy should be no different to any other woman. However, midwives should be aware that seizures are more likely to occur as a result of sleep deprivation, hypoglycaemia, anaemia, stress and hyperventilation, all of which can occur in labour. AEDs should be maintained in labour and the midwife should, therefore, carefully observe the woman for any early signs of a possible seizure.

### Postnatal and neonatal care

Midwives can provide essential support to women with epilepsy and their families in order for them to develop strategies to cope safely with their baby, and avoid the baby/woman being harmed should a seizure occur. Epilepsy Action (2004) has published written guidance on safety regarding minimizing risks when feeding, bathing, changing and transporting the baby. All midwives should be conversant with these guidelines and incorporate them in their parent education whenever caring for women with epilepsy in the postnatal period. AED therapy should be reviewed at 6 weeks and the dosage reduced to pre-pregnancy levels. The midwife should offer family planning and contraceptive advice to the couple. All methods of contraception are available to women with epilepsy, but oral contraceptives are less effective with some AEDs, as they induce hepatic enzymes that metabolize oestrogens faster. Consequently, these women would need a higher dosage of oestrogen ($>50$ mg) should this method be their choice.

In the fetus and neonate, many AEDs have been shown to inhibit prothrombin precursors, resulting in deficiency of vitamin K-dependent clotting factors. It is, therefore, essential that the midwife advises parents of this so that they can give consent for their baby to receive prophylactic vitamin K at birth. In the postnatal period women should not only be encouraged to rest as much as possible, as a marked loss of sleep can predispose to convulsions, but also to comply with their drug regime following the baby's birth. All AEDs are secreted in breast milk and, provided that the maternal dosage is not excessively high, there is no contraindication to breast feeding. If the woman has received high doses of phenobarbital, primidone or benzodiazepines during pregnancy, the baby may be hyperactive, restless, reluctant to suckle and experience vomiting and diarrhoea for up to a month. Although a minority of women with epilepsy will require careful monitoring from the midwife, obstetrician and neurologist, in the majority of cases, most women with this condition will have uncomplicated pregnancies, normal births and healthy babies.

## Autoimmune disease

## Systemic lupus erythematosus

Systemic lupus erythematosus (SLE) is a chronic autoimmune inflammatory disorder of the connective tissue that forms the fibrous, elastic fatty or cartilaginous matrix that connects and supports other tissues. It affects $<1:1000$ people but is 5–10 times more common in women, particularly from black and Asian populations. As connective tissue is found throughout the body and in almost every organ, SLE produces multisystem disorders affecting muscles, joints, skin, blood, eyes, heart, lungs, kidneys and the nervous system. The initial manifestation of SLE is often arthritis accompanied by fever, fatigue, malaise, weight loss, anaemia and photosensitivity. A wide range of skin lesions are seen and, depending on the organs involved, inflammatory conditions, such as pericarditis, neuritis, pleuritis, glomerulonephritis and gastritis, may also arise. Renal disease and neurological abnormalities are the most serious complications of the disorder.

Diagnosis of SLE is based on a collection of the signs and symptoms and may occur prior to conception, or may be suspected for the first time during pregnancy or the postnatal period, usually as a result of complications. SLE is a relapsing condition and pregnancy increases the risk of disease flare, pre-eclampsia and worsening nephropathy. Approximately one-third of women with SLE will experience an exacerbation during pregnancy. The diagnosis is confirmed by a positive serum assay for antinuclear antibodies.

Antiphospholipid syndrome (APS) is found in conjunction with SLE in 30 per cent of cases. A blood test will detect antiphospholipid antibodies, lupus anticoagulant and anticardiolipin antibodies, if APS is present. This will identify a group of women with SLE at particular risk of thromboembolic disorders and a high rate of fetal loss during pregnancy that includes recurrent miscarriages <10 weeks' gestation or pre-term birth before 34 weeks due to IUGR or pre-eclampsia.

Neonatal lupus syndrome is rare but may arise as a result of the transplacental passage of maternal anti-Ro/anti-La antibodies. The baby presents with a mild form of SLE that is transient and resolves when the antibodies are cleared a few months following birth. However, in the more severe cases, fetal anaemia, leucopenia and thrombocytopenia can result. The baby may also develop congenital heart block that is permanent and carries significant mortality and morbidity.

### Antenatal management

Owing to these significant risks, pregnant women with SLE and APS require intensive monitoring by specialists in caring for people with lupus disorders for both maternal and fetal indications. The frequency of antenatal visits is dependent on the severity of the woman's condition, but women with SLE may also require consistent social and psychological support from the midwife. Baseline haematological, immunological blood tests and renal studies including a 24-hour urine collection for creatinine clearance and total protein should be performed at the first antenatal visit. Blood pressure should also be monitored closely because of the increased risk of pre-eclampsia. Serial ultrasonography is performed to assess fetal growth, placental size and amniotic fluid volume.

If antenatal treatment is required for SLE, steroids and azathioprine may be given safely. However, NSAIDs should be avoided in pregnancy because of the adverse effects on the fetus. In women with APS

who have suffered repeated pregnancy loss or severe obstetric complications, the use of aspirin ± heparin has been shown to reduce the pregnancy loss rate.

### Management of labour and birth

The timing of labour and birth is dependent on the degree of severity of the condition affecting maternal and fetal well-being. If there are no complications such as pre-eclampsia or renal disease present, birth should be at term. It is recommended that there should be a hospital protocol for intrapartum management of women with lupus disorders and there be close liaison between the midwife, obstetrician, rheumatologist, anaesthetist, paediatrician and haematologist.

Women who have been on long-term steroid therapy will require parenteral steroid cover during labour. As women with SLE are susceptible to infection, it is important that midwives and other health professionals adhere to strict hand-washing and aseptic techniques and ensure invasive procedures such as vaginal examinations remain at a minimum. In addition, close monitoring of the maternal condition is required by the midwife, obstetrician and anaesthetist to assess cardiac, pulmonary and renal function. Haematological tests to assess if there are any clotting disorders and the wearing of TED stockings are measures that should be undertaken to prevent the development of deep vein thrombosis. Owing to SLE compromising the uteroplacental circulation, it is recommended that continuous fetal monitoring is undertaken along with fetal blood gas estimation.

### Postnatal and neonatal care

It is important that the midwife observes for signs of SLE flare occurring in the immediate postnatal period owing to the stress of labour. The midwife should also observe for signs of infection, pre-eclampsia, renal disease, thrombosis and neurological changes. As most of the drugs used to treat SLE are excreted in breast milk, careful consideration needs to given to breast feeding. Low-dose steroids, such as prednisolone, are considered safe, but immunosuppressive therapy is contraindicated and should be avoided when breast feeding. Large doses of aspirin and NSAIDs are contraindicated when breast feeding jaundiced babies. Paracetamol is, therefore, the recommended choice for analgesia in the postnatal period.

When advising the woman with SLE and her partner about suitable contraception following the birth of their baby, it is important that they realize the choices available may be limited. The combined oral contraceptive pill increases the risk of hypertension, thrombosis and SLE flares, and so low-dose oestrogen combined pills may be considered in women with mild forms of SLE where there is no history of thromboembolic disorders or APS. Furthermore, as intrauterine contraceptive devices are associated with an increased risk of infection, this method may not be deemed suitable for women with SLE. Progestogens and barrier methods, therefore, present the safest options and may be suitable for those women where other methods are considered unsuitable.

## Liver disorders

### Acute fatty liver of pregnancy

This is a rare but very serious disorder of liver function occurring in approximately one in 10 000 pregnancies. The aetiology of the condition is unknown, but histologically a perilobular fatty infiltration of the liver cells is noted. The condition typically develops in the third trimester or within a few days of a stillbirth. It is more common in obese women who present with abdominal pain, headache, nausea and vomiting. Progressive jaundice, encephalopathy, hypoglycaemia, coagulopathy and renal failure may develop and 50 per cent of these women also have symptoms of pre-eclampsia. There is, therefore, a risk that pre-eclampsia will mask the presentation of the condition. There is a significant risk of maternal or fetal death and a prompt diagnosis is, therefore, essential to ensure the correct treatment is given. Maternal death results from encephalopathy or overwhelming haemorrhage associated with disseminated intravascular coagulation. Fetal death is not uncommon and is considered to be related to maternal liver failure and the metabolic disturbance.

#### Antenatal management
Liver function tests are undertaken; diagnosis is made on the liver enzymes being moderately raised and the woman showing signs of renal failure. A liver biopsy is contraindicated owing to the risks of coagulopathy. Consequently management involves correcting any clotting deficiencies before the birth of the baby is contemplated. This may involve blood transfusions, fresh-frozen plasma, vitamin K, platelets, 50 per cent glucose, acetylcysteine and dialysis during the antenatal period and in the immediate postnatal period.

#### Management of labour and birth
Although it would be considered that Caesarean section has many advantages for the baby, the safest mode for the woman to give birth is vaginally, should this be possible. Epidural analgesia is contraindicated in all but the mildest of forms owing to coagulopathy problems. In severe cases, the management should include liaison with specialists from a regional liver unit.

#### Postnatal care
During the postnatal period, although recovery can be prolonged, the liver function usually returns to normal over a few weeks. Although in the majority of cases there is no long-term liver dysfunction, in the few cases where women have achieved a subsequent pregnancy, the recurrence of acute fatty liver of pregnancy appears to be low.

### Intrahepatic cholestasis of pregnancy

Intrahepatic cholestasis of pregnancy (ICP) is a condition occurring in approximately 0.5–1 per cent of pregnancies that presents most commonly in the third trimester, usually between 32 and 36 weeks. Its incidence varies widely geographically and it is especially common in certain South American countries, particularly Chile. ICP presents initially with generalized pruritus at night that is worst on the palms of the hands and soles of the feet, and women may complain of fatigue and insomnia because of this. Anorexia, pale stools, dark urine and steatorrhoea may develop. There is no rash except marks resulting from skin scratching; however, mild jaundice may develop in some cases and persist until the baby is born.

The condition is thought to arise from a genetic hypersensitivity to oestrogen. It is associated with an increased risk of fetal mortality and morbidity, particularly sudden unexplained intrauterine fetal deaths at term, and with maternal clotting defects owing to the inability to absorb vitamin K, which is fat soluble. Bile acids are considered to cause placental vasoconstriction, resulting in fetal hypoxia and in up to 40 per cent of pregnancies complicated with ICP, there will be meconium in the amniotic fluid, with the risk of neonatal meconium aspiration.

#### Antenatal management
Midwives should be suspicious of ICP should a woman present with severe itching in pregnancy and refer them for liver function tests. Cholestasis must be

differentiated from other causes of liver dysfunction in pregnancy, including viral hepatitis, extrahepatic obstruction from gall stones, autoimmune hepatitis, pre-eclampsia, HELLP syndrome or acute fatty liver of pregnancy, sepsis and drug-induced hepatitis. Diagnosis is made on serum testing of liver function with raised transaminases and bile acids being the most sensitive finding. In addition, a full haematological and clotting profile should be undertaken, including tests of renal function, hepatitis serology, autoimmune antibodies and liver ultrasound. Serial ultrasound scans to monitor fetal growth and amniotic fluid volume as well as Doppler blood flow studies and CTG are important features of assessing fetal well-being in pregnancies complicated with ICP.

Management includes the symptomatic relief of pruritus with emollients and antihistamines, such as oral chlorpheniramine. In cases where ursodeoxycholic acid has been used to reduce maternal itching, liver function has also been notably improved in most women. Careful monitoring is required to detect and prevent coagulation defects and prophylactic oral vitamin K is usually given during pregnancy to reduce the risk of postpartum haemorrhage.

## Management of labour and birth
As the risk of intrauterine death increases after 38 weeks, if labour has not occurred spontaneously by this time, it is normally induced between 35 and 38 weeks, when the fetus is considered mature. However, if the fetal condition appears to be compromised, the birth of the baby should be earlier.

## Postnatal care
After the baby is born, the itching normally subsides and maternal liver function returns to normal within 3–14 days. However, in subsequent pregnancies, the recurrence risk of cholestasis can be as high as 50 per cent. Bearing in mind that ICP is related to oestrogen, midwives should advise women to avoid oral contraceptives that contain oestrogen.

---

## REFLECTIVE ACTIVITY

Consider a woman with a medical disorder to whom you have recently provided midwifery care
- What were the clinical features of the disorder when first presented?
- How was the diagnosis made?
- What factors determined the subsequent management and care?
- To what extent did the management and care reflect national guidelines and/or local Trust guidelines/policies regarding this medical condition?

- What role did midwives, like yourself, play in the woman's management and care during the antenatal period, labour and postnatal period?
- Depending on the maternal and fetal outcome, could the management and care have improved in any way:
  - from the woman's perspective?
  - from your own/the midwife's perspective?
  - from the perspective of other health professionals involved in this case?
- How may this experience help to inform your own knowledge and clinical practice?

---

## Key Points

- Counselling prior to conception allows women who have a pre-existing medical condition to understand the possible risks in pregnancy and the level of antenatal care they will require.
- The role of the midwife is fundamental in identifying women with pre-existing medical conditions and those who are at risk of developing such conditions during pregnancy.
- A collaborative multidisciplinary approach to the management and care that emphasizes the need to treat the woman as an individual is essential to optimize maternal and fetal outcome.
- The midwife should be knowledgeable about medical disorders and aware of contemporary management and care, both at local and national level.

- The midwife has an important role in health education and support to women and families in order to develop strategies to minimize risk, and prevent further problems and complications that their medical condition may present.
- Midwives can empower women by involving them in making decisions and the planning of their care as far as their condition allows.
- The midwife has a responsibility to ensure the woman has full information about infant feeding and all available methods of contraception in relation to her medical condition in order that an informed decision can be made.

# References

British Thoracic Society. The British guidelines on asthma management 1995. Review and position statement. Thorax 1997; **52**(2)Suppl:1–21.

Epilepsy Action. *Epilepsy information: epilepsy and women.* Leeds: British Epilepsy Association, 2004.

Lewis G, Drife J (eds). *Confidential Enquiry into Maternal and Child Health; why mothers die 2000–2002.* Sixth report of the confidential enquiries into maternal deaths in the UK. London: RCOG Press, 2004.

National High Blood Pressure Education Program Working Group on High Blood Pressure in Pregnancy. Report of the National High Blood Pressure Education Program Working Group on high blood pressure in pregnancy. *American Journal of Obstetrics and Gynaecology* 2000; **183**:S1–S22.

Public Health (Control of Disease) Act 1984. London: HMSO.

World Health Organisation. *Definition, diagnosis and classification of diabetes mellitus and its complications.* Report of a WHO consultation. Part 1: Diagnosis and classification of diabetes mellitus. Geneva: WHO, 1999.

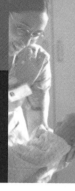

# Perinatal infections

## OVERVIEW

Infection presents a major challenge to the midwife and obstetrician both in developed and developing countries. The extremely high rates of maternal mortality due to puerperal sepsis during the nineteenth and early twentieth centuries were mainly due to transmission of infection within the hospital. Group A streptococcus was the commonest pathogen. Semmelweis, working in mid-nineteenth century Vienna, was the first to demonstrate the value of aseptic technique and hand-washing between patients. With improved infection control measures and the availability of intravenous antibiotics, maternal death from sepsis is now rare in the UK although the incidence has risen in the last 3 years (Lewis and Drife 2004). Altered maternal physiology during pregnancy places the mother at additional risk of certain infections. Unfortunately, neonatal death still occurs from infections, such as group B streptococcal meningitis, septicaemia and viral infections, such as herpes encephalitis.

## Infections associated with congenital infections

The infections that cause congenital abnormality are summarized by the acronym TORCH (toxoplasmosis, rubella, cytomegalovirus, herpes). Many other infections may adversely affect a fetus or neonate and these have been resummarized as STORCH5 (see box on page 194). However, pregnancy loss may occur in the first trimester in association with any acute infections in the mother (e.g. influenza).

## Syphilis

Syphilis is a sexually transmitted infection caused by the spirochete *Treponema pallidum*. It is common in many developing countries where up to 10 per cent of pregnant women may have positive serological tests. In Western Europe and the USA, the incidence fell progressively over the course of the second half of the twentieth century.

Primary syphilis presents as a painless genital ulcer (Figure 13.1) 3–6 weeks after the infection is acquired, with local lymphadenopathy. In women, the ulcer is most often on the cervix and may pass unnoticed. At this stage, the infection is highly contagious. Secondary manifestations of syphilis occur 6 weeks to 6 months after infection, often just as the primary chancre is regressing, and present as a non-itchy maculopapular rash affecting the palms of the hands and soles of the feet. Lesions affecting the mucous membranes are warty growths called condylamata lata. Other manifestations include alopecia, uveitis and sensorineural deafness. If no specific treatment is administered, the

## STORCH5: specific infections that adversely affect a fetus, neonate or pregnant woman

| | |
|---|---|
| S | Syphilis |
| T | Toxoplasmosis |
| O | Other |
| | Bacterial vaginosis |
| | *Trichomonas vaginalis* |
| | Group B streptococcus |
| | *Escherichia coli* |
| | *Ureaplasma urealyticum* |
| | *Haemophilus influenzae* |
| | Varicella |
| | *Listeria monocytogenes* |
| R | Rubella |
| C | Cytomegalovirus |
| H5 | Herpes |
| | Human immunodeficiency virus (HIV) |
| | Hepatitis B |
| | Human papillomavirus |
| | Human parvovirus |

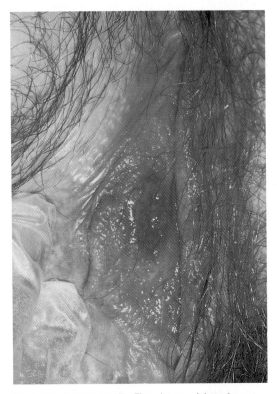

**Figure 13.1** Primary syphilis. There is one painless ulcer on each side of the labia minora. (Courtesy of Dr Raymond Maw, Royal Victoria Hospital, Belfast.)

lesions regress after 2–4 weeks, but the infected woman may suffer relapses during the following 2 years when lesions may reappear. At this stage, the infection is called early latent, as it may be transmitted during relapses. Subsequently, late infection ensues and syphilis cannot be transmitted sexually. Ultimately 20 per cent of untreated patients will develop symptomatic cardiovascular tertiary syphilis and 5–10 per cent will develop symptomatic neurosyphilis.

Up to 70 per cent (the highest risk) of fetuses become infected if the mother has primary or secondary syphilis during pregnancy. With later stages of syphilis, the risk is smaller, being approximately 14 per cent 5 years after the mother has acquired infection. The spectrum of congenital syphilis varies from a severe fetal infection causing intrauterine death to a neonate with symptomatic disease (early congenital syphilis), a child who subsequently develops the stigmata of congenital syphilis (late congenital syphilis) to a child who is asymptomatically infected. The key features are summarized in the box. Any woman presenting during pregnancy with small genital ulcers should be screened for syphilis and herpes, and the midwife should make the appropriate referral (Nursing and Midwifery Council 2004).

Syphilis can be detected during antenatal screening offered to pregnant women at the initial booking discussion. As for all screening tests, the midwife needs to ensure that the woman is given appropriate information and advice to be able to make an informed choice and give informed consent.

### Treatment

For early syphilis (primary, secondary or early latent), penicillin is the treatment of choice, given intramuscularly, for 12 days. Later stages of syphilis require 21 days of treatment. Treatment can cause a worsening of symptoms, and fever for 12–24 hours after starting treatment, and may be associated with uterine contractions and the onset of preterm labour. Close medical supervision is required.

Treatment can be difficult for women who are allergic to penicillin. Tetracycline is the usual second-line treatment but is contraindicated in pregnancy. Erythromycin is less reliable and resistance has been reported; it is best administered intravenously. It is essential that current and recent sexual partners of women with syphilis are screened. Older children may also need to be screened.

## Features of congenital syphilis

Severe intrauterine infection leading to miscarriage

**Early congenital syphilis**
- Maculopapular rash
- Hepatitis splenomegaly
- Mucus patches, lymphadenopathy
- Bone abnormalities, anaemia
- Active neurosyphilis

**Late congenital syphilis**
- Stigmata: Hutchinson's triad
  - interstitial keratitis,
  - sensorineural deafness
  - Hutchinson's teeth
  - Clutton's joints
- Active disease: general paresis of the insane (GPI), gummata

## Toxoplasmosis

The protozoan parasite, *Toxoplasma gondii*, may be acquired from exposure to cat faeces or from eating uncooked meat. The prevalence varies widely according to eating habits. In France, more than 70 per cent of pregnant women have been infected and acquired immunity before pregnancy, whilst in the UK only 10–20 per cent of women are immune. Despite this, it is estimated that approximately 1 in 140 pregnant women in France acquire the infection during pregnancy compared to 1 in 400 in the UK. Primary infection often passes asymptomatically. It may cause a glandular fever-like illness, but rarely it causes fulminating pneumonitis or fatal encephalomyelitis. Eye infections, presenting as chorioretinitis can occur from either congenital or acquired infection. In acquired immunodeficiency syndrome (AIDS), as immunity deteriorates, previously quiescent toxoplasma may recur, causing multiple brain abscesses.

Most infections are asymptomatic. Infection during the first trimester of pregnancy is most likely to cause severe fetal damage, but only 10–25 per cent of infections are transmitted to the fetus. In the third trimester, 75–90 per cent of infections are transmitted but the risk of fetal damage decreases from 65 per cent in the first trimester to almost zero for those infected near to the time of birth. Severely infected infants may have the classic tetrad of hydrocephalus or microcephaly, chorioretinitis, convulsions and cerebral calcifications. In such cases, extensive neurological damage occurs and the neonate may die. The majority of infected infants are asymptomatic at birth but develop sequelae several years later.

### Treatment

A combination of sulphadiazine and pyrimethamine is used in symptomatic adults. Pyrimethamine, is potentially teratogenic and should not be used during the first trimester. Spiramycin is less toxic and is devoid of teratogenic effects. A 3-week course of 2–3 g per day is administered during pregnancy. While this reduces the incidence of transplacental infection, it may not reduce the incidence of clinical congenital disease. Congenital toxoplasmosis should always be treated with pyrimethamine and sulphonamide.

### Prevention

As only ten or so severely affected babies are diagnosed per year in the UK, routine screening in pregnancy is not offered. It is important that pregnant women are advised about the risk factors and the mode of spread of toxoplasmosis from meat and cat faeces. They should avoid eating rare steaks or hamburgers, and take care when handling raw meat in the kitchen. Hand-washing with soap and water is essential. Pregnant women should avoid handling cats and particularly cat litter. Children's sandpits should be covered to prevent cats from defaecating in them.

## Cytomegalovirus

Cytomegalovirus (CMV) is a herpes virus and can establish latency. In the UK, approximately 40 per cent of women are susceptible when they become pregnant. It is spread through the respiratory and genitourinary tracts, and high levels of virus may be present in the urine. Primary infection often produces no symptoms or mild non-specific symptoms. The incidence of infection in pregnancy is estimated to be as high as 1 in 200 pregnancies, of which around 40 per cent will result in fetal infection. It is possible that infection later in pregnancy is more likely to result in fetal morbidity. Ninety per cent of infected infants are asymptomatic. Thus, of an estimated 1000 infected babies born per year in the UK, approximately 100 are damaged by the virus.

The principal features are microcephaly, blindness and deafness. Other manifestations include pneumonitis, chorioretinitis, cerebral calcification and developmental delay. As the primary infection in the mother is usually asymptomatic, the diagnosis is rarely made before birth. Probably about another 100 children are born each year with sensorineural hearing loss as the only sign of congenital CMV infection.

After infection, the virus is excreted for weeks or months by adults and by infants for years. It persists in the lymphocytes throughout life and can, therefore, be transmitted by blood transfusion or transplantation. Reactivation occurs intermittently with shedding in the genital, urinary or respiratory tract. In temperate countries, infection is usually transmitted by close contact, kissing or sexual contact; and approximately 1–2 per cent of the population become infected each year. In tropical countries, most infections take place in childhood and 60–70 per cent of individuals are infected within 6 months of birth. The remainder are mostly infected by the age of 5 and, therefore, there are few susceptible pregnant women. Clinical features in infected infants include hepatosplenomegaly, jaundice and purpura.

### Diagnosis

A definitive diagnosis of congenital infection can be made by isolating the virus from throat swabs, urine, blood or cerebrospinal fluid (CSF) in the first 3 weeks of life. Serological diagnosis is made by demonstrating a rising titre of immunoglobulin G (IgG) antibody or specific CMV IgM antibody. Specific IgM antibodies persist for a few weeks to a few months, and specific IgA antibodies from a few months to a year. The diagnosis may be made *in utero* by amniocentesis and polymerase chain reaction (PCR), as the virus is concentrated in the urine. The congenital manifestations need to be differentiated from other congenital infections, such as toxoplasmosis, rubella, herpes simplex and syphilis.

### Treatment

Specific antiviral agents are available for CMV, such as ganciclovir and foscarnet. These are not used in pregnancy, and have to be given by intravenous infusion. Assistance with rehabilitation for congenital abnormalities may be required.

# Rubella

Rubella causes a usually insignificant infection in adults or adolescents, but can cause devastating congenital infection. In most countries, between 70 and 90 per cent of young adults are immune to rubella. In some parts of Asia, only 50 per cent are immune. In temperate climates, acquired disease is most common in the spring and early summer, with an increase in local incidence every 3–5 years.

The incubation period is 2–3 weeks and clinical manifestations include mild fever, sore throat, enlarged cervical glands and a rash that may be discrete or give a general pink flush to the trunk. Painful joints are common in adults and symptoms persist for 3–7 days. However, infection in children often passes unnoticed. Any symptoms suggestive of rubella during pregnancy should lead to investigation. Similar clinical pictures (except those of congenital infection) are produced by many other viral infections.

Congenital infection involves cardiovascular defects, eye defects and deafness. In addition, hepatitis, thrombocytopenia, bone involvement, microcephaly, behavioural change and mental retardation have been reported. Abortions and stillbirths can occur as can preterm birth. The diagnosis should be suspected in any small-for-gestational-age baby with congenital abnormalities. The congenital syndrome occurs most commonly in early pregnancy; the incidence is 50 per cent following infection in the first month, dropping to 10 per cent, if infection occurs in the fourth month of pregnancy. The virus can be isolated from over 90 per cent of embryos of infected pregnancies and it appears that approximately half the cases are able to clear the infection as only 50 per cent of proven maternal infections result in infants with persistent IgG or IgM antibodies.

Diagnosis is based on serological tests. At booking, maternal antibody levels are measured and, if the antibody titre is low, a booster vaccination should be given after the birth. A very high IgG antibody titre is suggestive of recent infection but specific IgM is only detectable for 4–6 weeks in most cases. Non-immune women should be advised to stay away from known cases of rubella, as there is no specific treatment available. Congenital rubella can be diagnosed by detecting the virus and secretions from the throat, urine and faeces. It can also be found in CSF, blood, eyes and ears. Excretion diminishes slowly and has ceased by the age of 6 months in 70 per cent of cases. The presence of

IgG antibody after 6 months of age is confirmatory. Rubella-specific IgM may be found for 3–9 months.

Many children are so handicapped by deafness or blindness that they are unable to attend mainstream schools. If rubella is diagnosed during the first trimester, the risk of congenital infection is so high that many women elect to have a termination of pregnancy. In the past, adolescent girls were vaccinated against rubella and, in the last decade, vaccination has been incorporated in infancy within the measles, mumps, rubella (MMR) vaccine. Controversy related to the measles vaccine has caused a reduction in uptake and women susceptible to rubella will continue to present in pregnancy. However, a vaccination programme has led to a significant reduction in the incidence of congenital rubella to two per year for the UK.

## Varicella zoster

The herpes virus, varicella zoster, is transmitted easily from adults with chicken pox or shingles (herpes zoster) and 90 per cent of adults in the UK are immune to chickenpox. Shingles is a reactivation that can occur during pregnancy but does not pose any threat to the fetus. Transmission occurs through droplet spread, with an incubation period of about 2 weeks. In children, the illness is often mild and there may be only a handful of lesions. In adults, symptoms include headache, general aches and pains, and malaise. Clusters of vesicles emerge at different stages: usually most are densely grouped centrally. Once the infection clears, latent infection of both sensory and motor nerve cells is established. This infection can reactivate with dissemination of the virus into a dermatome, causing the eruption recognized as shingles. Pregnant women are more vulnerable to chickenpox and may develop pneumonitis, which can be fatal. Early administration of intravenous acyclovir may ameliorate the severity but intensive care support may be needed.

Varicella zoster can affect the fetus in two ways. If infection occurs prior to 20 weeks' gestation, there is a small risk (approximately 1 per cent) of a congenital varicella syndrome. This consists of hypoplastic limbs, scarring and central nervous system (CNS) anomalies. If a pregnant woman is exposed to chickenpox or shingles, she should be tested for varicella zoster antibody. If she is not immune, varicella zoster immune globulin (VZIG) should be administered. The possible role of antiviral agents has not yet been evaluated.

Neonatal chickenpox can occur if the mother presents with infection from 2 days before to 5 days after birth, as the fetus is exposed to virus in the absence of maternal antibody. Neonatal varicella may be very severe. VZIG should be given to the neonate immediately, if the mother develops chickenpox. If chickenpox develops during the first month of life, intravenous acyclovir should be given.

## Parvovirus B19

This infection is asymptomatic in 25 per cent of adults and over 50 per cent of children. It may be associated with only mild symptoms of malaise or present with a macular rash, and it can be associated with severe arthralgia. In approximately 15 per cent of infections occurring during pregnancy, the fetus becomes chronically infected. This leads to persistent anaemia *in utero*, which may develop into non-immune hydrops fetalis. This can resolve spontaneously or may require intrauterine blood transfusion.

The diagnosis of parvovirus infection is confirmed by demonstrating virus-specific IgM in maternal serum or demonstrating seroconversion with a specimen that previously proved negative. It should be sought in mothers who have the clinical features, or when hydrops fetalis develops. There is no specific treatment for parvovirus infection but the baby should be monitored carefully with repeat ultrasound examinations. The virus is not teratogenic.

## Listeria monocytogenes

This bacterium has been isolated from more than 50 species of domestic and wild animals including birds, fish, insects and crustaceans. It is found in sewage, water and mud, and can grow in refrigerated food including meat, eggs and dairy products, particularly soft cheeses. Cooking destroys it and, therefore, the risk of infection is greatest with uncooked food. Most infections are probably subclinical but pregnant women are more vulnerable to the infection. In the UK, the incidence of *Listeria* infection is approximately 1 in 37 000 births.

In adults, listeriosis may be confused with glandular fever and, in pregnancy, an episode of malaise, headache, fever, backache, conjunctivitis and diarrhoea associated with abdominal or loin pain may occur. In 40 per cent of cases, fever is not marked at any time and the disease presents as a mild flu-like illness.

*Listeria* infection of the newborn occurs in two forms: the early-onset type from *in-utero* infection that manifests as septicaemia within 2 days of birth. Usually the infant is born premature with signs of respiratory distress and there may be a rash. The late form presents predominantly as meningoencephalitis after the fifth day. Approximately 30 per cent of babies with early-onset disease are stillborn. The organism can infect the CNS in the newborn and also in immuno-suppressed adults. There may be only a low-grade fever and focal neurological signs may develop.

Diagnosis in the neonate requires a high index of suspicion. Specimens from affected sites including throat, liver, CSF, vagina, placenta, urine, faeces and blood can be used for culture.

The organism is susceptible to penicillins, macrolides and tetracyclines, and ampicillin is the treatment of choice. Without recognition of the diagnosis, the mortality for infantile listeriosis is as high as 90 per cent and the prognosis is worse in preterm babies. Early diagnosis and prompt treatment has reduced this figure to only 50 per cent.

## Malaria

Malaria is prevalent throughout the tropics and is a major cause of mortality in both children and adults. Major polymorphisms, such as thalassaemia and sickle cell trait, provide a selection advantage in these areas because affected individuals are more resistant to severe manifestations of malaria. *Plasmodium falciparum* causes the most severe type of malaria, which can present with hepatic and cerebral forms of infection. It is transmitted between human hosts by the female *Anopheles* mosquito. *P. falciparum* has been able to develop resistance to most antimalarials, creating a need for new agents to be developed. The other strains of malaria (*P. ovale* and *P. vivax*) seldom cause fatal disease and have not so far developed chloroquine resistance, but cause considerable morbidity. The development of the parasite in the mosquito only occurs at warm temperatures; therefore, infection is rarely transmitted at altitudes above 2200 m.

The principal feature of malaria is episodes of temperatures associated with rigors as the temperature rises, followed by sweating as the temperature falls. There is headache, nausea and vomiting and, with *P. falciparum* malaria, the pyrexia may be continuous. The incubation period is approximately 2 weeks. In severe infections, 20 per cent or more of the red cells may be infected and haemolysis occurs, leading to anaemia. This may result in haemoglobinuria (black-water fever), associated with acute renal failure. Hyponatraemia and disseminated intravascular coagulation may also occur. Cerebral malaria presents with disturbances in consciousness owing to obstruction of cerebral capillaries by infected red cells that have reduced deformability. Pregnant women are at increased risk of severe manifestations of malaria; infection may trigger a miscarriage or premature labour. Even non-falciparum malaria has been associated with intrauterine growth restriction.

The diagnosis should be suspected in anyone who has been to the tropics and presents with a febrile illness. A history of taking prophylaxis does not exclude the diagnosis, as no prophylaxis is 100 per cent effective. Fever in the tropics or in those recently returned may be caused by many other infections including typhoid, food-poisoning organisms and viral infections, such as dengue fever.

Malaria is usually treated with quinine sulphate, initially administered intravenously. Individuals with *P. falciparum* malaria should be admitted to hospital and monitored closely, as sudden deterioration requiring intensive care may occur. Non-falciparum malaria establishes chronic infection of the liver. If the individual is not returning to an endemic area, acute treatment should be followed by a course of fansidar to eradicate infection. Individuals living in endemic areas acquire immunity to malaria but this is lost within a few months of moving away; therefore, anyone travelling from the UK to an endemic area should consider taking prophylaxis.

A combination of chloroquine and proguanil taken weekly provides protection against non-falciparum malaria and falciparum in some areas. Malaria resistant to many antimicrobials is present in sub-Saharan Africa and South East Asia, where even mefloquine resistance has been reported. The choice of prophylactic agent should, therefore, be made after consulting current recommendations giving details of resistance patterns. Chloroquine is probably the least toxic prophylactic agent for pregnant women and those travelling to areas of chloroquine resistance must balance the risk of malaria against the potential toxicity of prophylactic agents. It is safest to avoid travel to such areas when pregnant but, if the mother cannot be persuaded to delay travel, the potential risks and benefits of chemoprophylaxis must be discussed with her.

## Chlamydia psittaci

This organism causes epidemic abortion in ewes. In humans, it causes an atypical pneumonia. Exposure to lambing ewes and the products of conception can lead to infection in pregnant women, resulting in intrauterine infection and abortion. It has occurred most commonly in vets and farm workers, and all pregnant women should be advised to avoid sheep during the lambing season.

## Bacterial vaginosis

Bacterial vaginosis (BV) is the commonest cause of vaginal discharge in women of childbearing age. The principal symptom is an offensive fishy-smelling vaginal discharge that is often more apparent during menstruation or following unprotected intercourse. In some populations, its prevalence is greater than 50 per cent, although in the UK it is found in 10–15 per cent of women. It is thought to represent a disturbance of the vaginal ecosystem in which the usually dominant lactobacilli are overwhelmed by an overgrowth of predominantly anaerobic organisms including *Gardnerella vaginalis*, *Bacteroides* spp., *Mycoplasma hominis* and *Mobiluncus* spp. Some of these organisms produce polyamines and trimethylamine, which are responsible for the fishy smell. There is also a rise in the vaginal pH from the normal level, below 4.5, to levels as high as 6 or 7. It is not a sexually transmitted infection and there is no benefit from treating male partners.

Bacterial vaginosis is not usually associated with vaginal soreness. However, it may coexist with either candidiasis or trichomoniasis, both of which cause irritation and soreness. A white or yellow thin homogenous discharge is produced. Examination of a 'wet mount' of vaginal fluid microscopically shows the presence of many small bacteria. A strong fishy smell is produced if the woman has BV. The condition may also be recognized on Papanicolaou-stained cervical smears. Culture of vaginal fluid is not useful for making the diagnosis, as the organisms can be found in more than 50 per cent of normal women.

Trichomoniasis or candida can both coexist along with BV, and the discharges they produce can look similar to those of BV. Microscopy and culture of vaginal fluid can confirm both of these alternatives. Discharge due to cervicitis is usually more mucoid or mucopurulent, and there should be signs of clinical cervicitis on examination. Many observational studies have confirmed that women with BV have an increased risk of second trimester loss and preterm birth: indeed, it may be the most important cause of idiopathic preterm birth. It is associated with chorioamnionitis, which can progress to deciduitis or amniotic fluid infection. Fetal pneumonitis and ultimately fetal death may follow this from sepsis. Symptomatic women should be treated with metronidazole 400 mg twice a day for 5 days. This produces resolution within a few days but relapse can occur, and as many as 30 per cent of women have BV again within 1 month.

## Infections affecting the neonate at birth

### Herpes simplex virus

Herpes simplex is a virus well adapted to its human host. Primary infection usually presents within 7 days of exposure and may be accompanied by widespread lesions around the mouth and oropharynx and, in the case of genital herpes, around the vulva, vagina and cervix. If inoculation occurs on skin, such as occupational exposure for a health care worker, a herpetic whitlow may result. In many populations more than 70–80 per cent are exposed to oral herpes, herpes simplex virus type 1 (HSV1), during childhood. This gives some degree of cross-protection against herpes simplex virus type 2 (HSV2), traditionally the causative agent of genital herpes, and primary infection may be mild. With less exposure to childhood infections in Western societies, fewer young adults have been exposed to HSV1 and, at present, 50 per cent of cases of genital herpes are now due to this strain of virus. Primary infection may, therefore, follow orogenital contact. Seroprevalence studies suggest that 15–70 per cent of the population have antibodies to HSV1 and approximately 20 per cent to HSV2.

Primary genital herpes presents with soreness and irritation of the affected part (Figure 13.2). It may, however, pass completely unnoticed or be manifest with a widespread eruption of painful ulcers preceded by vesicles. Severe dysuria and peripheral nerve involvement may lead to urinary retention in women requiring admission for analgesia and a temporary suprapubic catheter. In pregnancy with altered T-helper cell immunity, recurrent herpes may be more severe than usual and mimic primary herpes. In

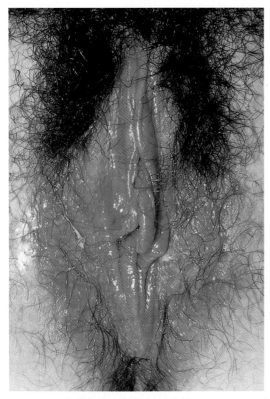

**Figure 13.2** Primary genital herpes. Multiple ulcers are seen with a wide distribution and confluent in some areas. In pregnancy, recurrent herpes can resemble a primary episode. (Courtesy of Dr Richard Lau, St George's Hospital, London.)

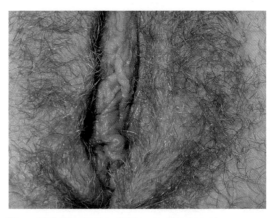

**Figure 13.3** Recurrent genital herpes. (Courtesy of Dr Colm O'Mahony, Countess of Chester Hospital.)

primary herpes, the lesions heal during the course of 2–3 weeks. Recurrences (Figure 13.3) usually last 3–7 days and are more localized, in a similar manner to an oral cold sore.

On examination, vesicles and ulcers are seen. The cervix may be severely inflamed and haemorrhagic. Cases of severe herpes mimicking pelvic inflammatory disease (PID) have been described, particularly in postnatal human immunodeficiency virus (HIV)-infected women.

More than half the men and women infected with genital herpes are unaware of its presence. Close and careful questioning may reveal a history of transient, almost trivial, sores occurring sporadically, usually in the same site. HSV2 is more likely to cause symptomatic recurrences than HSV1. The frequency of recurrences varies from person to person and a small minority will have more than six recurrences per year; some are incapacitated due to neurological symptoms, such as pains going down the legs.

The initial diagnosis is clinical but should always be confirmed by taking a swab from a vesicle or ulcer for culture or electron microscopy. Specific viral transport medium is essential. Serological tests have not been useful, as assays have not been able to distinguish between antibodies to HSV1 and HSV2.

Herpes simplex needs to be differentiated from other causes of genital ulcers. These include infections, such as syphilis and tropical genital ulcer disease (see later). Genital ulcers can occur in association with systemic diseases, such as sarcoidosis or systemic lupus erythematosus.

In the non-pregnant woman, a first presentation of herpes should be treated with a 5-day course of acyclovir 200 mg five times a day. This will stop further lesions developing and allow those that are present to heal. In many cases, it will be a recurrent rather than a true primary infection that is being treated, but it is not possible to differentiate reliably unless there was a history of herpes infection. There is insufficient data to confirm that acyclovir is safe during pregnancy. However, to date, there is no excess of birth defects associated with its use. Topical acyclovir cream is not effective in the treatment of genital herpes.

It is important to diagnose herpes in pregnancy because a devastating neonatal infection can occur with involvement of skin, liver and CNS. Neonatal mortality is 75 per cent. However, if acyclovir is administered rapidly, this can be reduced to 40 per cent. The vast majority of these cases are associated with a primary herpes infection in the mother in the weeks prior to the birth. The baby then has no protective antibody and is vulnerable to disseminated infection, or localized herpes encephalitis. If primary herpes presents around the time of birth, the case should be discussed with the paediatrician. Caesarean section will provide protection to the infant as long as the membranes have not ruptured for more than 4 hours. Genital swabs should be cultured from the mother and throat swabs from the baby, and intravenous acyclovir should be administered to the neonate. Women known to have recurrent herpes have also been offered Caesarean section, if a recurrence occurs at the time of the birth. It has been found that the risk of infection to the neonate from a maternal recurrence of herpes is very small and many units have now abandoned Caesarean section for this indication. The potential role of acyclovir administration for the last 2–4 weeks of pregnancy in women with recurrent herpes has not been fully evaluated because neonatal herpes in such cases is so rare.

Infection during the first trimester may cause miscarriage. A congenital syndrome has also been described, associated with micro-ophthalmia, chorioretinitis and microcephaly.

## Group B streptococcus

This organism is a commensal in the gut and genital tract and found in 20–40 per cent of women. It may cause severe neonatal infection leading to neonatal death and can cause upper genital tract infection progressing to septicaemia and occasionally maternal death.

Carriage of the organism is asymptomatic. It colonizes the vagina from the gut and then ascends into the uterus. It can be detected on culture of vaginal swabs but colonization of the vagina can occur at any stage of pregnancy. Attempts have been made to screen for infection in early pregnancy and eradicate the organism with penicillin; however, recolonization frequently occurs and this approach has not been shown to reduce the incidence of neonatal infection. The current recommendation is, therefore, that the organism should be sought by culture of vaginal swabs in complicated pregnancies or those with a prior preterm birth. If the organism is present, penicillin should be administered intravenously at birth. The infants most at risk are premature, and those who undergo prolonged rupture of membranes, are growth restricted or have birth asphyxia. Early disease presents as overwhelming septicaemia and pneumonia. Occasionally, an infant colonized in the perinatal period may develop

secondary disease between 1 and 4 weeks of age, presenting as meningitis.

## Chlamydia trachomatis

*Chlamydia trachomatis* is an obligate intracellular parasite. Genital infection with serotypes D–K is the commonest bacterial sexually transmitted infection in developed countries. It is also very common in developing countries. In many tropical countries, trachoma, caused by serotypes A–C, is endemic and transmission is thought to occur amongst household contacts; it leads to blindness in the most severe cases. *Chlamydia trachomatis* is important in pregnancy because it causes neonatal eye infection (ophthalmia neonatorum) and neonatal pneumonitis.

The organism is detected much more commonly in young sexually active women and women under the age of 25. The spectrum of disease varies from chronic asymptomatic infection to cervicitis, endometritis, salpingitis (PID) and intraperitoneal spread leading to perihepatitis. In men, it causes non-gonococcal urethritis, which may present with urethral discharge and dysuria. Many male partners of women with *Chlamydia trachomatis*, however, are asymptomatic.

Pelvic inflammatory disease is uncommon during pregnancy and many pregnant women carrying *Chlamydia trachomatis* are only diagnosed after the neonate develops clinical disease. Where screening is undertaken, in communities with a high prevalence of *Chlamydia trachomatis*, asymptomatic infection will be detected. An infected cervix is friable and bleeds easily on contact, with an associated purulent discharge from the cervical os, termed 'mucopurulent cervicitis'. The changes induced by pregnancy may be similar, so that the specificity of such findings is lower than in the non-pregnant woman. Tubal damage associated with previous chlamydial infection is an important predisposing factor for ectopic pregnancy.

Approximately 50 per cent of babies born to women with chlamydial infection develop ophthalmia neonatorum. This usually presents about a week after birth with a red sticky eye, which may be bilateral. Chloramphenicol drops, which are commonly prescribed, will only produce partial resolution. A swab for *Chlamydia trachomatis* should be taken from the baby's eye. The organism can also be sought in nasopharyngeal aspirates. Diagnosis of chlamydial infection is made by detecting the organism. Enzyme-linked immunosorbant assay (ELISA) tests are easily used to screen large numbers of samples but, unfortunately, the sensitivity is only 60 per cent. For this reason, culture, DNA detection-based tests or direct immuno-fluorescence must be used. Tests that rely on ampli-fication of DNA provide greater sensitivity and specificity and will be used increasingly as routine. The organism can be detected with such tests in endocervical swabs, first-pass urine samples and even self-administered vaginal swabs. The most important differential diagnosis for cervicitis is gonorrhoea.

The treatment of choice for *Chlamydia trachomatis* is tetracycline, usually doxycycline. However, tetra-cycline should be avoided in the second and third trimester of pregnancy because it binds to developing bones and teeth in the fetus, causing brown staining of the teeth and dysplastic bones. Erythromycin 500 mg twice a day for 2 weeks is, therefore, prescribed. This causes nausea and, as the pharmacokinetics are not reliable in pregnancy, a test of cure 2 weeks after com-pleting treatment is obligatory. It is essential that male partners are screened and treated before sexual intercourse is resumed. Definitive treatment with a tetracycline should be administered after birth and breast feeding. Neonates with ophthalmia neonato-rum should be treated with tetracycline eye ointment. As there is a risk of subsequent chlamydial pneu-monitis, they should also be treated with a 2-week course of erythromycin syrup.

Many women with *Chlamydia trachomatis* have sub-clinical endometritis, which may predispose to early pregnancy loss, chorioamnionitis and preterm birth and clinical postpartum endometritis. It has been asso-ciated with failure of implantation in women under-going *in-vitro* fertilization. Such women and their partners should be screened.

## Gonorrhoea

*Neisseria gonorrhoeae* is a sexually transmissible agent causing cervicitis, urethritis, endometritis, salpingitis (PID) and perihepatitis in women. In men, it causes urethritis and epididymitis, and in both men and women, it causes proctitis and pharyngitis. It is com-mon worldwide, although the incidence has decreased in developed countries since the Second World War. Infection in both sexes is frequently asymptomatic.

Like chlamydia, gonorrhoea is commonest in young sexually active women with the incidence declining over the age of 25. Its importance in obstetrics and midwifery is due to a neonatal eye infection, which, if untreated, can progress to blindness owing to corneal scarring.

The diagnosis of gonorrhoea is established by micro-scopy and culture. Gram-stained microscopy of cer-vical urethral and rectal swabs is performed. If clinical suspicion is high, a second set of cultures should be taken. It is routine practice to perform two sets of cul-tures as a test of cure following treatment. DNA detection-based tests are now available and these offer superior sensitivity to culture; however, at present, they do not allow the opportunity for antibiotic resistance testing for which culture remains necessary.

*Neisseria gonorrhoeae* has demonstrated a great abil-ity to acquire resistance to antibiotics. In many develop-ing countries, the price of antibiotics is prohibitive, so that suboptimal doses are used. This encourages the development of resistant strains, which are then exported worldwide. Chromosomal mutation has also produced moderate levels of penicillin resistance and is responsible for resistance to quinolones. Quinolones are contraindicated in pregnancy; there-fore, in a penicillin-allergic woman or a woman with penicillin-resistant infection, a cephalosporin, such as cefotaxime 2 g in a single intramuscular dose, should be administered.

---

### Commonly used antibiotics in pregnancy

**Thought to be safe**
- Penicillins (e.g. amoxicillin)
- Cephalosporins (e.g. cefotaxime)
- Erythromycin
- Nitrofurantoin in first and second trimesters

**Probably safe but limited experience**
- Co-amoxiclav
- Azithromycin

**Significant caution required**
- Quinolones (e.g. ciprofloxacin)
- Folate reductase inhibitors (e.g. cotrimoxazole)

**Contraindicated**
- Tetracyclines

Neonates may present with ophthalmia neonatorum owing to gonorrhoea a few days after birth. If *Neisseria gonorrhoeae* is cultured, topical and systemic treatment should be administered according to antibiotic sensitivities. In a similar way to *Chlamydia trachomatis*, gonorrhoea is associated with chorioamnionitis and preterm birth.

## Trichomoniasis

*Trichomoniasis vaginalis* causes severe vulvovaginitis in susceptible women. It is generally sexually transmitted, although infection may persist asymptomatically for many months in women and in some men. In men, it may cause urethritis but is frequently asymptomatic. Transient infection can be transmitted to female infants who will present with purulent vaginal discharge.

The incidence of trichomoniasis has fallen in developed countries. It remains highly prevalent in many developing countries where as many as 20–30 per cent of pregnant women carry the infection. It presents with a purulent vaginal discharge and may be associated with severe inflammation causing soreness and itching with a tide mark extending on to the thighs. The diagnosis is made by detecting the organism on wet-mount microscopy, with a sensitivity of approximately 50–60 per cent.

Newborn girls have stratified squamous epithelium in the vagina, similar to that of an adult due to the influence of high levels of maternal oestrogen *in utero*. They are, therefore, susceptible to infection and may develop asymptomatic discharge. As the influence of maternal oestrogen wanes over the first few weeks of life, such infection usually resolves spontaneously and specific treatment is rarely necessary.

Trichomoniasis frequently coexists with disturbed vaginal flora that develops into BV. The only established treatments for trichomoniasis are metronidazole or tinidazole, but these have been considered to carry a risk of teratogenicity. Retrospective studies of women who have taken metronidazole during pregnancy have shown no excess of fetal abnormalities and, therefore, symptomatic women may be treated with a 5-day course of metronidazole 400 mg twice a day. It is sensible that the potential risks of any treatment are discussed with the mother so that she can make an informed decision. Clotrimazole has some activity against trichomoniasis and application of intravaginal clotrimazole pessaries may control symptoms until the end of the first trimester, if a woman is particularly concerned about systemic treatment.

## Infections affecting the mother

## Vaginal candidiasis

Over three-quarters of women have at least one episode of vaginal candidiasis during their lifetime. A few women get frequent recurrences. The organism is carried in the gut, under the nails, in the vagina and on the skin. The yeast *Candida albicans* is implicated in more than 80 per cent of cases. *Candida glabrata*, *C. krusei* and *C. tropicalis* account for most of the rest. Sexual acquisition is rarely important, although the physical trauma of intercourse may be sufficient to trigger an attack in a predisposed individual. Candida is an opportunist, growing under favourable conditions. Symptomatic episodes are common in pregnancy. Its growth is favoured by the high levels of oestrogen, increased availability of sugars and subtle alterations in immunity.

The classical presentation is itching and soreness of the vagina and vulva with a curdy white discharge that may smell yeasty but not unpleasant. Not all candida presents in the same way; in some cases, there may be itching and redness with a thin watery discharge. Diagnosis can be confirmed by microscopy and culture of the vaginal fluid. Asymptomatic women from whom candida is grown on culture do not require treatment.

Recurrent candida, or resistance to treatment, is relatively uncommon. If this appears to be the case, it is important that other infections are considered, particularly herpes simplex, which causes localized ulceration and soreness, and dermatological conditions, such as eczema and lichen sclerosis.

In general, it is better to use a topical rather than systemic treatment. This minimizes the risk of systemic side effects and exposure of the fetus. Vaginal creams and pessaries can be prescribed at a variety of doses and duration of treatment. For uncomplicated candida, a single dose treatment, such as clotrimazole 500 mg, is adequate. If oral therapy has to be used, a single 150 mg tablet of fluconazole is usually effective, but its activity is limited to *Candida albicans* strains and its role in pregnancy is not yet defined.

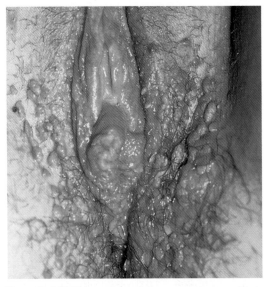

**Figure 13.4** Multiple genital warts in a pregnant woman. Warts often increase in size and number during pregnancy. (Courtesy of Dr Richard Lau, St. George's Hospital, London.)

## Genital warts

Warts are caused by human papillomavirus (HPV) infections. More than 100 strains have so far been identified and certain strains are generally transmitted sexually, producing genital warts on the mucosa of the genital tract. Most symptomatic infections develop within 8 months of starting a sexual relationship with a new partner but the incubation period may be a few years in some cases. It is thought that cell-mediated immunity is important for suppressing wart virus infections. With the alterations in maternal immunity that occur during pregnancy, a previously asymptomatic infection may start to produce genital warts or established infections may become more florid (Figure 13.4).

Topical application of podophyllin or podophyllotoxin is often used as first-line treatment, but these are contraindicated in pregnancy. The risk of fetal damage from administration of a small amount of such chemicals to genital warts in a woman who does not realize she is pregnant is so low that it is not an indication for termination of pregnancy, unless applied to a very large area. Surgical methods, such as cryotherapy or excision, therefore, are the only treatments available for pregnant women. Even so, the warts may not fully resolve until the woman has given birth. Male partners should be advised to attend a genitourinary medicine clinic for screening and treatment of any warts that they may have, and condoms should be used during sexual intercourse. In an established relationship, it is likely that wart virus transmission has already occurred and, therefore, it is no longer necessary to give such advice unless a new relationship has started.

Any baby born to a mother with wart virus will be exposed to such virus during birth. It appears, however, that few neonates acquire infection from their mothers. Rarely, infants may present with laryngeal warts due to a genital strain of wart virus, but transmission appears to occur from less than 1 per cent of infected mothers. It is unlikely that maternal transmission leads to established infection in the genital tract of boys or girls.

## Other vertically transmissible viral infections

### Hepatitis A

This is caused by an RNA virus, which is spread through the oral–faecal route. Approximately 50 per cent of the UK population have antibodies from childhood infection but the prevalence is falling. The majority of individuals in developing countries acquire infection during childhood. It is usually a benign illness, but occasionally fulminating hepatitis has been described in pregnant women; however, this has not been associated with congenital abnormalities. Individuals are most infectious before they develop jaundice. Some degree of protection may be provided through vaccination or administration of human immune globulin during the incubation period.

### Hepatitis B

Hepatitis B is a more severe infection that may be followed by chronic carriage and disease ending in cirrhosis. It is transmitted sexually, through blood products and through vertical transmission from an infected mother. A majority of acute infections are not clinically recognized as only 20 per cent of individuals develop jaundice. The earlier in life the infection occurs, the more likely the person is to become a carrier; 80 per cent of infants infected perinatally become carriers. Infection is particularly common in China and South East Asia, but prevalent in most tropical countries.

Pregnant women are screened for hepatitis B at booking.

## Hepatitis C

This is another RNA virus that causes chronic hepatitis. Again acute infection often passes asymptomatically, but more than 50 per cent of infected individuals have active hepatitis, which will progress to cirrhosis and possibly hepatocellular carcinoma. In the UK, infection is highly prevalent in those with a history of intravenous drug use. It may be transmitted sexually but transmission is not very efficient with only 1–2 per cent of long-term partners becoming infected. Vertical transmission again occurs uncommonly, although the risk is increased in those co-infected with HIV.

## HIV infection

HIV infection is a major challenge for the obstetric team and for midwifery care. There is a need to reduce the risk of vertical transmission to the fetus and to maintain optimal health of the mother. This usually involves the use of interventions, such as drugs of known or unknown fetal toxicity, performing Caesarean section and advice not to breast feed. It is best managed through a multidisciplinary team incorporating obstetricians, midwives, paediatricians and HIV specialists.

AIDS is caused by infection with HIV. More than 20 million individuals are now infected worldwide and, in countries with a high prevalence, it is the leading cause of death in young adults. It is a particularly devastating disease because of the stigma of sexual transmission, the risk of vertical transmission to children and the likelihood that other family members are infected. Even if a child is not infected, the death of one or both parents threatens their development and survival in many parts of the world. At present, HIV is increasing in prevalence in most parts of the world.

### Natural history and principles of treatment of HIV infection
Twenty per cent of those infected with HIV experience an acute seroconversion illness a few weeks after acquisition. Clinical features include fever, generalized lymphadenopathy, a macular erythematous rash, pharyngitis and conjunctivitis. A steady decline in immune function over the first few years may be

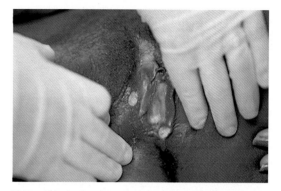

**Figure 13.5** Genital ulcers in a woman with HIV infection. These persistent painful ulcers were due to herpes simplex. Persistence for more than 1 month is AIDS defining. In the tropics, the differential diagnosis includes chancroid and Donovanosis.

manifest by non-life-threatening opportunistic conditions, such as recurrent oral and vaginal candidiasis, single dermatome herpes zoster (shingles), frequent and prolonged episodes of oral or genital herpes, persistent warts and genital ulcers (Figure 13.5). Furry white patches on the sides of the tongue, termed oral hairy leukoplakia, may come and go. Persistent generalized lymphadenopathy may be present. Skin problems include seborrhoeic dermatitis, folliculitis, dry skin, tinea pedis and a high frequency of allergic reactions.

Without antiretroviral treatment, the average time for the development of AIDS is 10 years. Essentially, AIDS is defined by the onset of life-threatening opportunistic infections or malignancies associated with immunodeficiency. The commonest presentations are listed (see box). There are two strategies used in treatment. Combinations of antiretroviral drugs are prescribed. The acronym HAART has been adopted for highly active antiretroviral therapy. Combinations may include two or more nucleoside analogue reverse transcriptase inhibitors, such as zidovudine or didinasine, a non-nucleoside reverse transcriptase inhibitor, such as nevirapine, or one or more protease inhibitors, such as nelfinavir. If successful, the immune system improves after a few months.

If immunodeficiency has already occurred, treatment and prevention of opportunistic infections is needed. This may include cotrimoxazole to prevent *Pneumocystis carinii* pneumonia and, in severely immunosuppressed individuals, azithromycin to prevent disseminated *Mycobacterium avium intracellulare* complex infection, and ganciclovir to prevent cytomegalovirus infection. Regular administration of

## Common acquired immunodeficiency syndrome (AIDS)-presenting illnesses

**Pulmonary**
- *Pneumocystis carinii* pneumonia
- Tuberculosis – pulmonary or extrapulmonary

**Neurological**
- Cerebral toxoplasmosis
- Cryptococcal meningitis
- AIDS dementia

**Gastrointestinal**
- Diarrhoea and wasting syndrome, which may be due to infection with *Cryptosporidium, Microsporidium* or *Isospora*
- Oesophageal candidiasis

**Ophthalmic**
- Cytomegalovirus retinitis

**Malignancy**
- Kaposi's sarcoma
- Non-Hodgkin's lymphoma

**Systemic**
- *Mycobacterium avium intracellulare* complex infection

antifungal agents may be necessary to control oral and vaginal candidiasis.

### Diagnosis

As the consequences of receiving a diagnosis of HIV are serious, a test should only be performed with informed consent from the patient. She may wish to discuss it with a partner, for whom the test may have major implications. To avoid the serious consequences of incorrect labelling or other human errors, it is good practice to confirm correct labelling of the sample and request form with another health care worker.

### Transmission

In most developing countries, HIV is principally spread through vaginal intercourse, with approximately equal numbers of men and women infected. In developed countries, the majority of infections have been acquired through homosexual sex or intravenous drug use, although the incidence of heterosexual transmission is increasing. Genital infections are risk factors for HIV transmission and acquisition, including genital ulcer disease, chlamydia and gonorrhoea. BV may also be a risk factor, and is very common in some African countries, with a prevalence of 50 per cent or greater. Good control of sexually transmitted infections should reduce the incidence of HIV infection.

### Vertical transmission

Vertical transmission occurs in 25–40 per cent of pregnancies, if no interventions are used to reduce the risk. It is thought that a minority of infections occur during gestation. These babies can present with AIDS in the neonatal period. The majority of infections occur during parturition. Breast feeding accounts for transmission in up to 15 per cent of pregnancies, corresponding to 37 per cent of infected infants. Transmission by this route may occur even after several months. The risk of vertical transmission is increased if there is a high HIV viral load or a preterm birth. The role of genital infections in vertical transmission is still being assessed. Many children infected with HIV will survive into adolescence.

Three interventions have been shown to reduce the risk of vertical transmission of HIV:
- avoiding breast feeding;
- elective Caesarean section;
- antiviral medication prescribed during the latter half of pregnancy, and to the neonate for 6 weeks.

If all three interventions are undertaken, the risk of transmission is probably less than 3 per cent.

## 🔍 Key Points

**HIV and pregnancy**
As a minimum the following information needs to be discussed before a test is performed:
- The antibody test may take 3 months to become reactive after exposure.

- If there has been a recent high-risk exposure, the test should be repeated 3 months and 6 months after the event.
- A confirmatory sample should always be taken if the first test is reactive.

- Without specific treatment, the average time to develop AIDS is 10 years. It is possible to remain healthy even 15 years after initial infection.
- In countries with adequate health-care resources, the prognosis is greatly improved by treatment.
- In pregnancy, the risk of vertical transmission is about 1 in 4, if no interventions are undertaken.

- A combination of antiretroviral medication, Caesarean section and avoidance of breast feeding reduce the risk to <3 per cent.
- Who, if anyone, does the woman plan to tell about the test and its result?

## References

Lewis G, Drife J (eds). *Confidential Enquiry into Maternal and Child Health; why mothers die 2000–2002*. Sixth report of the confidential enquiries into maternal deaths in the UK. London: RCOG Press, 2004.

Nursing and Midwifery Council (NMC). *Midwives' rules and standards*. London: NMC, 2004.

## Key additional reading

National AIDS Manual 2004. *Fact sheets* (available on www.aidsmap.com).

Wright H. Breastfeeding and the transmission of HIV. *British Journal of Midwifery* 2004; **12**:88–92.

# Labour

## OVERVIEW

Labour can be defined as the process by which regular, rhythmic, painful contractions bring about effacement and dilatation of the cervix and descent of the presenting part, ultimately leading to expulsion of the fetus and the placenta from the mother. Social, psychological, biological and ethical factors combine together in a complex interplay, which makes the midwifery management of labour a significant challenge. A midwife or doctor who manages labour must be aware of the normal anatomy and physiology of the mother and fetus, what distinguishes normal from abnormal labour and, when it is appropriate, whether to await events or to intervene.

## Introduction

Labour and delivery is the focus and climax of the reproductive process. It is both a physical and emotional challenge for the mother. There is interplay between the 'powers' of the uterus (the contractions), the 'passages' of the birth canal (the bony pelvis and the soft tissues of the pelvic floor and perineum) and the 'passenger' (the fetus). Each contraction promotes dilatation of the uterine cervix and descent of the fetus.

Before exploring the process of labour in detail, an understanding of the anatomy of the female pelvis and the fetus are essential. The mechanism of labour will be presented here.

## Anatomy of the female pelvis and the fetus relevant to labour

### The pelvis

The female pelvis is adapted for childbearing and, owing to its features, does not cause any problems in labour if the pelvis is adequate and the baby's size is normal.

#### The pelvic brim or inlet

The pelvic brim is the inlet of the pelvis and is bounded anteriorly by the symphysis pubis (the joint separating the two pubic bones), on each side by the upper

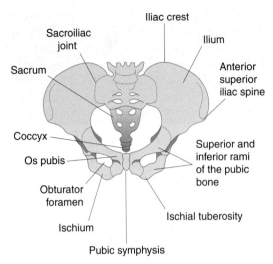

Figure 14.1 The bony pelvis.

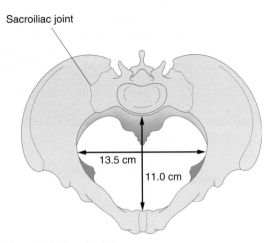

**Figure 14.2** The pelvic brim.

margin of the pubic bone, the ileopectineal line and the ala of the sacrum, and posteriorly by the promontory of the sacrum (Figure 14.1). The normal transverse diameter in this plane is 13.5 cm and is wider than the anterior–posterior diameter, which is normally 11 cm (Figure 14.2). The angle of the inlet is normally 60° to the horizontal in the erect position but in Afro-Caribbean women this angle may be as much as 90° (Figure 14.3). This increased angle may delay the head entering the pelvis until the second stage of labour.

*The pelvic mid-cavity*

This pelvic mid-cavity can be described as an area bounded in front by the middle of the symphysis pubis, on each side by the pubic bone, the obturator fascia and the inner aspect of the ischial bone and spines, and posteriorly by the junction of the second and third sections of the sacrum. The cavity is almost round as the transverse and anterior diameters are similar at 12 cm. The ischial spines are palpable vaginally and are used as landmarks to assess the descent of the fetal head on vaginal examination (station). They are also used as landmarks for providing an anaesthetic block to the pudendal nerve. The pudendal nerve passes behind and below the ischial spine on each side. The pelvic axis describes an imaginary curved line, which shows the path that the centre of the fetal head takes during its passage through the pelvis.

*The pelvic outlet*

The pelvic outlet is bounded in front by the lower margin of the symphysis pubis, on each side by the

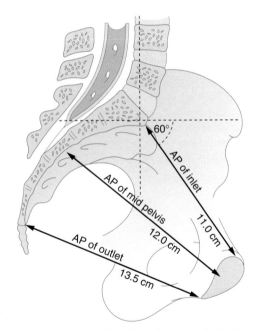

**Figure 14.3** Sagittal section of the pelvis demonstrating the anterior–posterior (AP) diameters of the inlet and outlet.

descending ramus of the pubic bone, the ischial tuberosity and the sacrotuberous ligament, and posteriorly by the inferior aspect of the sacrum. The anterior–posterior diameter of the pelvic outlet is 13.5 cm and the transverse diameter is 11 cm (Figure 14.4) Therefore, the transverse is the widest diameter at the inlet but at the outlet it is the anterior–posterior. Recognizing this is crucial to the understanding of the mechanism of labour.

The pelvic measurements given here are obviously average values and relate to bony points. Maternal stature, previous pelvic fractures and metabolic bone disease, such as rickets, may all be associated with measurements less than these population means. Furthermore, as the pelvic ligaments at the pubic ramus and the sacroiliac joints soften towards the end of the third trimester, the pelvis often becomes more flexible to allow these diameters to increase during labour.

A variety of pelvic shapes have been described and these may contribute to difficulties in labour. The gynaecoid pelvis is the most favourable for labour and the most common (Figure 14.5a–c). Other pelvic shapes are shown in Figures 14.6–14.8. An android-type pelvis is said to predispose to deep transverse arrest (Figure 14.6) and the anthropoid shape encourages persistence of the occipitoposterior (OP) position. A platypelloid pelvis also is associated with an increased risk of obstructed labour.

### The pelvic floor

This is formed by the two levator ani muscles, which, with their fascia, form a musculofascial gutter during the second stage of labour (Figure 14.9).

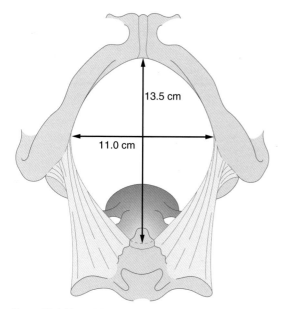

**Figure 14.4** The pelvic outlet.

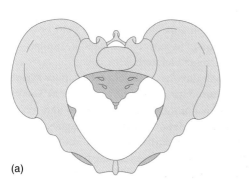 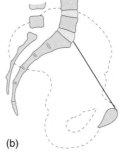 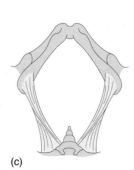

**Figure 14.5** The gynaecoid pelvis: (a) brim; (b) lateral view; (c) outlet.

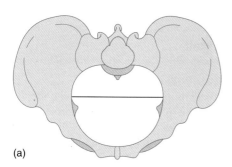 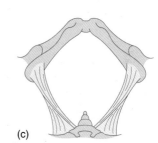

**Figure 14.6** The android pelvis: (a) brim; (b) lateral view; (c) outlet.

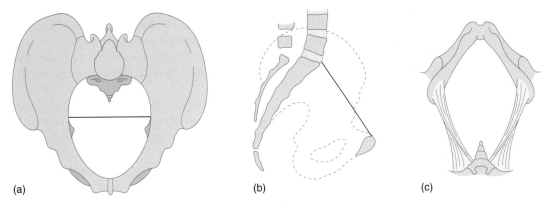

**Figure 14.7** The anthropoid pelvis: (a) brim; (b) lateral view; (c) outlet.

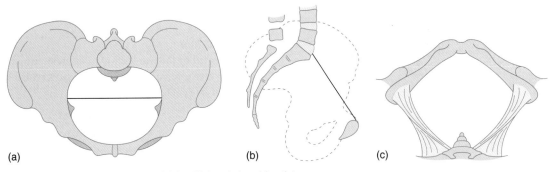

**Figure 14.8** The platypelloid pelvis: (a) brim; (b) lateral view; (c) outlet.

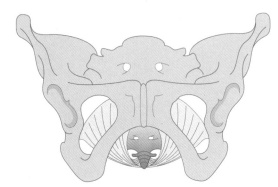

**Figure 14.9** The musculofascial gutter of the levator sling.

### The perineum

The perineal body is a condensation of fibrous and muscular tissue lying between the vagina and the anus (Figure 14.10). It receives attachments of the posterior ends of the bulbocavernous muscles, the medial ends of the superficial and deep transverse perineal muscles, and the anterior fibres of the external anal sphincter. It is always involved in a second-degree perineal tear and an episiotomy.

## The fetal skull

### The bones, sutures and fontanelles

The fetal skull is made up of the vault, the face and the base. The sutures are the lines formed where the individual bony plates of the skull meet. At the time of labour, the sutures joining the bones of the vault are soft, unossified membranes, whereas the sutures of the face and the skull base are firmly united (Figure 14.11). The bones that form the vault are the parietal bones, and parts of the occipital, frontal and temporal bones. Between these bones are four membranous sutures: the sagittal, frontal, coronal and lambdoidal sutures.

Fontanelles are the junctions of the various sutures. The anterior fontanelle or bregma (diamond shaped) is at the junction of the sagittal, frontal and coronal sutures. The posterior fontanelle (triangular shaped) lies at the junction of the sagittal suture and the lambdoidal sutures between the two parietal bones and the occipital bone. The fact that these sutures are not united is important for labour. It allows these bones to

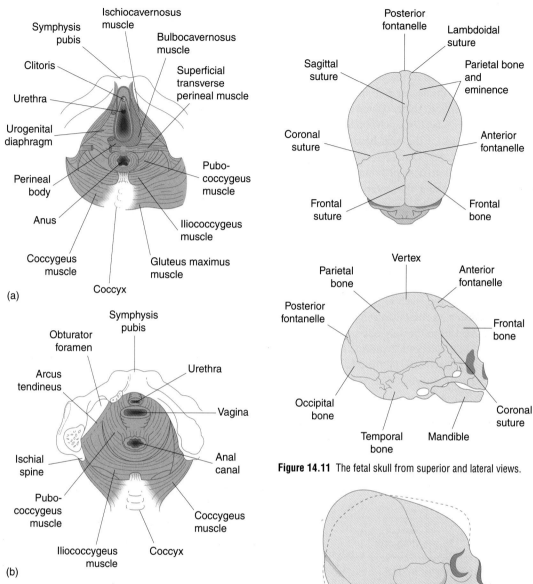

Figure 14.11 The fetal skull from superior and lateral views.

**Figure 14.10** The perineum, perineal body and pelvic floor from below, showing superficial (a) and deeper (b) views. The pelvic floor muscles are made up of the levator ani (pubococcygeus and ileococcygeus).

move together and even to overlap. The parietal bones usually tend to slide over the frontal and occipital bones. Furthermore, the bones themselves are compressible. Together, these characteristics of the fetal skull allow a process called *moulding* (the change in shape of the fetal skull during labour), to occur, which effectively reduces the diameters of the fetal skull and encourages progress through the bony pelvis, without harming the underlying brain (Figure 14.12). Severe

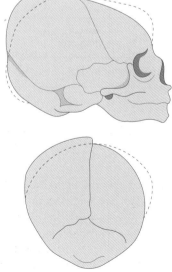

**Figure 14.12** A schematic representation of moulding of the fetal skull.

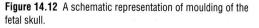

or abnormal moulding, however, can be a sign of cephalopelvic disproportion.

## The diameters of the skull

The fetal head is ovoid in shape. The *attitude* of the fetal head refers to the degree of flexion and extension at the upper cervical spine. Different longitudinal diameters are presented to the pelvis in labour, depending on the *attitude* of the fetal head (Figures 14.13 and 14.14).

The area of the fetal skull bounded by the two parietal eminences and the anterior and posterior fontanelles is termed the *vertex*. The longitudinal diameter that presents in a well-flexed fetal head (vertex presentation) is the *suboccipitobregmatic diameter*. This is usually 9.5 cm and is measured from the suboccipital region to the centre of the anterior fontanelle (bregma). The longitudinal diameter that presents in a less well-flexed head, such as is found in occipitoposterior position, is the *suboccipitofrontal diameter*, and is measured from the suboccipital region to the prominence of the forehead. It measures 10 cm.

With further extension of the head, the *occipitofrontal diameter* presents. This is measured from the root of the nose to the posterior fontanelle and is 11.5 cm. The greatest longitudinal diameter that may present is the *mentovertical*, which is taken from the chin to the furthest point of the vertex and measures 13 cm. This is known as a brow presentation and it is usually too large to pass through the normal pelvis. Extension of the fetal head beyond this point results

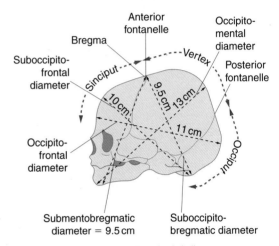

**Figure 14.13** The diameters of the fetal skull.

| | Flexed ⟶ Extended | | | |
|---|---|---|---|---|
| **Attitude** | Well flexed | Less well flexed (partially extended) or deflexed | Extended 'brow presentation' | Hyperextended 'face presentation' |
| **Diameter** | Suboccipito-bregmatic | Occipitofrontal | Occipitomental | Submento-bregmatic |
| **Measurement** | 9.5 cm | 11.5 cm | 13.0 cm | 9.5 cm |

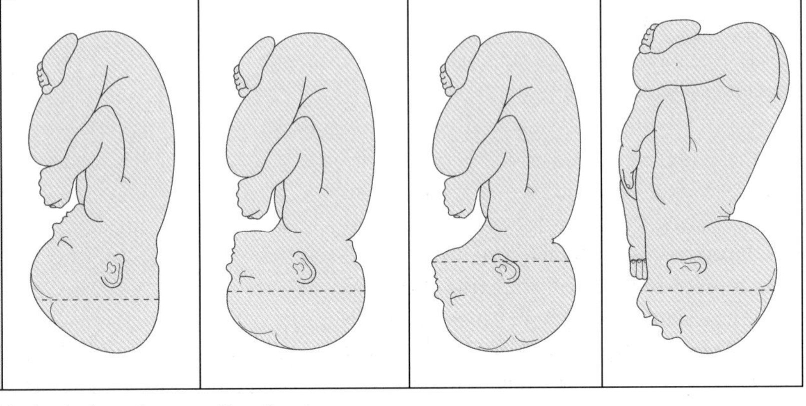

**Figure 14.14** The effect of fetal attitude on the presenting diameter.

in a smaller diameter. The *submentobregmatic diameter* is measured from below the chin to the anterior fontanelle and measures 9.5 cm. This is clinically a face presentation. The incidence of face presentation is about 1:500.

## The process of labour

### The onset of labour

The onset of labour can be defined as regular contractions bringing about progressive cervical change. The loss of a 'show' (a blood-stained plug of mucus passed from the cervix) or spontaneous rupture of the membranes (SROM), do not define the onset of labour, although they may occur at the same time. Labour can be well established before either of these events occur and both may precede labour. Although much is understood about the physiology of labour in humans, the initiating biological event is partly unclear.

### The stages of labour

The important events in normal labour are the onset of labour and the maternal urge to push, which usually corresponds with full dilatation of the cervix and the baby's head resting on the perineum. Defining the three stages of labour becomes more relevant if the labour does not progress normally or is delayed.

*First stage*

The first stage describes the time from the onset of labour to full dilatation of the cervix (10 cm). The first stage of labour can be divided into two phases. The *latent phase* is the time between the onset of labour and 3–4 cm dilatation. During this time, the cervix becomes *fully effaced*. Effacement is a process by which the cervix shortens in length as it becomes incorporated into the lower segment of the uterus. The process of effacement may begin during the weeks preceding the onset of labour but will be complete by the end of the latent phase. The cervical os cannot usually begin to dilate until effacement is complete. Effacement and dilatation should be thought of as consecutive events in the nulliparous woman, but may occur simultaneously in the multiparous woman. Dilatation is expressed in centimetres between 0 and 10.

The duration of the latent phase is variable and time limits are unhelpful. However, it usually lasts between 3 and 8 hours, being shorter in multiparous women. The second phase of the first stage of labour is called the *active phase* and describes the time between the end of the latent phase (3–4 cm dilatation) to full dilatation (10 cm; Figure 14.15). It is also variable in length, usually lasting between 2 and 6 hours. Again, it is usually shorter in multiparous women.

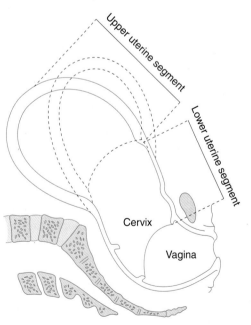

**Figure 14.15** The thick upper segment and the thin lower segment of the uterus at the end of the first stage of labour. The dotted lines indicate the position assumed by the uterus during contraction.

### Second stage

The second stage describes the time from full dilatation of the cervix to delivery of the fetus. The second stage of labour may also be subdivided into two phases. The *passive phase* is where there is no maternal urge to push and the fetal head is still relatively high in the pelvis. The second phase is rather confusingly called *active* second stage. There is a maternal urge to push because the fetal head is low, causing a reflex need to 'bear down'. In normal labour, the second stage is often diagnosed at this point. Conventionally, the upper duration for normal second stage is 2 hours in a primiparous and 1 hour in a multiparous woman, but this may vary.

### Third stage

The third stage is the time from delivery of the fetus until delivery of the placenta. Bleeding is controlled. The placenta is usually delivered within a few minutes of the birth of the baby depending on the management employed.

## The duration of labour

It has now been acknowledged that the available evidence does not support arbitrary time limits, which had been previously set for the first and second stages of labour. The presence of a doula/partner/supporter has a very considerable effect on the woman's experience and on the outcome of the labour. This one-to-one support does a lot to minimize the need for pain relief and to improve the woman's experience of childbirth. Evidence also shows that the length of labour is shortened. The midwife should not limit the time of the labour so long as the mother is comfortable, and the fetus is well and there are reassuring signs of this. The essential criterion is that of progress. Contemporary midwifery practice maintains that the woman remains the focus of care. One birthing unit in London advocates removing the clock in the birthing room in order to do away with the constant surveillance of time.

## The mechanism of labour

This refers to the series of changes in position and attitude that the fetus adopts during its passage through the birth canal. It is described here for the vertex presentation and the gynaecoid pelvis. The relation of the fetal head and body to the maternal pelvis changes as the fetus descends through the pelvis. This is essential so that the optimal diameters of the fetal skull are present at each stage of the descent.

### Engagement

The head normally enters the pelvis in the transverse position or some minor variant of this, so taking advantage of the widest diameter. Engagement is said to have occurred when the widest part of the presenting part has passed successfully through the brim of the pelvis. Engagement has occurred in the vast majority of nulliparous women prior to labour but not so for the majority of multiparous women.

The number of fifths of the fetal head palpable abdominally is often used to describe whether engagement has taken place. If more than two-fifths of the fetal head is palpable abdominally then the head is not engaged.

### Descent

During the first stage of labour, contraction and retraction of the uterine muscle exerts pressure on the fetus to descend. This process accelerates with the rupture of membranes and maternal efforts to push (Figure 14.16).

### Flexion

As the head descends into the narrower mid-cavity, flexion increases. This is probably a passive movement, in part due to the surrounding structures, and is important in minimizing the presenting diameter of the fetal head to facilitate its passage through the birth canal. Pressure exerted down the fetal axis will be more readily transmitted to the occiput, thus increasing flexion.

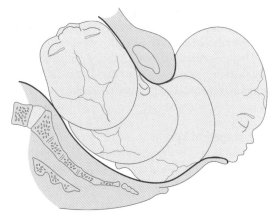

**Figure 14.16** Descent and flexion of the head followed by internal rotation and ending in the birth of the head by extension.

Internal rotation

If the head is well flexed, then the occiput will be the leading point and, on reaching the sloping gutter of the levator ani muscles, will be encouraged to rotate anteriorly so that the sagittal suture now lies in the anterior–posterior diameter of the pelvic outlet (i.e. the widest diameter). Resistance is an important dynamic of rotation. If the fetus has engaged in the occipitoposterior position, internal rotation can occur from an OP position to an occipitoanterior position. This long internal rotation, together with the larger presenting diameters of the fetal skull, explains the increased duration of labour associated with this malposition. Alternatively, an OP position may persist, resulting in a 'face to pubes' delivery. More often, the persistent OP position is associated with extension of the fetal head with a resulting increase in the diameter presented to the pelvic outlet. This may lead to obstructed labour and the need for instrumental delivery or even Caesarean section.

### Extension

Following completion of internal rotation, the occiput is underneath the symphysis pubis and the bregma is near the lower border of the sacrum. The soft tissues of the perineum still offer resistance, and may be traumatized in the process (see Chapter 15). The well-flexed head now extends, with the occiput escaping from underneath the symphysis pubis and starting to distend the vulva. This is known as the crowning of the head. The head extends further and the occiput underneath the symphysis pubis almost acts as a fulcrum point as the bregma, face and the chin appear in succession over the posterior vaginal opening and perineal body. This extension and movement minimize soft tissue trauma by utilizing the smallest diameters of the head for the birth.

### Restitution

Restitution is the undoing of the twist of the fetal head, which resulted from the internal rotation. It is the slight rotation of the occiput through one-eighth of a circle. When the head is delivering, the occiput is directly anterior. As soon as it escapes from the vulva, the head aligns itself with the shoulders, which have entered the pelvis in the oblique position.

### External rotation

In order to be delivered, the shoulders have to rotate into the anterior–posterior plane, the widest diameter

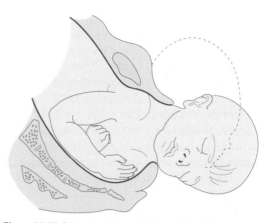

**Figure 14.17** External rotation of the head after delivery as the anterior shoulder rotates forward to pass under the subpubic arch.

at the outlet. When this occurs, the occiput rotates through a further one-eighth of a circle to the transverse position. This is called external rotation (Figure 14.17).

### Delivery of the shoulders and fetal body

When restitution and external rotation have occurred, the shoulders will be in the anterior–posterior plane. The anterior shoulder is under the symphysis pubis and delivers first, and the posterior shoulder delivers subsequently. Although this process may occur without assistance, often 'lateral traction' is exerted by gently pulling the fetal head in a downward direction to help release the anterior shoulder from beneath the pubic symphysis.

Normally, the rest the fetal body is delivered easily with the posterior shoulder guided upwards, over the perineum by traction in the opposite direction, so sweeping the baby on to the maternal abdomen.

## Understanding the physiology

### Hormonal factors

Progesterone maintains uterine quiescence during pregnancy by suppressing prostaglandin production, inhibiting communication between myometrial cells and preventing oxytocin release. Oestrogen opposes the action of progesterone. Prior to labour, there is a reduction in progesterone receptors and an increase in the concentration of oestrogen relative to the progesterone. Oxytocin release from the pituitary, and prostaglandin synthesis by the chorion and the decidua increases, leading to an increase in calcium influx into myometrial cells. This change in the hormonal milieu also increases gap junction formation between individual myometrial cells, creating a functional syncytium, which is necessary for coordinated uterine activity. Maternal corticotrophin-releasing hormone increases in concentration toward term and potentiates the action of prostaglandins and oxytocin on myometrial contractility.

Fetally produced cortisol may contribute to the conversion of progesterone to oestrogen. Which of these hormonal steps initiates labour is unclear. As labour becomes established, the output of oxytocin increases through the Ferguson reflex. Pressure from the fetal presenting part against the cervix is relayed via a reflex arc involving the spinal cord and results in increased oxytocin release form the posterior pituitary.

### The myometrium

Myometrial cells contain filaments of actin and myosin, which are the two key proteins for contraction. The interaction of myosin and actin brings about contraction, while their separation brings about relaxation. An increase in intracellular free calcium ions results in the formation of the contractile entity of actin-phosphorylated myosin. Beta-adrenergic compounds and calcium-channel blockers decrease intracellular calcium. Prostaglandins and oxytocin increase intracellular free calcium ions.

Individual myometrial cells are laid down in a mesh of collagen. There is a cell-to-cell communication system by means of gap junctions, which facilitates the passage of various products of metabolism and electrical current between cells. Of interest is that these gap junctions are absent for most of the pregnancy but appear in significant numbers at term. It also appears that the gap junctions increase in size and number with the actual labour process and tend to disappear afterwards. Prostaglandins stimulate their formation, while beta-adrenergic compounds possibly inhibit them from being formed. The probability of a uterine pacemaker, from which contractions originate, is likely but has not been proven histologically.

Retraction is a major feature of uterine contractility during labour. This is the progressive shortening of the uterine smooth muscle cells in the upper portion of the uterus as labour progresses. After the cells contract, they relax but they do not return to their original length. The result of this retraction process is the development of the thicker, active, contracting upper segment of the uterus. At the same time, the lower segment of the uterus becomes thinner and more stretched. Eventually, this results in the cervix being taken up into the lower segment of the uterus and forming a continuum with the lower uterine segment (see Figure 14.15).

### The cervix

A spectacular alteration takes place in the cervix. The structure of the cervix softens and dilates during labour. The cervix consists mainly of fibrous tissue and collagen, bound together by a ground substance. The precise mechanism involved in the softening of the cervix is not understood, but is compared to an inflammatory response, mainly caused by prostaglandins, which causes a reduction in the amount of collagen. This is due to the activation of collagenolytic enzymes and the increase in the water content of the cervix at the end of pregnancy.

## Management of normal labour

*The actions, or lack of interventions on the part of the midwife reflect a philosophy of care that is oriented to the enhancement of the woman's capabilities to give birth (Roberts 2002:2)*

At term, women are advised to contact their midwife, local labour suite or their community midwife either when they have spontaneous rupture of membranes or when their contractions are occurring every 5 minutes or more. Whether at home, or in hospital, the midwife will then make an assessment of the situation based on the history and on clinical examination. She will also assess the need for comfort strategies and support for the woman.

### History

Important points to note in the admission history are:
- details of previous births and the size of previous babies;
- the frequency, duration and perception of strength of the contractions;
- whether the membranes have ruptured/colour and amount of amniotic fluid;

- the presence of abnormal vaginal discharge or bleeding;
- the activity of the fetus or the occurrence of fetal movement;
- any medical issues of note that may influence the labour and delivery (e.g. pregnancy-induced hypertension, fetal growth restriction, previous Caesarean section)

## General examination

The temperature, pulse and blood pressure must be recorded and a sample of urine tested for protein, blood, ketones and glucose.

## Abdominal examination

Abdominal examination is carried out to confirm the lie, presentation, that the fetal size corresponds to the gestational age and also to listen to the fetal heart. The examination also includes an assessment of the contractions. This takes time (at least 10 minutes) and is done by palpating the uterus directly, to give an accurate account of the length, strength and frequency of these and, most importantly, asking the woman how she perceives and experiences them.

## Vaginal examination

A full explanation of the purpose and technique of vaginal examination is given to the woman and her consent is obtained. The index and middle fingers are passed to the top of the vagina and the cervix. The cervix is examined for dilatation, effacement and application to the presenting part. The dilatation is estimated digitally in centimetres. When no cervix can be felt, this means the cervix is fully dilated (10 cm). The length of the cervix should be recorded. The cervix at 36 weeks is about 3 cm long. It then gradually shortens by the process of effacement. In early labour, it may still be uneffaced. At about 3 cm of dilatation, the cervix should be fully effaced.

Providing the cervix is at least 3 cm dilated, it should be possible to determine both the position and station of the presenting part. In normal labour, the vertex will be presenting and the position can be determined by locating the occiput. The occiput is identified by feeling for the triangular posterior

fontanelle, with three sutures running into it. Failure to feel the posterior fontanelle may be because the head is deflexed, the occiput is posterior or because there is so much caput that the suture cannot be felt. All of these indicate the possibility of a prolonged labour. Normally, the occiput will be transverse (OT position) or anterior (OA).

Relating the lowest part of the head to the ischial spines will give an estimation of the station. This vaginal assessment of station should always be taken together with assessment of the degree of engagement, by abdominal palpation. If the head is at or below the ischial spines (0 to +1 or more) and the occiput is anterior, the outlook is favourable for vaginal delivery. The condition of the membranes should also be noted. If they have ruptured, the colour and amount of fluid draining should be noted. Goodly amounts of clear fluid are a good prognostic feature; scanty, heavily blood-stained or meconium-stained fluid needs to be considered by the midwife.

The admission history and review act as an initial screening. If features are normal, the woman will remain under midwifery care. A flow chart for this is shown in Figure 14.18.

## Fetal assessment

Fetal assessment in labour is by:
- observation of the colour of the liquor – fresh meconium staining and heavy bleeding are markers of potential fetal compromise (Figure: 14.19);
- intermittent auscultation of the fetal heart using a Pinard stethoscope or a hand-held Doppler;
- continuous external fetal monitoring using the cardiotocograph (CTG);
- fetal scalp blood sampling.

Meconium is often passed by a healthy fetus at or after term as a result of maturation of gastrointestinal physiology. In this scenario, it is usually thin and a very dark green or brown colour. It may, however, also be expelled from a fetus exposed to marked intrauterine hypoxia or acidosis. In this scenario, it is often thicker and much brighter green in colour.

Insufficient oxygen delivery to the fetus causes a switch to fetal anaerobic metabolism and the generation of lactic acid and hydrogen ions. In excess, these saturate the buffering systems of the fetus and cause a metabolic acidosis, which, in the extreme, can cause

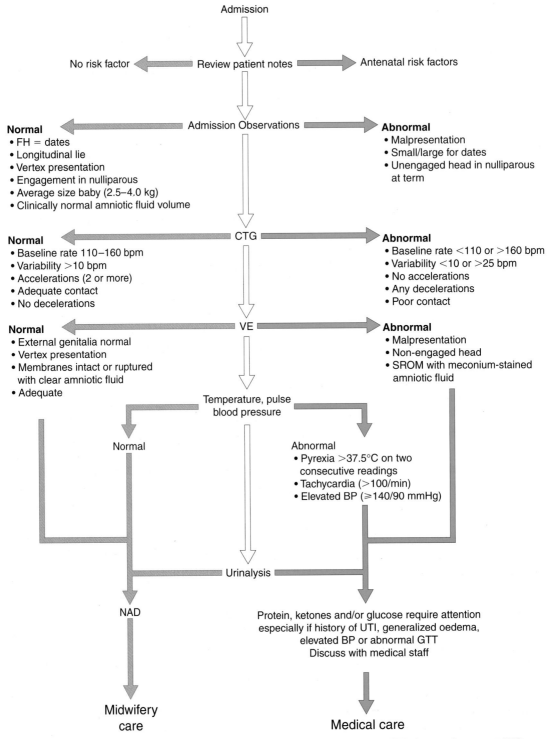

**Figure 14.18** Admission management flow chart. BP, blood pressure; CTG, cardiotocograph; GTT, glucose tolerance test; NAD, no abnormality detected; SFH, symphysis–fundal height; SROM, spontaneous rupture of the membranes; UTI, urinary tract infection; VE, vaginal examination.

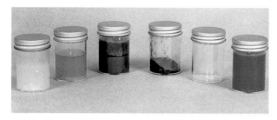

**Figure 14.19** Samples of amniotic fluid. From left to right: clear/whitish amniotic fluid; slight meconium staining (grade 1); moderate meconium staining (grade 2); thick meconium (grade 3); no fluid obtained; blood-stained amniotic fluid.

neuronal damage and permanent neurological injury. Hypoxia and acidosis cause a characteristic change in the fetal heart rate pattern, which can be detected by the CTG. Unfortunately, these CTG changes can be difficult to interpret and carry a significant false-positive rate (i.e. they often suggest fetal compromise), when in fact the fetus is still in good condition. In order that the use of CTG does not lead to unnecessary intervention, a fetal scalp blood sample may be performed during labour to measure fetal pH and base excess directly [National Institute for Clinical Excellence (NICE) 2001]. Often these results are normal, even when CTG shows suspicious signs.

## Records

The midwife's record of labour is a legal document and, as such, can be scrutinized in court for up to 25 years, examined by the midwifery supervisor or during any audit process. These records are a summary of the woman's physical, psychological, social and spiritual state, and an accurate synopsis of the midwife's response to these.

## Partogram

The partogram is a chart, which provides an overview of the elements of labour (Figure 14.20). Early deviation from the norm can then be identified. The observation chart provides such comments as: name, age parity, gestational age/date of expected birth, blood group, any risk factors present (e.g. previous stillbirth, previous Caesarean section), together with the following:
- fetal heart rate;
- temperature;
- pulse;
- blood pressure;
- vaginal examination (any loss per vaginum or bleeding, caput, state of the membranes);
- length/strength/frequency of contractions (over a period of 10 minutes);
- intake/output;
- medication;
- pain relief.

## The first stage

The key principles of management are as follows:
- provision of continuity of care and emotional support to the mother;
- observation of the progress of labour with timely intervention, if indicated;
- monitoring of fetal well-being;
- adequate and appropriate pain relief consistent with the woman's wishes;
- adequate hydration to prevent ketosis.

### Mobilization and care

Women in labour should be encouraged to mobilize and should be able to birth in the setting they have chosen. Encouragement and reassurance is extremely important. Intervention is avoided unless there is a need or request for this. Women should be given the message that, given the right environment and circumstances, they will be able to cope with the pain of normal labour. There is no reason to restrict eating and drinking, although lighter foods and clear fluids may be better tolerated. Vaginal examinations are usually performed every 4 hours; however, evidence shows that many other signs may be used to confirm that progress in labour is being made. The descent of the fetal head and the baby abdominally, uterine contractions that are stronger and longer, the presence of show and the spontaneous rupture of membranes, maternal breathing pattern changes, and pelvic pressure all show that labour is progressing.

Descent of the presenting part through the pelvis is another crucial component of progress and should be recorded at each vaginal examination. Full dilatation may be reached but, if descent is inadequate, then vaginal delivery will not occur. If the membranes are intact, it is not necessary to rupture them if the progress of labour is satisfactory.

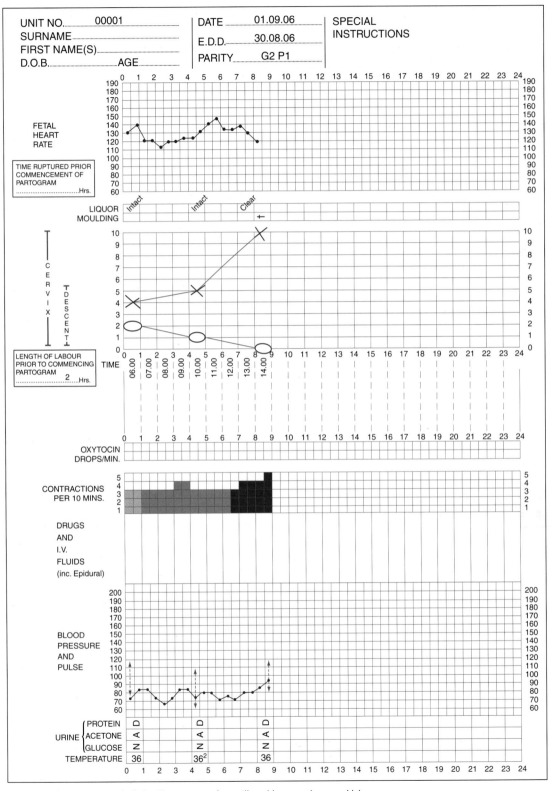

**Figure 14.20** A partogram depicting the progress of a mutligravid woman in normal labour.

## Second stage

If the labour has been normal, the first sign of the second phase of the second stage is an urge to push by the mother. Full dilatation of the cervix should be confirmed. The woman will get an expulsive reflex with each contraction. Early in the second stage, it does not matter what position the woman adopts but, if she is well propped up with her head upright and her hands behind her knees, she will be in a comfortable position to push effectively with some assistance from gravity. Alternatively, pushing can be quite effective in the left lateral position, which has the advantage of removing the weight of the uterus from the inferior vena cava and aorta (so maximizing cardiac output and uterine artery blood flow). There may be requests by women to deliver in different positions, or in water. In general, as long as mother and baby are well, and there is good progress in labour, then the outcome will be good.

### Descent and delivery of the head

The progress of the descent of the head can be judged by watching the perineum. At first there is a slight general bulge as the woman strains. When the head stretches the perineum, the anus will begin to open and, soon after this, the baby's head will be seen at the vulva at the height of each contraction. Between contractions, the elastic tone of the perineal muscles will push the head back into the pelvic cavity. The perineal body and vulval outlet will become more and more stretched, until eventually, the head is low enough to pass forwards under the subpubic arch. When the head no longer recedes between contractions (crowning), this indicates that it has passed through the pelvic floor and delivery is imminent. Therefore, at this stage, the midwife must control the head to prevent its being born suddenly. Once the head has crowned, the woman should be discouraged from bearing down to enable the baby to be born gradually. The head may now be delivered carefully. The head will extend as it does this.

### Delivery of the shoulders and rest of the body

Once the fetal head is born, a check is made to see whether the cord is wound tightly around the neck, thereby making delivery of the body difficult. If this is the case, the cord may need to be clamped and divided before delivery of the rest of the body. If there is meconium staining of the amniotic fluid, nasopharyngeal suction may be performed, if necessary. With the next contraction, external rotation of the head occurs and the shoulders can be delivered. To aid delivery of the shoulders, the head should be pulled gently downwards and forwards until the anterior shoulder appears beneath the pubis. The head is then lifted gradually until the posterior shoulder appears over the perineum and the baby will be born in a movement of lateral flexion.

## Immediate care of the neonate

When the baby is born, the time of birth is noted, and baby usually takes its first breath within the first minute. The baby is then given to its mother. There is no need for immediate clamping of the cord and, indeed, about 80 mL of blood will be transferred from the placenta to the baby before cord pulsations cease, reducing the chances of neonatal anaemia and iron deficiency. After clamping the cord, the baby should have a 1-minute Apgar score assessed. Skin to skin contact should be encouraged and the baby may attempt suckling at the breast. This will help establish the bonding process and also encourage the release of oxytocin, which will stimulate uterine contractions as well as promoting lactation. The baby is identified, weighed and vitamin K may be given with the mother's consent.

## Third stage

The third stage of labour is continuous with the second in that, as labour progresses, retraction of the uterine muscle reduces the placental area. The placenta itself becomes compressed and the blood in the intervillous space is pushed into the spongy layer of the decidua. The retraction of the oblique fibres of the myometrium constricts the vessels supplying the placenta, thus preventing the blood from draining back into the maternal vascular tree. As pressure inside the vessels increase, these eventually rupture and blood collects between the spongy layer of the decidua and the maternal side of the placenta, thus instigating the process of separation, aided by the ongoing process of retraction of the myometrium.

In summary, the three mechanisms that aid the process of placental separation are:
- the placental site is reduced by the action of retraction;

- the blood vessels supplying the placenta are constricted, then rupture, and blood collects behind the placenta;
- the formation of a retroplacental clot, usually centrally.

The placenta then peels away from the uterus, stripping itself from the centre laterally, owing to the increased weight, the fetal side appearing first in the vulva, and encapsulating the blood and clot in the bag of membranes as it is expelled. This mechanism is known as the Schultze method. The other mechanism is called the Duncan method of expulsion whereby the retroplacental blood formation does not form a clot, but escapes from the lower border of the placenta, thus the placenta is delivered in a side-on fashion, sliding down into the lower uterine segment and appearing at the vulva (i.e. membranes, blood and placenta are expelled together). The blood loss is greater and may be mistaken for the onset of haemorrhage. There is also greater risk of retained parts, placenta or membranes.

### Control of bleeding

Four mechanisms control the bleeding:

- the action of the living ligatures, the oblique fibres of the myometrium;
- the strengthening uterine contractions;
- clot formation in the ruptured vessels is increased and the placental area is covered by a fibrin mesh;
- the baby suckling at its mother's breast stimulates the release of oxytocin, increasing contraction–retraction of the myometrium.

### Midwifery care

The midwife's role is dependant on an adequate knowledge of the physiology of this process. Therefore, the principles of good management must be adhered to: awaiting the signs of placental separation (hardening and rising of the fundus, lengthening of the cord and a trickle of blood); and not interfering in the physiology and allowing the process to complete itself (i.e. no unsolicited touching and rubbing of the fundus, which inhibits and indeed interrupts the process; Figure 14.21).

*Active management* is a procedure whereby prophylactic uterotonics are given, usually intramuscularly, to control postpartum haemorrhage despite the assessed obstetric risk to the woman. This is usually carried out in conjunction with the clamping and cutting of the cord, shortly after the birth of the baby, and followed by controlled cord traction (Figure 14.22) in

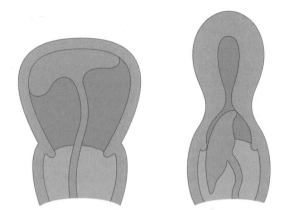

**Figure 14.21** Signs of separation and descent of the placenta. After separation, the uterine upper segment rises up and feels more rounded.

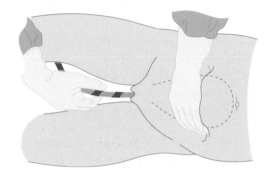

**Figure 14.22** Delivering the placenta by controlled cord traction.

a backwards and downwards motion, thus expediting the expulsion of the placenta.

*Physiological management* is, as the name suggests, awaiting the physiological occurrence of the expulsion of the placenta and membranes, and normal haemostasis. Here the midwife awaits the signs of placental separation, encourages the woman to push (either an upright or squatting position will aid the descent and separation of the placenta) and the placenta is expelled using gravity.

There still is much debate around the research carried out on active versus physiological management of the third stage. The studies done, however, agree on many issues, which are listed below (Begley 1990, Prendiville et al. 2002).

- The practitioner must be familiar with the technique of physiological management.
- Women require antenatal information on the physiological third stage.
- Active management of the third stage of labour is justified.

- Active management is associated with unpleasant side effects, such as nausea and vomiting, and hypertensive incidents.

After completion of the third stage, the placenta should be inspected for missing cotyledons or a succenturiate lobe. If these are suspected, then manual removal of the placenta (possibly under ultrasound guidance) should be arranged, as in this situation, the risk of postpartum haemorrhage is high. Finally, the vulva of the mother should be inspected for any tears or lacerations. Minor tears do not require suturing, but tears extending into the perineal muscles (or, indeed, an episiotomy) will require careful repair (see Chapter 15).

There is much debate around the definition of normal and normality in labour today. The thinking is that midwifery is struggling to determine what is normal, as 'normal' is a vast and variable concept, being understood individually and differently by midwives and women. The skill is knowing when and how to intervene but, even more so, when not to interfere in the normal process.

## Key Points

**Key features of normal labour**
- Spontaneous onset
- Single cephalic presentation
- 37–42 weeks' gestation
- No artificial interventions
- Unassisted spontaneous vaginal delivery
- Duration of less than 12 hours in nulliparous women, and less than 8 hours in multiparous women

## CASE HISTORY 1

Mrs RW is a 32-year-old para 1 (previous normal vaginal delivery at term) with no medical or obstetric history of note. She realized she was pregnant at approximately 6 weeks' gestation and organized an appointment with her general practitioner, who confirmed the pregnancy and referred her on to one of the community midwives attached to the practice. Owing to the absence of risk factors for complications, she was booked under midwifery care. A dating scan organized by the midwife agreed with the menstrual expected day of delivery (EDD) and screening tests in the second trimester were all reassuring. Regular visits through the second and third trimesters did not reveal any new problems.

At 39 weeks' gestation, after a week of increasing uncomfortable but irregular uterine tightenings, Mrs W experienced a 'show'. Her contractions remained irregular for a further 24 hours. Finally, they began to come frequently and when they reached every 5 minutes, she phoned her midwife who recommended assessment at the local maternity unit. Mrs W called her own parents who came to look after her first child, and she and her husband drove to the hospital.

On admission, the midwife took a history and performed an abdominal examination. The head was well engaged and the contractions were coming now every 3 minutes. A cardiotocograph on admission was normal, as were the maternal observations. A vaginal examination showed the membranes to be intact and the cervix to be fully effaced and 4 cm dilated. The vertex was found to be 1 cm above the spines. Mrs W, therefore, remained 'low risk' and under the care of the midwives.

She remained mobile and continued to drink whilst in labour but did not desire anything to eat. She spent some time in the bath, as this helped her cope with the contraction pains. The midwife listened regularly to the fetal heart with a Pinard stethoscope, during and after contractions, and this remained steady and of a normal rate. Maternal observations also remained normal. Three hours later her membranes ruptured. Permission was given for an internal examination and the cervix was found to be 9 cm dilated. She was finding the contractions much more painful, but with support and reassurance from her partner and the midwife did not require anything more than nitrous oxide for analgesia.

One hour later, she was aware of a strong urge to defaecate and began involuntarily pushing. Mrs W elected to lie in a supine position on the bed from this point onwards. The fetal heart was listened to during and after each and every contraction during the second stage. Twenty minutes later, the maternal anus began to dilate slightly and the vertex became visible soon after. Three further contractions and the head had delivered and, with the fourth, the rest of the baby's body. The midwife delivered the baby on to the maternal chest, and clamped and cut the cord a few minutes later. An intramuscular (IM) injection of Syntometrine was given as the mother had chosen this method of management of the third stage. The baby was born and the placenta delivered 8 minutes later. Vitamin K 1 mg IM was given to the baby with the consent of the mother. The baby made a good attempt to suckle. A baby check suggested all was well and Mrs W left hospital 7 hours later with her husband and new baby.

## Abnormal labour

### Poor progress in labour

Progress in labour is dependent on three variables:
- the powers, i.e. the efficiency of uterine contractions;
- the passenger (i.e. the fetus, with particular respect to its size, presentation and position);
- the passages (i.e. the uterus, cervix and bony pelvis).

Abnormalities in one or more of these factors can slow the normal progress of labour. It is essential that accurate observations and good-quality midwifery care are carried out. This will enable effective communication and accurate information to be exchanged, thus improving outcomes for the mother and the baby.

### Inefficient uterine action

This is the most common cause of poor progress in labour. It is more common in primigravidae and is characterized by weak, irregular or infrequent contractions. The assessment of uterine contractions is most commonly carried out by clinical examination. This must be done accurately, noting the length, strength and frequency of these. A frequency of three contractions in 10 minutes is usually considered ideal. Fewer contractions than this does not necessarily mean progress will be slow. Treatment is by maternal hydration and mobilization to promote uterine activity and improve the Ferguson reflex. An upright or position where women bend forwards, can make a posterior position turn to an anterior, if this is the cause of inefficient uterine action. Rupture of the membranes and intravenous oxytocin (Syntocinon) may be used to correct the ineffective contractions. Cephalopelvic disproportion must be ruled out before doing so.

### Cephalopelvic disproportion

Cephalopelvic disproportion (CPD) implies anatomical disproportion between the fetal head and maternal pelvis. This can be due to a large head, small pelvis or, usually, a combination of the two. Women of small stature (<1.60 m) with a large baby in their first pregnancy are likely candidates to develop this problem. The pelvis may be unusually small because of previous fracture or metabolic bone disease. Relative CPD can also occur with malposition of the fetal head together with deflexion, as occurs in the occipitoposterior

position (this is categorized as either direct OP, right OP or left OP; Figure 14.23).

Cephalopelvic disproportion is suspected in labour if:
- progress is slow or arrested despite efficient uterine contractions;
- the fetal head is not engaging;
- vaginal examination shows significant moulding and caput formation is present relatively early on in labour;
- the head is poorly applied to the cervix.

Oxytocin can be given cautiously to a primigravida with mild to moderate CPD as long as the CTG is reactive (NICE 2001). Relative disproportion may be overcome if the malposition is corrected (i.e. an occipitoanterior position is effected). Using oxytocin in a multiparous woman with slow or obstructed labour carries the risk of causing uterine rupture and must be used with caution.

### Malpresentations

Vital to good progress in labour is the tight application of the fetal presenting part on to the cervix. Breech and face presentations (see later) may fail to do this and the resulting progress in labour may be poor. Brow presentations are associated with the mentovertical diameter, which is simply too large to fit through the bony pelvis unless flexion occurs or

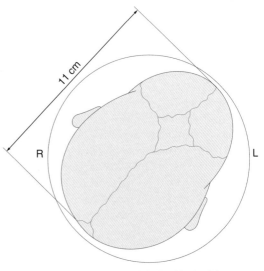

**Figure 14.23** Vaginal palpation of the head in the right occipitoposterior position. The circle represents the pelvic cavity, with a diameter of 12 cm. The head is poorly flexed so that the anterior fontanelle is easily felt.

hyperextension to a face presentation. Brow presentation, therefore, often presents as poor progress in first stage, often in a multiparous woman. Shoulder presentations cannot deliver vaginally and, once again, poor progress will occur. Malpresentations are more common in women of high parity and they carry a risk of uterine rupture, if the labour is allowed to become obstructed.

### Abnormalities of the passages

The bony pelvis may cause delay in progress of labour as discussed earlier under 'Cephalopelvic disproportion'. Abnormalities of the uterus and cervix can also delay labour. Unsuspected fibroids of the lower uterine segment can prevent descent of the fetal head. Delay can also be caused by cervical dystocia, a term used to describe a non-compliant cervix, which effaces but fails to dilate because of severe scarring, usually as a result of a previous cone biopsy. Caesarean section may be necessary.

## Poor progress in the second stage of labour

Delayed progress may occur as a result of the following:
- inefficient uterine action;
- inefficient maternal effort;
- full bladder or rectum;
- rigid perineum;
- contracted pelvis;
- big baby;
- fetal abnormality;
- persistent occipitoposterior position;
- deep transverse arrest (Figure 14.24);
- malpresentations.

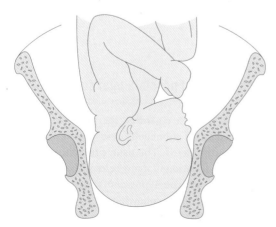

**Figure 14.24** Deep transverse arrest of the head.

The condition of the mother and baby must be assessed circumspectly and, if progress is advancing, time may be allowed, with continued and careful vigilance from the midwife. Mobilization, hydration, bladder care and adequate pain relief are all prerequisites to a positive maternal experience and a healthy outcome for the baby. These are even more essential when labour becomes prolonged and team members rely on each other for good communication and exact accounts of the women's situation, in order to make expedient decisions.

## Patterns of abnormal progress in labour

NICE (2004) states that the use of a partogram to plot the progress of labour, including the action line, improves the detection of poor progress, thus reducing the need for Caesarean section. Indeed, three patterns of abnormal labour are commonly described on the partogram (Figure 14.25).

### Prolonged latent phase

This occurs when the latent phase is longer than the arbitrary time limits discussed previously. It is more common in primiparous women and probably results from a delay in the chemical processes, which occur within the cervix that soften it and allow effacement. Prolonged latent phase can be extremely frustrating and tiring for the woman; however, intervention in the form of an artificial rupture of membranes (ARM) or oxytocin infusion will increase the likelihood of poor progress later in the labour and the need for Caesarean birth. It is best managed away from the labour suite with simple analgesics, mobilization and support.

### Primary dysfunctional labour

This is the term used to describe poor progress in the active phase of labour (<1 cm/hour cervical dilatation) and is also more common in primiparous women. It is most commonly caused by inefficient uterine contractions, but can also result from CPD and malposition of the fetus.

### Secondary arrest

This occurs when progress in the active phase is initially good but then slows, or stops altogether, typically after 7 cm dilatation. Although inefficient uterine contractions may be the cause, fetal malpositions, malpresentations and CPD are more common.

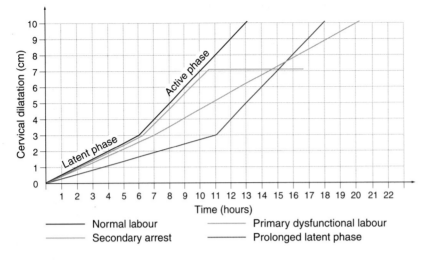

**Figure 14.25** Abnormalities of the partogram.

## Presumed fetal compromise in labour

Concerns for the well-being of the fetus is one of the most common reasons for medical intervention during labour. The fetus may already be compromised before labour, and the reduction in placental blood flow associated with contractions may uncover this and ultimately lead to fetal hypoxia and eventually acidosis. Fetal compromise may present as fresh meconium staining to the amniotic fluid or an abnormal CTG. However, neither of these circumstances confirm fetal hypoxia/acidosis. Meconium can be passed for benign reasons, such as fetal maturity, and it is well recognized that the abnormal CTG carries a very high false-positive rate for the diagnosis of fetal compromise; therefore, the use of the term 'fetal distress' as a reason for intervention is often inaccurate. In fact, intervention often occurs only because of *presumed* fetal compromise. After delivery, the condition of the baby is often found to be good. Only a fetal blood sample can definitely diagnose fetal hypoxia and acidosis in labour.

## Management of possible fetal compromise

If there is concern regarding the well-being of the fetus in labour, a number of resuscitative measures should be considered. The main procedure that will improve the situation in many cases will be to put the mother in the left lateral position, then to correct the situation by use of the following:
- Maternal dehydration and ketosis can be corrected with intravenous fluids.

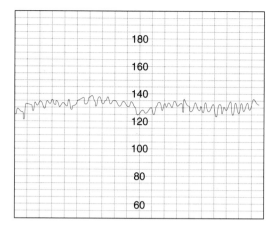

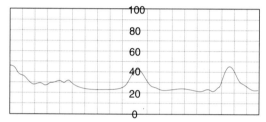

**Figure 14.26** Normal trace. The upper record is of the fetal heart rate and the lower record shows uterine activity.

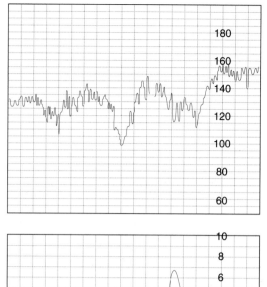

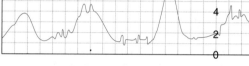

**Figure 14.27** Fetal heart rate: late decelerations.

- Maternal hypotension secondary to an epidural can be reversed by a fluid bolus, although a vasoconstrictor, such as ephedrine, is occasionally necessary.
- Uterine hyperstimulation from excess Syntocinon can be reduced by turning off the infusion temporarily and using tocolytic drugs, such as salbutamol and ritodrine.
- Venocaval compression and reduced uterine blood flow will also be eased by turning the woman into a left lateral position.
- Oxygen is often given to the mother by a face mask; however, there is conflicting evidence as to whether this improves fetal oxygenation.

If meconium staining to the liquor is noted, then a CTG must be commenced. Fresh thick meconium in the presence of a reassuring CTG is still cause for concern and, although the labour should be allowed to continue, the threshold for intervention will be lowered and a neonatologist should be present at delivery. The airways will be aspirated at birth.

If a CTG becomes suspicious or abnormal (Figures 14.26–14.30), then it is important to carry out an

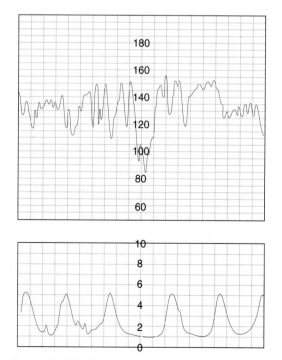

**Figure 14.28** Fetal heart rate: variable decelerations.

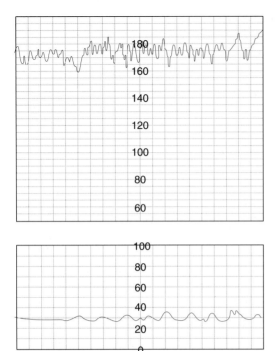

**Figure 14.29** Fetal tachycardia.

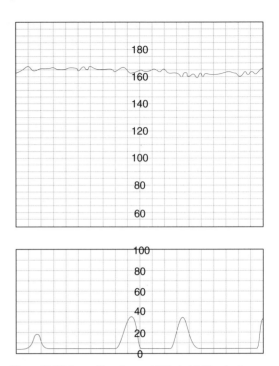

**Figure 14.30** Loss of baseline variability in fetal heart rate.

immediate vaginal examination to exclude malpresentation and cord prolapse, and to assess the progress of the labour. If the cervix is fully dilated, then it may be possible to deliver the baby vaginally using the forceps or ventouse. Alternatively, if the cervix is not fully dilated, fetal scalp blood sampling can be considered, although this is usually only possible at 2–3 cm dilatation or more (see box). A normal result will permit labour to continue, although it may

need to be repeated every 45–60 minutes if the CTG abnormalities persist or worsen. If there is another indication for Caesarean section, such as failure to progress, a normal result will allow the delivery to be performed with slightly less urgency, allowing a spinal anaesthetic. An abnormal result mandates immediate delivery by Caesarean section, if the woman is not fully dilated.

## Fetal blood sampling: the technique

- An amnioscope is inserted into the vagina and its distal end is placed at right angles on to the fetal head. The scalp is cleaned using a dry swab and a small cut is made using a blade with a guard. The resulting blood is collected into a microtube. The amount of blood required is approximately 25 μL.
- The normal pH would be above 7.25. A pH below 7.20 would be considered confirmation of fetal compromise.
- The base deficit can also be useful in interpretation of the fetal scalp pH. A base excess or more than −10

demonstrates a significant metabolic acidosis with increasing risk of fetal neurological injury beyond this level.
- One fetal scalp pH in labour is not very useful. A downward trend in the fetal scalp pH values is significant and should be assessed together with how the labour is progressing, and whether birth is imminent.
- If an abnormal CTG persists in labour, then despite normal values, fetal scalp sampling should be repeated every 30–60 minutes.

## CASE HISTORY 2

Mrs TS is a 30-year-old gravida 2 para 1. She is 153 cm tall. Her previous baby weighed 3.2 kg at term and was delivered by forceps after a prolonged second stage. The father of this second baby is a new partner.

Mrs TS has been admitted in spontaneous labour 10 days past her due date. Her hand-held records show concern from her midwife that this is a significantly larger baby than last time. Indeed, a scan at 36 weeks' gestation placed the abdominal and head circumference measurements on the 97th centiles. A subsequent glucose tolerance test was normal. Despite good progress in the earlier part of the labour, dilatation has arrested at 7 cm. On examination, the head is found to be 3/5 palpable per abdomen, the position is left occipitotransverse and the contractions are poor. There is meconium-stained amniotic fluid.

### What are the risk factors present here?

The large fetal size and the short maternal stature raise the possibility of cephalopelvic disproportion. The previous need for a forceps delivery of only an average size baby may have resulted from small pelvic diameters. There is a risk of obstructed labour, poor progress and the need for a Caesarean section. The meconium may simply be a sign of fetal maturity but it may also indicate a degree of fetal compromise. At the very least, it poses the risk of meconium aspiration at delivery.

### What care should Mrs TS receive?

She should be informed of the concerns and provided with adequate pain relief. Fetal monitoring with a continuous CTG should begin. (This, fortunately, proves to be reactive and, therefore, reassuring.) There is no need for a fetal blood sampling at this point.

Mrs TS should then be assessed by an experienced obstetric registrar, who must make a diagnosis as to the cause of this secondary arrest in the first stage. Has the delay in labour occurred simply because of poor uterine contractions? Is there CPD exacerbated by the fetal malposition?

If there is no caput or moulding, and the contractions indeed prove to be poor and infrequent, then a cautious trial of oxytocin can be considered. However, this woman has significant risk factors for CPD, and augmenting the labour with Syntocinon risks uterine rupture if the labour becomes truly obstructed.

### What subsequent assessment should be undertaken?

Two hours later, a vaginal examination should be performed, preferably by the same obstetrician. If the augmentation has been unsuccessful and the cervix is no further dilated, then a Caesarean section is indicated. Even if full dilatation is reached, a vaginal birth may not be possible. The obstetrician must be confident that the head has descended sufficiently, without the development of excessive moulding or caput.

## Women with a uterine scar

Women who have a uterine scar and who go into labour spontaneously, have a greater likelihood of birthing normally. A trial of scar is carried out when there is doubt about the outcome owing to a previous Caesarean section. The criteria necessary before attempting this are:

- it has been confirmed that the presenting part is capable of flexion, to enable it to engage;
- all the necessary equipment for an assisted birth is available;
- progress of both the presenting part and the cervical dilatation is made;
- time limits as to the duration of the trial are set.

## Malpresentations

### Face presentation

This malpresentation occurs in about 1:500 labours and is due to complete extension of the fetal head (Figures 14.31 and 14.32). In the majority of cases, the cause for the extension is unknown, although it is frequently attributed to excessive tone of the extensor muscles of the fetal neck. Certainly, during the antenatal period, full extension of the fetal neck can frequently be identified by ultrasound, which may last for a few hours. Rarely, extension may be due to a fetal anomaly, such as a thyroid tumour. The presenting diameter is the submentobregmatic, which measures 9.5 cm, that is, approximately the same as the suboccipitobregmatic (vertex) presentation. Despite this, engagement of the fetal head is late and progress

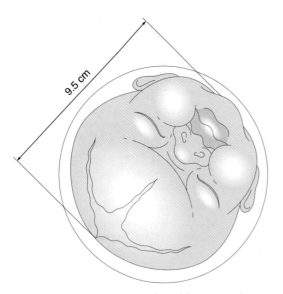

**Figure 14.31** Vaginal examination in the left mentoanterior position. The circle represents the pelvic cavity, with a diameter of 12 cm.

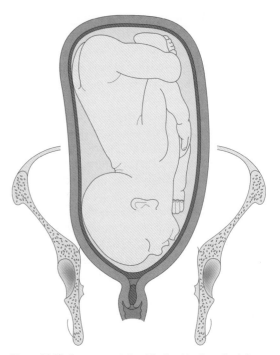

**Figure 14.33** Brow presentation. The head is above the brim and not engaged. The mentovertical diameter of the head is trying to engage in the transverse diameter at the brim.

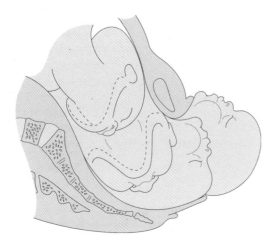

**Figure 14.32** The mechanism of labour with a face presentation. The head descends with increasing extension. The chin reaches the pelvic floor and undergoes forward rotation. The head is born by flexion.

in labour is frequently slow, possibly because the facial bones do not mould. It is diagnosed in labour by palpating the nose, mouth and eyes on vaginal examination. If progress in labour is good and the chin remains mentoanterior, then vaginal delivery is possible, the head being delivered by flexion (Figure 14.32). If the chin is posterior (mentoposterior position), then delivery is impossible, as extension over the perineum cannot occur. In these circumstances, Caesarean section is performed. Oxytocin should not

be used and, if there is any concern regarding the fetal condition, Caesarean section should be performed.

### Brow presentation

This arises when there is less extreme extension of the fetal neck than is seen with a face presentation (Figure 14.33). It can be considered a mid-way position between vertex and face. It is the least common malpresentation, occurring in 1:2000 labours. The causes of this are similar to face presentation, although some brow presentations will arise as a result of exaggerated extension associated with occipitoposterior position. The presenting diameter is mentovertical (measuring 13.5 cm). This is incompatible with a vaginal delivery. It is diagnosed in labour by palpating the anterior fontanelle, supraorbital ridges and nose on vaginal examination (Figure 14.34). If this presentation persists, Caesarean section is required.

### Shoulder presentation

This is frequently reported as occurring in 1:300 deliveries but few of these women will go into labour. Shoulder presentation occurs as the result of a transverse or oblique lie of the fetus. Possible causes include placenta praevia, pelvic tumour or uterine anomaly.

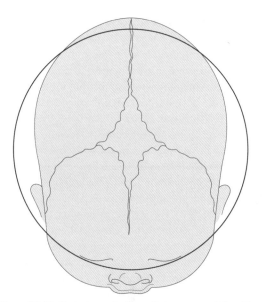

**Figure 14.34** Vaginal examination with brow presentation. The circle represents the pelvic cavity, with a diameter of 12 cm. The mentovertical diameter of 13 cm is too large to permit engagement of the head.

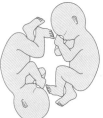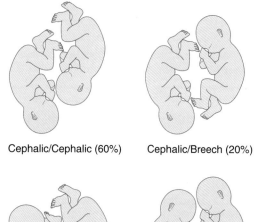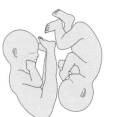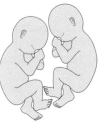

Cephalic/Cephalic (60%)   Cephalic/Breech (20%)

Breech/Cephalic (10%)   Breech/Breech (10%)

**Figure 14.35** The four major presentations of twin pregnancy.

Occasionally, a woman, usually of high parity, will present in labour with a shoulder presentation as a result of an uncorrected unstable lie due to uterine laxity. Normally, the antenatal problem of unstable lie will have been recognized and the woman admitted for observation. Delivery should be by Caesarean section. Delay in making the diagnosis risks cord prolapse when the membranes rupture or uterine rupture.

## Multiple gestations

About 1:80 pregnancies at term are multifetal. High-order multiples, such as triplets and quadruplets, are now invariably delivered by Caesarean section because of the risks to the last fetus, if vaginal delivery is attempted. Elective (i.e. planned) Caesarean section is frequently performed in twin pregnancies also, mostly for fetal reasons. These include the following:

- malpresentation of the first twin;
- second twin larger than the first;
- evidence of intrauterine growth restriction in one or both twins;
- monochorionic twins;
- history of fertility treatment.

There are four principal combinations of presentation (Figure 14.35):

- cephalic/cephalic – 60 per cent;
- cephalic/breech – 20 per cent;
- breech/cephalic – 10 per cent;
- breech/breech – 10 per cent.

Essentially, the lie and the presentation of the second twin is not crucially important. Planned Caesarean section will usually be performed, however, if the first twin presents by the breech and certainly if it is transverse. The ideal criteria for a twin labour are:

- spontaneous onset;
- cephalic presentation of twin 1;
- twin 1 larger than twin 2;
- dichorionic pregnancy.

The mechanics of the delivery of twins is discussed in greater detail in Chapter 9. Suffice to say that CTG abnormalities, fetal compromise, malpresentations, cord prolapse, the need for emergency Caesarean section and postpartum haemorrhage are all experienced more commonly than in singleton labours.

### Key Points

- Most labour is uncomplicated and the outcomes are good.
- Abnormalities of the uterine contractions ('the powers'), the fetus ('the passenger') and the pelvis and lower genital tract ('the passages') can cause abnormal labour.
- The term 'fetal distress' is unhelpful, and often misleading. If there are concerns for fetal well being in labour, 'presumed fetal compromise' should be used instead.

- Augmentation of labour with oxytocin will often correct poor uterine contractions and fetal malposition.
- Augmentation of labour with oxytocin must be used with caution in multiparous women, those with a uterine scar and in cases of malpresentation.

## Induction of labour

Induction of labour is the planned initiation of labour prior to its spontaneous onset. Between 15 and 25 per cent of all pregnancies in the UK end as an induction of labour (IOL). The reasons for IOL are listed below (see box). Broadly speaking, an IOL is performed when the risks to the fetus and/or the mother of the pregnancy continuing outweigh those of bringing the pregnancy to an end. IOL should only be performed if there is a reasonable chance of success, and if the risks of the process to the mother and/or fetus are acceptable. If either of these is not the case, a planned Caesarean section should be performed instead. Contraindications include placenta praevia, cephalopelvic disproportion, oblique or transverse lie, severe fetal compromise and, of course, lack of maternal consent.

### Common indications for induction of labour

- 'Post dates' (i.e. 12 days or more beyond expected day of delivery)
- Fetal growth restriction
- Other evidence of placental insufficiency (e.g. oligohydramnios)
- Pre-eclampsia
- Other maternal hypertensive disorders
- Deteriorating maternal illnesses
- Prolonged prelabour rupture of membranes
- Unexplained antepartum haemorrhage
- Diabetes mellitus
- Twin pregnancy continuing beyond 38 weeks
- Rhesus isoimmunization
- Maternal choice/request

The most common reason for IOL is 'post dates' or 'post maturity'. There is evidence that prolonged pregnancies extending beyond 42 weeks' gestation are associated with a higher risk of stillbirth, fetal compromise in labour, meconium aspiration and mechanical

problems at delivery. Because of this, women are usually recommended IOL at 10–12 days past their EDD. Another common indication for IOL is prolonged prelabour rupture of membranes. It is not uncommon for the membranes to rupture but for the subsequent onset of labour to be significantly delayed. The longer this situation is left to continue, the greater the risk of ascending infection (chorioamnionitis). Women who rupture their membranes at term before going into labour are usually advised to undergo IOL if their labour has not commenced within the next 24–72 hours (opinions vary as to how long women can be safely left). For premature labours, this period of time may be longer, but close fetal and maternal surveillance for signs of infection is necessary. Pre-eclampsia is another common indication for IOL; however, if the pre-eclampsia is severe and/or early in onset, Caesarean section may be indicated.

### The Bishop score

Bishop (1964) observed that, as the time of spontaneous labour approached, the cervix changed. It became softer, shortened, came forward and started to dilate. This reflects the natural preparation for labour. If labour is induced before this, then the induction process will tend to be correspondingly longer or may even fail. Bishop produced a scoring system (Table 14.1) to quantify the state of readiness of the cervix and fetus. High scores (a 'favourable' cervix) are associated with an easier shorter induction and one that is less likely to fail.

### Methods

Various routes and various preparations of prostaglandins have been used (gel or vaginal tablets), but the most common formulation in current use is prostaglandin gel (prostaglandin E; PGE), which is inserted vaginally into the posterior fornix. This is stored in the fridge. Recent work has proven the efficacy of Misoprostol tablets, which now feature as an alternative to PGE gel (NICE 2001).

Sweeping the membranes from the lower uterine segment possibly produces increased amounts of prostaglandin. Studies show that membrane stripping was a safe and effective way of avoiding induction by promoting spontaneous onset of labour at term.

**Table 14.1** – Modified Bishop score

| | Score | | | |
|---|---|---|---|---|
| | 0 | 1 | 2 | 3 |
| Dilatation of cervix (cm) | 0 | 1 or 2 | 3 or 4 | 5 or more |
| Consistency of cervix | Firm | Medium | Soft | – |
| Length of cervical canal (cm) | >2 | 2–1 | 1–0.5 | <0.5 |
| Position of cervix | Posterior | Central | Anterior | – |
| Station of presenting part | −3 | −2 | −1 or 0 | Below spines |

Women with an unfavourable cervix will require between one and three doses of vaginal prostaglandin. It is usually possible after this to perform an ARM and then to commence Syntocinon, if this is necessary. Women with a more favourable cervix may not require pretreatment with prostaglandin, and an ARM with or without Syntocinon may be sufficient to instigate labour.

## Complications of induction of labour

A CTG should be performed at the start of every induction and is normally continued throughout the process, as only pregnancies perceived to be at risk are induced. Many indications for IOL will be associated with a higher risk of fetal compromise in labour. The main risks of induction of labour include failure of induction, hyperstimulation with Syntocinon and long labours, which may predispose to postpartum haemorrhage owing to uterine atony.

## Comfort in labour

The provision of pain relief in childbirth varies in different cultures and according to women's preferences. Just as one woman's labour can be made into an unhappy experience by unsolicited and unnecessary analgesia, pain relief that is inadequate or offered too late can ruin another's experience. It should be remembered that the final decision rests with the woman, although there are certain circumstances when particular forms of analgesia are contraindicated and should not be offered to the woman.

## Non-pharmacological methods

*Relaxation* and controlling breathing may be of benefit to some women, as hyperventilation may occur when a woman becomes anxious. The environment is important and an ambiance that is tranquil and replicates that of the home is conducive to promoting well-being, therefore, maintaining the neurohormonal reflex and the effect of this on the woman and her labour. Homeopathy, acupuncture and hypnosis are sometimes employed.

*Transcutaneous electrical nerve stimulation* is frequently used. It works on the principle of blocking pain fibres in the posterior ganglia of the spinal cord by stimulation of small afferent fibres (the 'gate' theory). The advantages have been shown to be involvement of the husband/partner/companion, making this person feel useful. One of the main benefits is that it reduces and delays the need for other analgesia.

*Hydrotherapy* and relaxation in warm water during the first stage of labour often leads to a sense of well-being and allows women to cope much better with the pain. This therapy has been used for many years. The two-fold action of heat, which reduces muscle spasm, and hydrokinesis, the doing away with the effect of gravity, eradicates the discomfort and stretching felt in the pelvic region.

## Pharmacological methods

*Inhalational analgesia*
'Entonox' is an odourless premixed gas made up of 50 per cent nitrous oxide and 50 per cent oxygen (laughing gas). This is available by either piped supply

or cylinder, and is administered by four types of apparatus: Entonox, Pneupac, SOS Notronox and Peacemaker. As the gases separate below a temperature of $-7°C$, the cylinders must be stored at a temperature of 10°C, on their side, and inverted several times to remix the contents. Entonox takes effect within 20 seconds; therefore, the woman is instructed to inhale this just before the contraction commences, as the maximum effect occurs after around 45 seconds. Hopefully, this coincides with the height of the contraction, thus providing effective pain relief. This method is also advantageous in that the woman can administer it herself. Evidence shows that a high percentage of women stated satisfaction with this technique.

The excretion of the gas is rapid, via the lungs; therefore, toxic levels do not develop.

### Epidural analgesia

The pain relief from an epidural is achieved by blocking the conduction of nerve impulses along sensory nerves as they enter the spinal cord. The woman may not experience the pain of contractions, but she is able to move her lower limbs, pass urine and feel the need to push. However, there is an increased probability of interventions during labour.

The decision to have an epidural sited should be a combined one between the woman, her midwife, the obstetric team and the anaesthetist. The final decision in most cases rests with the woman unless there is a definite contraindication.

Indications
Tests for clotting factors and platelets are carried out prior to the siting of the epidural. It is particularly indicated for preeclamptic women, because of its hypotensive effect. Other indications include:

- preterm labour, to avoid use of drugs;
- prolonged labour, to enable the woman to rest;
- malpresentations (e.g. breech) to preclude premature pushing, and to allow intervention, if necessary;
- multiple pregnancy, to allow intervention and reduce the need for narcotic drugs;
- occipitoposterior position, to prevent pain and early pushing;
- cardiac and respiratory conditions (maternal);
- for operative delivery.
  The main contraindications are:
- coagulation disorders;
- local or systemic sepsis;
- hypovolaemia;

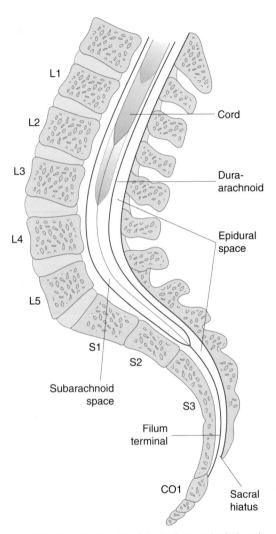

**Figure 14.36** Sagittal section of the lumbrosacral spinal cord.

- lack of trained staff (both anaesthetic and midwifery);
- spinal deformity.

Advanced cervical dilatation on its own is not a contraindication to an epidural. It is more important to assess the rate of progress, the anticipated length of time to delivery and the type of delivery expected.

Technique
Intravenous (IV) access is required prior to the insertion of the epidural. The need for preloading with IV crystalloid fluids has decreased, as low-dose epidurals are now used. The epidural catheter is normally inserted at the L2–L3, L3–L4 or L4–L5 interspace, and should come to lie in the epidural space which contains blood vessels, nerve roots and fat (Figure 14.36). The

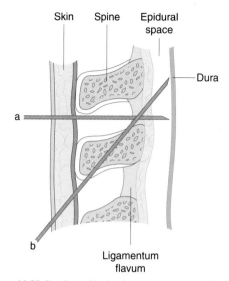

Skin    Spine    Epidural space

a

b

Dura

Ligamentum flavum

**Figure 14.37** Needle positioning for an epidural anaesthetic. Midline (a) and paramedian (b) approaches.

catheter is aspirated to check for position and, if no blood or cerebrospinal fluid is obtained, a test dose is given to confirm the catheter position (Figure 14.37). This test dose is a small volume of dilute local anaesthetic (e.g. 2 ml 0.5 per cent bupivacaine). If it has no obvious effect on sensation in the lower limbs, then the catheter is correctly sited. If there is a sensory block, leg weakness and peripheral vasodilatation, then the catheter has been inserted too far and into the subarachnoid (spinal space). Inserting the normal dose of local anaesthetic into the spinal space by accident would risk complete motor and respiratory paralysis. If none of these signs are observed 5 minutes after injection of the test dose, then a loading dose can be administered.

After the loading dose is given, the mother should be kept in the right or left lateral position, and her blood pressure should be measured every 5 minutes for 30 minutes. A fall in blood pressure may result from the vasodilatation caused by blocking of the sympathetic tone to peripheral blood vessels. This hypotension is usually short lived but may cause a fetal bradycardia owing to redirection of maternal blood away from the uterus. It should be treated with intravenous fluids and, if necessary, vasoconstrictors, such as ephedrine. The woman should lie in the left lateral position or be seated for the siting of the epidural, as this improves placental circulation. Opioids, such as fentanyl, may be used to supplement the epidural block and allow a reduction in the amount of local anaesthetic required. This has the added advantage of impairing

motor function in the lower legs to a lesser degree. Regional analgesia can be maintained throughout labour with either intermittent boluses or continuous infusions, or, occasionally, a combination of both.

### Spinal analgesia

In spinal anaesthesia, the local anaesthetic solution is injected into the subarachnoid space, directly into the cerebrospinal fluid, rather than into the epidural space. It is rapid and easy to perform, and usually effective. It produces a total motor and sensory block beyond the anaesthetized region but there is an increased risk of profound hypotensive incidents. It is, therefore, useful for shorter procedures, such as birth by forceps and manual removal of placenta, and repair of complicated vaginal or perineal tears. It can also be used for Caesarean section but may well be combined with epidural for this.

### Complications of regional analgesia

Patchy blocks result from the ineffective block on one area of the woman's body. The anaesthetist must be kept informed and will attempt to render the block more effective by resiting it, changing the position of the woman or injecting more anaesthetic. Other complications include the following.

- *Hypotension* is a fairly common complication and is usually easily treated.
- *Accidental dural puncture* during the search for the epidural space should occur in less than 1 per cent of cases. Because the needle used for an epidural is wider bore than that used for a spinal, if the subarachnoid space is accidentally reached with an epidural needle, then there is a risk that the hole left afterwards in the dura will be large enough to allow the leakage of cerebrospinal fluid. This results in a 'spinal headache', which is characterized by relief when lying flat but exacerbation by sitting upright. If the headache is severe or persistent, a blood patch may be necessary. This involves injecting a small volume of the woman's blood into the epidural space at the level of the accidental dural puncture. The resulting blood clot is thought to block off the leak of CSF.
- *Accidental total spinal anaesthesia* (injection of epidural doses of local anaesthetic into the subarachnoid space) causes severe hypotension, respiratory failure, unconsciousness and death if not recognized and treated immediately.
- *Neurological complications* are rare and are usually associated with other factors.

- *Drug toxicity* can occur with accidental placement of a catheter within a blood vessel. This is normally revealed by aspiration prior to injection.
- *Bladder care* is fundamental in these cases, as control and sensation is impaired. The midwife must maintain an accurate fluid balance and catheterize, if so indicated.
- *Backache* during and after pregnancy is not uncommon.
- *The effect of epidural analgesia on labour* and the operative delivery rate has become controversial, as the effect of epidural is to reduce the muscle tone of the pelvic floor, which needs to maintain a certain resistance, in order to increase flexion of the presenting part. The fetal head then does not fully flex, becomes arrested and intervention follows.

## Care by the midwife

Following administration of the first dose of bupivacaine and any further top-up doses, the blood pressure and pulse should be taken and recorded every 5 minutes for half an hour, and subsequently, half hourly. The woman can sit up, tilted to one side to avert aortocaval compression, once it has been ascertained that her blood pressure is stable. Regular changing of position will ensure comfort and avoid pressure areas from developing. The woman is encouraged to empty her bladder frequently. Uterine activity will be monitored by the midwife, but also by cardiotocography, as will the fetal heart rate.

## Summary

- An epidural can be a valuable form of pain relief for women in labour.
- Teamwork and cooperation are essential to optimize care and to site the epidural in a timely fashion.
- The midwife's role is important both at the epidural siting and during the continuing care.

## References

Begley CM. A comparison of active and physiological management of the third stage of labour. *Midwifery* 1990; **6**:3–17.

Bishop EH. Pelvic scoring for elective induction. *Obstetrics and Gynaecology* 1964; **24**:266–8.

National Institute for Clinical Excellence. *The use of electronic fetal monitoring.* London: NICE, 2001.

National Institute for Clinical Excellence. *Quick reference guide – clinical guideline 13 caesarean section.* London: NICE, 2004.

Prendiville WJ, Elbourne D, McDonald S. Active versus expectant management of the third stage of labour. *The Cochrane Library*, Issue 1. Oxford: Update Software, 2002.

Roberts JE. The push for evidence: management of the second stage. *Journal of Midwifery and Women's Health* 2002; **47**:2–14.

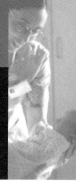

# Operative and assisted birth

## OVERVIEW

Operative vaginal delivery is carried out for three basic reasons, that is, to manage, expedite or shorten the second stage of labour, when there are problems with the maternal or fetal condition, or they are presumed to be at risk. It is also used to protect the fetal head in premature or breech delivery. The majority of Caesarean section births are for hypertensive disorders of pregnancy, antepartum haemorrhage or fetal compromise, and the main reasons for the increase in Caesarean section rates are breech presentation, repeat Caesarean section or dystocia. The role of the midwife is to be with the woman, supporting, encouraging and informing her of events, and to facilitate choice in all issues pertaining to her care. The most important factor is that of making sure that the woman is feeling in control of events, as this is shown to be a major feature of maternal satisfaction. The interactions and the exchanges, which provide support and appropriate information to the woman, have been shown to be the most influential features of quality and appreciated care.

## Episiotomy

Episiotomy is a surgical incision of the perineum made to increase the diameter of the vulval outlet during childbirth.

## History and epidemiology

By the 1970s, episiotomy rates were as high as 90 per cent. Further research carried out over the last 20 years has shown the problems associated with the procedure, which include unsatisfactory anatomical results, increased blood loss, perineal pain and dyspareunia. These studies have concluded that the routine use of episiotomy should be abandoned. The World Health Organisation recommends an episiotomy rate of 10 per cent for normal deliveries.

## How to avoid an episiotomy/perineal trauma

Alternating positions of the woman during labour may prevent perineal damage (e.g. kneeling, a supported squat or all fours). Physiological pushing and an upright position may allow the presenting part to descend and stretch the perineum gently, thus thinning it out gradually. Fetal distress can sometimes be rectified by change of maternal position and may prevent a ventouse or forceps delivery. A constant caring companion reduces the incidence of episiotomy and perineal trauma. Alternatives to epidurals for pain relief should be considered. When instrumental delivery is required, the use of the vacuum extractor rather than forceps was believed to decrease the incidence in perineal trauma. However, recent studies show that there is a considerable merit still in using forceps and these have the capacity to lower Caesarean section rates. Evidence shows that forceps are associated with less failure and are quicker to use than the ventouse. One study found no significant difference between forceps delivery and vacuum extraction in the rates of urinary and bowel dysfunction (Johanson and Menon 2000). Other reports would disagree (Fitzpatrick et al. 2003). The smaller Kiwi ventouse is also more frequently being used by midwives who are trained in this skill.

## Technique of episiotomy

There are two different techniques that are widely used (Figure 15.1):
1. midline (common in USA) – this is cut vertically from the fourchette down towards the anus;
2. mediolateral (standard in the UK) – this starts in the midline position at the fourchette but is then directed diagonally outwards to avoid the anal sphincter.

The advantages of the midline episiotomy are:
- less blood loss;
- easier to repair;
- the wound heals quicker;
- there is less pain in the postpartum period;
- the incidence of dyspareunia is reduced.

However, the major disadvantage is that it carries a more than six-fold risk of extending to involve the anal sphincter (third/fourth-degree tear).

## Anaesthesia

Prior to an episiotomy being performed, adequate anaesthesia must be administered. If the woman has an epidural, it must be topped up accordingly or the perineum must be infiltrated with local anaesthetic. A pudendal block may also be used.

Possible indications for an episiotomy include:
- fetal distress;
- short, long or inelastic perineum;
- shoulder dystocia;

- fetal malposition (e.g. occipitoposterior);
- an instrumental or breech delivery;
- previous pelvic floor surgery.

## Performing the episiotomy

The episiotomy must be made in one single cut and should begin in the midline at the fourchette.

## Complications

Cuts that begin more laterally are likely to be more painful and more complicated to suture. Any episiotomy may extend and cause a third-degree tear to the anal sphincter. An episiotomy can bleed significantly, which is why the perineum should be thinned out before attempting to carry out the procedure. Haemostasis should be achieved, with pressure or arterial clamps if necessary. Prophylactic antibiotics may be indicated.

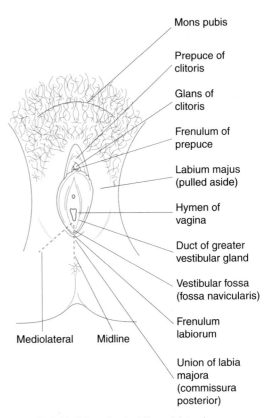

Mons pubis

Prepuce of clitoris

Glans of clitoris

Frenulum of prepuce

Labium majus (pulled aside)

Hymen of vagina

Duct of greater vestibular gland

Vestibular fossa (fossa navicularis)

Frenulum labiorum

Union of labia majora (commissura posterior)

Mediolateral    Midline

**Figure 15.1** Mediolateral and midline episiotomies.

- The episiotomy rate should be kept under 20 per cent
- Mediolateral are the method of choice – but this must begin in the midline
- Refer for an experienced opinion, if the episiotomy extends or appears complicated

## Perineal repair

Perineal injury is defined as follows (Figure 15.2).
- *First degree:* involves skin only.
- *Second degree:* involves perineal muscle and, therefore, includes episiotomy.
- *Third degree:* second-degree tear with disruption of the anal sphincter and is further subdivided into:
  - 3a: less than 50 per cent of external sphincter torn;
  - 3b: more than 50 per cent of external sphincter torn;
  - 3c: internal anal sphincter also torn.
- *Fourth degree:* third-degree tear with torn anal epithelium.

### History and epidemiology

Perineal injuries have occurred since childbirth began and surgical attempts at repair have been documented across a wide range of cultures, starting with crude juxtaposition described in ancient Egypt. In the UK today, approximately 750 000 women give birth each year and, of these, 525 000 (70 per cent) will sustain perineal trauma and will require stitches. The majority of these women will experience perineal pain in the immediate period following delivery and over 100 000 will have long-term problems, such as dyspareunia. If the repair is performed perfunctorily or inadequately, it may leave women suffering from perineal pain, which they describe as being far worse than the pain of childbirth.

Long-term perineal morbidity, associated with failure to recognize or to repair trauma to the external anal sphincter adequately, can lead to major physical, psychological and social problems for the woman.

### Technique

The skill of the operator, repair technique and suture material are contributing factors to perineal pain during the healing process. Some first-degree tears will not require suturing if in apposition, and others will simply require one or two interrupted sutures. A loose, continuous, non-locking suture technique to appose each layer (vaginal epithelium, perineal muscle and skin) is associated with less short-term pain.

### Complications

Missing the apex of the tear or episiotomy may allow continued bleeding or the development of a paragenital

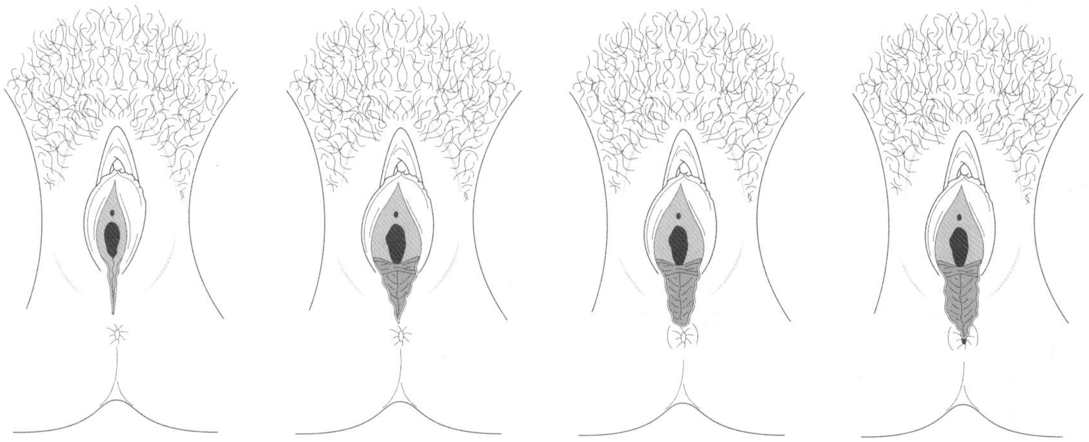

| 1st degree | 2nd degree | 3rd degree | 4th degree |

**Figure 15.2** Perineal anatomy with schematic graded injuries.

haematoma. Deep sutures including the rectal mucosa could lead to fistula formation. Overenthusiastic tight suturing can lead to significant later discomfort. Closure of the skin over the fourchette sometimes leads to formation of a bridge of tissue that can make intercourse very uncomfortable. Malaligned repairs lead to distortions in healing and increased scarring.

### Key Points

- Absorbable synthetic sutures are preferable
- The technique is the all-important factor
- If the tear is extensive, regional/general anaesthetic may be required
- Refer to an experienced person if necessary

### Third/fourth degree tear repair

#### History and epidemiology
Traditionally, this has been thought to be a complication affecting relatively small numbers of women (0.5–2 per cent). More recent work has shown that unrecognized complete disruption of the anal sphincter is much more common than this. Overall long-term incontinence affects 5 per cent of women.

#### Technique
As the anal sphincter (like the levator ani muscle) is normally in a state of tonic contraction even at rest, disruption will result in retraction of the muscle ends. In order to bring the muscle ends together, adequate muscle relaxation with regional or general anaesthesia is essential. Some surgeons juxtapose the ends of the sphincter (end-to-end) while others overlap them. Current evidence suggests that the short-term outcome is similar with either technique. Antibiotics and laxative agents are prescribed to prevent secondary infection and constipation.

#### Complications
Up to half the women who sustain a third/fourth degree tear develop bowel symptoms (including incontinence) despite a postpartum primary anal sphincter repair. The most probable explanation for the poor outcome is either inexpertise of the operator or inappropriate repair technique. It is for this reason that the most experienced person available should be involved.

## Instrumental and assisted birth

### History and epidemiology

Instrumental vaginal delivery is the hallmark of the specialty of obstetrics and the 'man-midwife'. Prior to the sixteenth century, childbirth was predominantly the domain of traditional (female) birth attendants. Barber-surgeons and others with appropriate skills were involved in the management of obstructed labour (usually by destroying the fetus). A variety of single-bladed instruments were also used as levers to deliver the fetal head. With the discovery of forceps (first used, and kept secret, by the Chamberlen family in London), a means to end the suffering of obstructed labour and a tool for delivering babies alive became available. Used exclusively by men, this allowed them to achieve and maintain a position of authority until the twentieth century.

Hundreds of different sorts of forceps have been invented and continue to be used around the world. Some forceps in current use were designed in Victorian times and others in the previous century, for example, Simpson's (Figure 15.3) and Neville-Barnes'. Although they have undoubtedly been used to save many lives, they are also associated with many maternal deaths. Particularly dangerous were 'high-forceps' deliveries; sometimes, these were attempted by general practitioner (GP) obstetricians at home. Where the delivery failed, the woman would be referred to the hospital as an FFO (failed forceps outside). To ensure that GPs did not try high deliveries, before the Second World War, Wrigley introduced a new design with short shanks/arms. Kjelland's

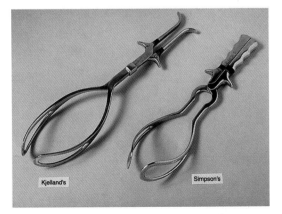

**Figure 15.3** Kjelland's (left) and Simpson's (right) forceps.

forceps are another important development from the turn of the century (Figure 15.3). These forceps did not have a 'pelvic curve' and could be turned around in the vagina to rotate an occipitoposterior position. These are not used today.

In the 1950s, the vacuum extractor (or ventouse) was invented in Sweden and is now more widely used worldwide than forceps.

Worldwide, assisted vaginal birth remains an integral part of the obstetrician's duties. Although it may occur as infrequently as 1.5 per cent of deliveries (Czech Republic), in other countries it occurs as often as 15 per cent (Australia and Canada). Discrepant rates may be related to differing management of labour.

## How to lower instrumental vaginal birth rates

Various techniques may help in achieving low instrumental delivery rates, for example, companionship in labour, upright positions and the use of exercise balls (now becoming more frequently used) and birthing stools, active management of the second stage with Syntocinon, and undertaking fetal scalp sampling when fetal heart rate decelerations occur. Letting the epidural wear off or having a more liberal attitude to the length of the second stage, when an epidural is being used, will also reduce the risks of needing an assisted birth.

## Ventouse delivery

The soft cups are smoothly applied to the contour of the baby's head. It has been shown that successful delivery is most likely with the ventouse when the cup is applied in the midline over the occiput. A well-placed cup will result in a well-flexed head and a good vacuum formation, whilst failure to put the cup far enough back will result in deflexion and failure to achieve the vacuum and birth.

### Technique

To minimize the chances of any fetal damage, the prerequisites and basic rules for delivery with the ventouse should be followed.

Indications for delivery with the ventouse are:
- delay in the second stage;
- fetal distress in the second stage;
- maternal conditions requiring a short second stage. Contraindications for delivery with the ventouse are:
- face presentation;
- gestation less than 34 weeks;
- marked active bleeding from a fetal blood sampling site.
  Prerequisites for delivery with the ventouse are:
- dilatation of the cervix and full engagement of the head;
- cooperation of the patient;
- good contractions should be ensured.
  Basic rules for delivery with the ventouse are:
- the delivery should be completed within 15 minutes of application;
- the head should descend with each pull;
- the cup should be reapplied no more than twice;
- if failure with the correctly placed ventouse occurs despite good traction, the forceps should not be tried.

### Examination

Firstly, the patient should be carefully examined. The size of the baby should be estimated per abdomen and the head should be fully engaged (none of the head should be palpable above the pubic symphysis). The position of the vertex and the amount of caput should be determined by vaginal examination and no attempt should be made to deliver the baby vaginally if the presenting part is above the ischial spines. In a 'flexed' attitude, only the posterior fontanelle can be felt, whilst any situation where the anterior fontanelle can be felt or where the posterior fontanelle cannot be found is 'deflexed'. The presence of excessive caput may also indicate relative cephalopelvic disproportion.

### Preparation

The bladder should be empty. No additional anaesthetic is required (perineal infiltration will suffice if an episiotomy is planned). Lithotomy is the commonest position used but delivery may be possible in dorsal, lateral or squatting positions. The appropriate cup should be chosen. It should be connected to the pump and a check should be made for leakages prior to commencing the delivery.

### Delivery with the ventouse

The vacuum extractor cup is gently inserted into the vagina with one hand whilst the other hand parts the labia (Figure 15.4). The pressure is taken to 0.8 kg/cm$^2$,

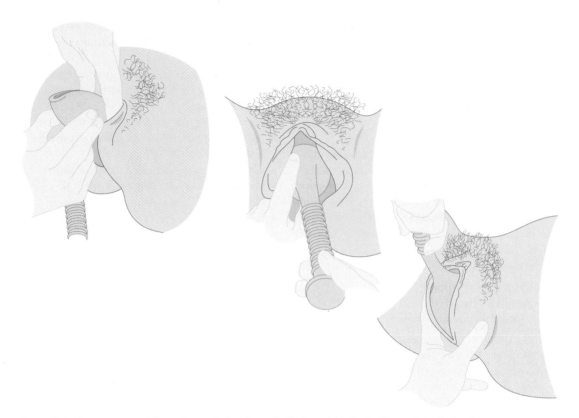

**Figure 15.4** Sil-cup ventouse delivery. The cup is placed over the flexion point in front of the posterior fontanelle.

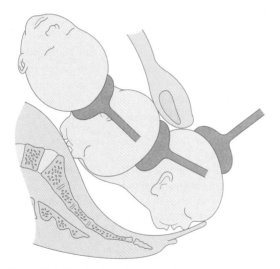

**Figure 15.5** Traction down the pelvic axis.

the cup whilst the other applies traction. Malmstrom, who invented the ventouse, emphasizes that 'vacuum extraction is a matter of cooperation between the traction hand and the backward-pressing hand'. The hand on the cup detects any early detachment and also indicates whether the head moves downwards with each pull. The fingers on the head can promote flexion and can help to guide the head under the arch of the pubis by using the space in front of the sacrum. As the head crowns, the angle of traction changes through an arc of over 90°. At this point, if the perineum is stretching, it is simply supported with the hand that was on the bell.

### The difficult ventouse
Each of the following factors contributes to failures.
- Failure to use the correct cup type. Failures with the silicone-rubber cup will be common, if used inappropriately (i.e. when there is deflexion of the head, excess caput, a big baby or a prolonged second stage of labour).

beginning traction with the next contraction after this pressure has been achieved.

Traction should be along the pelvic axis (downwards at 45°) for the duration of the contraction (Figure 15.5). One hand should rest on the bell of

- Inadequate initial assessment of the case:
  - the head being too high – a classic mistake is to assume that because caput can be felt below the ischial spines, the head must be engaged;
  - misdiagnosis of the position and attitude of the head – attention to simple detail will minimize the occurrence of this problem.
- Placements that are either too anterior or too lateral will increase the failure rate. If the cup placement is found to be incorrect, it may be appropriate to begin again with correct placement midline over the occiput.
- Failures due to traction in the wrong direction. These may be amenable simply to a change in angle of traction.
- Excessive caput. This may well be an indication for a Caesarean section.
- Poor maternal effort. There is no doubt that maternal effort can contribute substantially to the success of the delivery. Adequate encouragement and instruction should be given to the mother.

The incidence of (true) failure is low and usually secondary to outlet contraction.

### Complications

With good technique and adherence to guidelines, the risk of complications to mother or baby are small. Trauma to the genital tract is the commonest maternal complication. Unrecognized injury of the cervix leading to serious haemorrhage has been reported. Most babies will have a chignon (oedematous skin bump) at the site of the cup application. Some will also have a cephalhaematoma (subperiosteal bleed). Rare serious intracranial injuries will be more likely to occur if multiple attempts at delivery are made (especially if a variety of instruments are used).

### ⚲ Key Points

- Ensure the head is engaged abdominally and the presenting part is not above the ischial spines vaginally
- Unless the head is on the perineum, *do not* use an alternative instrument after failure with ventouse or forceps
- *Document* carefully and accurately

## Forceps delivery

### Technique

- It is essential the head is fully engaged on abdominal palpation. This is particularly true

with face presentation, which will appear to be engaged on vaginal examination sometime before the head is actually engaged.
- It is generally advised that catheterization and an episiotomy are required for forceps delivery.
- It is essential that the position of the head is carefully noted, if occipitotransverse or occipitoposterior, Caesarean section may be the birth method of choice.
- The operator must check the forceps are a matching pair.
- The left-handed blade is applied first.
- It is held in the operator's left hand (like a pen).
- Insertion (downwards, then inwards) is guided by the right hand.
- Exactly the same procedure is followed for the other blade.
- The blades must lock easily and they should not be forced to close.
- The first pull is downward and then upward (Figure 15.6). If the head does not descend, the station may be higher than first thought or the position may be occipitoposterior.

### Fetal and neonatal morbidity

There is some dispute concerning the neonatal morbidity rates following instrumental birth. Systematic reviews comparing vacuum birth with forceps birth found no significant difference in Apgar scores and few serious injuries to the neonate. The vacuum was associated with an increase in cephalhaematoma and retinal haemorrhage. It still remains difficult to establish

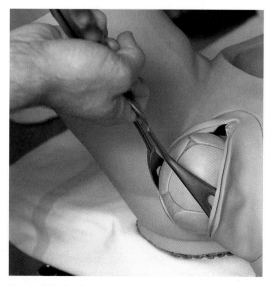

**Figure 15.6** Application of forceps (using model).

whether complications in labour result in operative birth or whether the mode of birth itself contributes to an unfavourable outcome. One study shows that neonatal trauma and fetal acidosis were more common after failed instrumental birth than following immediate Caesarean section (Murphy et al. 2003). Increased rates of neonatal encephalopathy, associated with cerebral palsy and neonatal death, have both been described following emergency Caesarean section and instrumental birth. Litigation is often associated with suboptimal care on the labour ward and also with diversions from protocol and guidelines. It is, therefore, imperative that the decision to assist birth is taken circumspectly and that guidelines are followed specifically.

## Breech delivery

### Definition
The three different types of breech presentation (extended, flexed and footling) are illustrated in Figure 15.7. Three per cent of all term pregnancies present as breech. This may be due to fetal (congenital abnormality), placental (cornual or praevia), amniotic fluid (increased) or uterine (bicornuate or septate) factors.

Clinicians skilled in the art of breech delivery are becoming more rare. Women with a term breech pregnancy now mainly have an elective Caesarean section. External cephalic version should now be offered to all antenatal women who have a breech presentation at term (see Chapter 8).

### Caesarean section or vaginal breech?
A recent large multicentre trial confirmed that planned vaginal birth of a breech presentation is associated with a 3 per cent increased risk of death or serious morbidity to the baby. Although this trial did not evaluate long-term outcomes for the baby or its mother, and has received some criticism, it has led to the recommendation that the preferred method of delivering a term breech singleton is by planned Caesarean section. Despite this, either by choice or as a result of a swift labour, a small proportion of women with breech presentations will give birth vaginally. It is, therefore, important that midwives, obstetricians and maternity units are prepared for vaginal breech births.

There is inadequate evidence to determine the appropriate mode of delivery in the preterm breech.

### Prerequisites for vaginal breech delivery
Fetomaternal
- The presentation should be either extended (hips flexed, knees extended) or flexed (hips flexed, knees flexed but feet not below the fetal buttocks).
- There should be no evidence of fetopelvic disproportion with a pelvis clinically thought to be adequate and an estimated fetal weight of <3500 g (ultrasound or clinical measurement).
- There should be no evidence of hyperextension of the fetal head and fetal abnormalities should be excluded.

Management of labour
- Fetal well-being and progress of labour should be carefully monitored.
- An epidural analgesia is not essential and may be associated with prolongation of the second stage; it can prevent pushing before full dilatation.

**Figure 15.7** Different breech types.

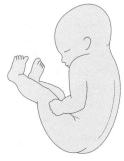
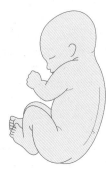
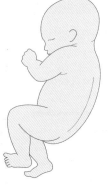

Extended breech          Flexed breech          Footling breech

- In selected cases, induction or augmentation may be justified.
- Fetal blood sampling from the buttocks provides an accurate assessment of the acid–base status

Skilled operator
- There should be an operator experienced in delivering breech babies available in the hospital.
- A symphysiotomy (division of the symphysis pubis) may be necessary should the head be entrapped; this is rare.

Although much emphasis is placed on adequate case selection prior to labour, a recent survey of outcome of the undiagnosed breech in labour managed by experienced medical staff showed that safe vaginal delivery can be achieved.

## Technique
Breech delivery epitomizes the position of 'masterly inactivity' (hands off). Problems are more likely to arise when attempts are made to speed up the process (by pulling on the baby).

### Delivery of the buttocks
In most circumstances, full dilation and descent of the breech will have occurred naturally. When the buttocks become visible and begin to distend the perineum, preparations for the delivery are made. The buttocks will lie in the anterior–posterior diameter. Once the anterior buttock is delivered and the anus is seen over the fourchette (and no sooner than this), an episiotomy may be carried out.

### Delivery of the legs and lower body
If the legs are flexed, they will deliver spontaneously. If extended, they may need to be delivered using 'Pinard's manoeuvre'. This entails using a finger to flex the leg at the knee and then extend at the hip, first anteriorly then posteriorly. With contractions and maternal effort, the lower body will be delivered. The accoucheur must avoid any traction on the cord; it is now recommended to leave this, if it is not problematic, as handling the vessels may induce spasm.

### Delivery of the shoulders
The baby will be lying with the shoulders in the transverse diameter of the pelvic mid-cavity. As the anterior shoulder rotates into the anterior–posterior diameter, the spine or the scapula will become visible. At this point, a finger gently placed above the shoulder will help to deliver the arm. As the posterior arm/ shoulder reaches the pelvic floor, it too will rotate anteriorly (in the opposite direction). Once the spine becomes visible, delivery of the second arm will follow. This can be imagined as a 'rocking boat' with one side moving upwards and then the other. Loveset's manoeuvre essentially copies these natural movements (Figure 15.8). However, it is unnecessary and meddlesome to do routinely (one risks pulling the shoulders down but leaving the arms higher up, alongside the head), and should only be employed if necessary.

### Delivery of the head
The head is delivered using the Mauriceau–Smellie–Veit manoeuvre – the baby lies on the accoucheur's arm with downward traction being levelled on the head via a finger in the mouth and one on each maxilla (Figure 15.9). Delivery occurs with first downward and then upward movement (as with instrumental deliveries). If this manoeuvre proves difficult, then forceps need to be applied. An assistant holds the baby's body aloft while the forceps are applied in the usual manner (Figure 15.10).

## Complications
The greatest fear with a vaginal breech is that the baby will get 'stuck'. Interference in the natural process by inconsiderate use of oxytocic agents or by trying to pull the baby out (breech extraction) will (paradoxically) increase the risk of obstruction occurring. When delay occurs, particularly with delivery of the shoulders or head, then the presence of an experienced obstetrician will reduce the risk of death or serious injury.

## Caesarean section

## History and epidemiology

Caesarean section to deliver the baby of a mother who has died has been documented in ancient Egypt, Asia and Europe. The first Caesarean carried out on a live woman is thought to be that of the wife of Jacob Nufer, a sixteenth-century Swiss pig-farmer. She was in obstructed labour and her life was saved by the procedure. The history of the operation thereafter is fascinating, with a wide range of isolated cases being documented with various techniques being investigated to try to lower the enormous risks of death due to haemorrhage and sepsis. By the early twentieth century, the

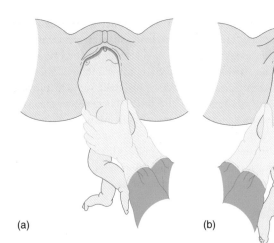

(a)

(b)

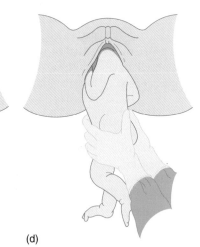

(c)

(d)

**Figure 15.8** Loveset's manoeuvre.

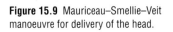

**Figure 15.9** Mauriceau–Smellie–Veit manoeuvre for delivery of the head.

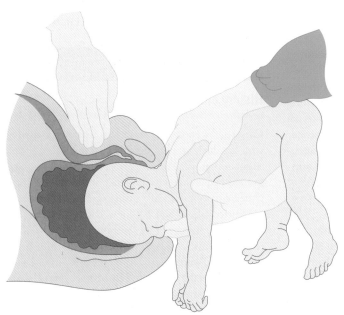

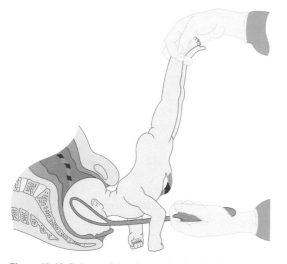

**Figure 15.10** Delivery of the after-coming head with forceps.

'classical' (midline vertical uterine incision) operation had become quite widespread for obstructed labour and placenta praevia. When Munro-Kerr introduced the concept of a 'lower segment operation' in the 1920s, some were derisive. Nevertheless he persisted with the new procedure, which has now become the standard intervention for complicated labour worldwide.

## Caesarean section rates

The rise in Caesarean section rates has been blamed on the increased use of induction, epidurals and instrumental birth, but the central issue is that of future mode of birth. Repeat Caesarean section is one of the main causes of the increase in rates. Therefore, by reducing primary Caesarean sections, the overall Caesarean section rate would decrease. Women who have vaginal birth have more positive psychological, physical and social outcomes, have higher breast feeding rates and also more positive interactions with their babies.

### National Institute for Clinical Excellence guidelines (2004): key priorities for implementation

#### Making the decision

- When considering a Caesarean section (CS), there should be discussion on the risks and benefits, and risks of CS compared with vaginal birth specific to the woman and her pregnancy.

- Maternal request is not on its own an indication for CS, and specific reasons for the request should be explored, discussed and recorded. When a woman requests a CS in the absence of an identifiable reason, the overall benefits and risks of CS compared with vaginal birth should be discussed and recorded.

#### Carrying out the procedure

- The following interventions should be used to decrease morbidity from CS:
  - regional anaesthesia
  - antibiotic prophylaxis
  - thromboprophylaxis
  - antacids
  - antiemetics.
- The risk of respiratory morbidity is increased in babies born by CS before labour but this risk decreases significantly after 39 weeks. Therefore, planned CS should not routinely be carried out *before 39 weeks*.

#### Reducing the likelihood of Caesarean section

- Women who have an uncomplicated singleton breech pregnancy at 36 weeks' gestation should be offered external cephalic version. Exceptions include women in labour, and women with a uterine scar or abnormality, fetal compromise, ruptured membranes, vaginal bleeding or medical conditions.
- Women should be informed that continuous support during labour from women with or without prior training reduces the likelihood of CS.
- Women with uncomplicated pregnancies should be offered induction of labour beyond 41 weeks because this reduces the risk of perinatal mortality and the likelihood of CS.
- A partogram with a 4-hour action line should be used to monitor progress of labour of women in spontaneous labour with an uncomplicated singleton pregnancy at term because it reduces the likelihood of CS.
- Consultant obstetricians should be involved in the decision-making for CS because this reduces the likelihood of CS.
- Electronic fetal monitoring is associated with an increased likelihood of CS. When CS is contemplated because of an abnormal fetal heart rate pattern, in cases of suspected fetal acidosis, fetal blood sampling should be offered, if this is technically possible and there are no contraindications.

## Preparation for Caesarean section

Premedication with antacid is standard. In theatre, the operating table must be kept in a left lateral tilt position until after the delivery. Thromboprophylaxis and prophylactic antibiotics should be considered for all women (National Institute for Clinical Excellence 2004). This is especially indicated for emergency Caesarean section.

## Operative procedure

Double gloving reduces the likelihood of needle puncture and use of a clear plastic shield reduces exposure of the face. A transverse suprapubic skin incision should be used. The bladder should be reflected inferiorly before incising the uterus. It is possible to injure the baby as the uterine wall is opened; accordingly, considerable care needs to be taken. Delivery of the placenta should be by continuous cord traction. The uterus should be left inside the abdomen for repair. Securing both angles of the uterine incision first will reduce the risk of 'missing an angle' and having post-surgical bleeding.

## Complications

Overall, the risks of both early and long-term complications are increased in women delivered by Caesarean section, when compared with the outcomes after normal vaginal delivery. The risks are surgical and anaesthetic. The main problems are thromboembolism, infection and haemorrhage, which can be minimized by appropriate prophylaxis and surgical skill. Women are increasingly demanding Caesarean section to minimize the risk of pelvic floor trauma and its sequelae. Although women have a right to choose their mode of delivery, they need to be counselled regarding the increased mortality and morbidity associated with Caesarean section.

## Indications for Caesarean section

Indications for Caesarean section are as follows:
- obstructed labour, malpresentation, malposition or multiple gestation;
- fetal distress/prolapsed cord;
- maternal medical conditions requiring urgent/controlled delivery;
- obstetric complications (e.g. placenta praevia);
- previous Caesarean section.

The 'classical' operation is still undertaken occasionally (less than 1 per cent of cases), for the following specific indications:
- preterm delivery with poorly formed lower segment;
- placenta praevia/abruptio with large vessels in lower segment;
- premature rupture of membranes, poor lower segment and transverse lie;
- transverse lie with back inferior;
- large cervical fibroid;
- severe adhesions in lower segment reducing accessibility;
- postmortem Caesarean section.

## Placental complications

### Retained placenta

Incidence

Retained placenta is found in 2 per cent of deliveries. The frequency of retained placenta is markedly increased (20-fold) at gestations <26 weeks and even up to 37 weeks it remains three times more common than at term. At term, 90 per cent of placentas will be delivered within 15 minutes. Once the third stage exceeds 30 minutes. there is a ten-fold increase in the risk of haemorrhage.

Management

When the placenta is delivered, it should be inspected for completeness because, if there is a suggestion of retained segments, manual exploration of the uterine cavity is required. This will need to be undertaken under anaesthesia.

If the placenta is retained as a whole, it is often worth checking prior to induction of anaesthesia that it has not detached spontaneously. Not infrequently, a placenta is found in the cervical canal or vagina at this time. If it is still within the uterus, the operator (wearing a 'gauntlet' glove) should use the fingers of one hand, held as a 'spatula', to lift the placenta, whilst the hand on the abdomen balances these movements with downward pressure on the uterus. If there are retained fragments, then further manual exploration (with a gauze swab around the exploring fingers) of the uterine cavity will need to be undertaken. Antibiotics should be routinely administered, as there is a significant association between manual removal of the placenta and postpartum endometritis.

## Placenta accreta

### Definition
Placenta accreta is a retained placenta that is morbidly adherent to the uterine wall.

### Epidemiology
Placenta accreta is a serious cause of haemorrhage. It is becoming more common, and over the last 40 years, the incidence has increased ten-fold. This phenomenon is due to the fact that lower segment Caesarean section appears to increase the risk of subsequent placenta praevia, and there is a well-documented association between placenta praevia and previous Caesarean section and placenta accreta. In recent reviews, up to a quarter of women undergoing Caesarean section for placenta praevia, in the presence of one or more scars, subsequently underwent Caesarean hysterectomy for placenta accreta.

### Management
If placenta accreta with haemorrhage is encountered, and if the woman has no intention to bear further children, hysterectomy is the procedure of choice. However, if hysterectomy is considered as a last resort, then other measures may be successful in up to 50 per cent of women. These procedures range from simple excision of the site of trophoblast invasion with oversewing of the area to uterine or internal iliac artery ligation.

### Key Points

- Anticipate haemorrhage, site intravenous infusion, take blood for full blood count, group, save and catheterize
- Check that placenta is not in the cervical canal or vagina prior to giving anaesthetic
- Give prophylactic antibiotics
- Carry out manual removal – call senior help if accreta and/or heavy bleeding
- Prompt recognition of the injury and action to control the bleeding is essential

## Rarely performed but important operative interventions

### Symphysiotomy

Symphysiotomy is considered of some value for the management of cephalopelvic disproportion in selected situations in developing countries and it has also been recommended as the treatment of choice for a trapped after-coming head of a breech.

It has a very low maternal mortality with no procedure-related deaths in a series of nearly 2000 women. In contrast, Caesarean section in rural developing world hospitals may be associated with a mortality of up to 5 per cent and a reported incidence of uterine scar rupture in subsequent pregnancies of up to 6.8 per cent. However, after a symphysiotomy, subsequent symptoms, such as pain in the symphysis pubis and groin, are common. A major advantage is that the majority of women (73 per cent) will have an uncomplicated vaginal delivery in a subsequent pregnancy.

### Indication
Symphysiotomy can be considered in cases of cephalopelvic disproportion with a vertex presentation and a living fetus. At least one-third of the fetal head should have entered the pelvic brim. It may also be indicated for the trapped after-coming head of a breech and has been described as an intervention in a 'desperate case' scenario of shoulder dystocia.

### Destructive operations

Destructive operations may be required where the fetus is dead, and where a vaginal delivery is either the only delivery that can be managed in that particular situation or it is the only route by which the mother wishes to be delivered. The three commonest destructive procedures are craniotomy, perforation of the after-coming head and decapitation.

### Craniotomy
Craniotomy is indicated for the delivery of a dead fetus when labour is neglected and obstructed in a cephalic presentation.

### After-coming head of the breech
This can be managed similarly, by craniotomy with perforation of the head through the occiput. Where

there is hydrocephalus and accompanying spina bifida, cerebrospinal fluid can either be withdrawn by exposing the spinal canal and passing a catheter into the canal and up into the cranium, or the hydrocephalic head can be decompressed transabdominally using a spinal needle.

## Decapitation

In cases of neglected obstructed labour with shoulder presentation and a dead fetus, decapitation might be the treatment of choice.

---

**C A S E   H I S T O R Y**

Miss MS
1.80 m tall, 76 kg at booking
First pregnancy: spontaneous labour at 39 weeks' gestation
Abdominal examination: average size baby, estimated around 3.6 kg
Vaginal examination: vertex presentation
After a slow labour, finally reached full dilatation of the cervix after 10 hours
Normal, reactive cardiotocograph baseline 135/minute; clear liquor draining
After one and a half hour's active pushing, the station of the head is +1 cm below the ischial spines (0/5 palpable on abdominal examination), there is caput and moulding. The position of the head is occipitoanterior.

### Should Miss S have an assisted delivery?

After a long labour and prolonged maternal efforts at pushing in the second stage of labour, an assisted delivery is quite appropriate. Hopefully, the baby can be delivered vaginally as there is no evidence of fetal compromise and the vertex is at station +1 below the ischial spines.

### What features suggest that an assisted delivery might be difficult?

Caput and moulding suggest that room and space in the pelvis is quite limited. This might mean an assisted delivery would be trickier than first thought and the operator must be sure of the exact position of the head, prior to attempting delivery.

### Which instrument should be chosen?

Either ventouse or forceps would be reasonable. Many obstetricians would use ventouse in the first instance to reduce maternal soft tissue trauma. Equally, it could be argued that the presence of caput would make ventouse more likely to fail, and a non-rotational forceps (such as Neville-Barnes') could be used.

### Should the delivery be performed in the obstetric theatre?

If there is any concern that the delivery might not succeed easily or there is fetal distress, then Miss S should be moved to the operating theatre for a 'trial of ventouse/forceps'. Should the delivery not be completed simply and rapidly, a Caesarean section might be required. In this situation, a Caesarean section would be most unlikely unless the fetus were to become compromised and attempted vaginal delivery was more difficult than at first thought. One important question depends on the skill of the obstetrician. Is the true position of the vertex (taking into account the boggy caput) at +1 cm and is the fetal head really occipitoanterior? If this was in fact occipitoposterior and the baby's head was at the spines (0 cm) then, in many cases, a Caesarean might be performed.

### What risks are there for Miss S after delivery?

Postpartum haemorrhage is always more common after an assisted delivery owing to the risk of uterine atony, and vaginal or cervical lacerations. In this situation, these risks are compounded by a long labour. The appropriate steps should be taken to anticipate and deal with this (i.e. intravenous access, blood sent for haemoglobin estimation and grouping and saving, oxytocin/ergometrine at delivery and an intravenous oxytocin infusion for 4 hours after delivery).

# References

Fitzpatrick M, Behan M, O'Connell PR , O'Herlihy C. Randomised clinical trial to assess anal sphincter function after forceps or vacuum assisted vaginal delivery *Obstetric and Gynecological Survey* 2003; **58**:647–8.

Johanson RB, Menon V. Vacuum extraction versus forceps for assisted vaginal delivery *The Cochrane Database Systematic Reviews* 1999, Issue 2. Article no. CD 000224. DOI: 10.1002/14651858.CD000224. Oxford: Update Software: 2000.

Murphy DJ, Liebling RE, Patel R, Verity L, Swingler R. Cohort study of operative delivery in the second stage of labour and standard of obstetric care. *British Journal of Obstetrics and Gynaecology* 2003; **110**:610–15.

National Institute for Clinical Excellence. *Caesarean section*. London: NICE, 2004.

# Key additional reading

Pregnancy and childbirth reviews. *The Cochrane Database of Systematic Reviews*. The Cochrane Library. Oxford: Update Software.

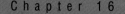
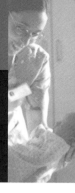

# Childbirth emergencies

## OVERVIEW

Emergencies in childbirth carry a high risk of morbidity and mortality to the woman and her baby, and may occur in both the home and hospital environment. In the majority of cases, the immediate management is dependent on the diagnosis and prompt action of the midwife to summon medical aid and undertake appropriate life-saving measures until that assistance arrives. In the UK, the maternal mortality rate is around 13.1 per 100 000 maternities (Lewis and Drife 2004), apparently representing relatively few deaths due directly to pregnancy complications. However, in many cases, care could and should have been better, resulting in fewer deaths. Worldwide the situation is much worse, with around 600 000 maternal deaths reported each year, which are mainly attributed to haemorrhage, sepsis, eclampsia and obstructive labour.

In the UK, the main causes of maternal death directly attributable to pregnancy are embolism (thrombotic and amniotic fluid), hypertensive disorders, haemorrhage and sepsis. Furthermore, as the childbearing population ages, coincidental medical conditions that may be associated with, or made worse by pregnancy (e.g. congenital heart disease or epilepsy) make a progressively larger contribution to mortality and morbidity, such that they may also present as an emergency.

## Definition of childbirth emergencies

An emergency is an occurrence of a serious and dangerous nature, developing suddenly and unexpectedly, demanding immediate attention. Although the actual emergency itself will occur without any warning, in some cases, pre-existing risk factors will be present. Depending on the type of emergency, when it occurs and the environment in which it occurs, will determine to what extent the health and well-being of the woman and/or fetus/neonate will be affected. This may not only involve the physical health, but also the psychological and sociological aspects of health of the woman, her baby and family.

## Management

The ideal management of a potential emergency situation is in its avoidance. Although it may not always be possible to anticipate every emergency, it is important that every midwife is competent to recognize risk factors promptly during all stages of the childbirth process and refer these potentially high risk cases to her medical colleagues in order to reduce the occurrence of an emergency. The midwife is also responsible to ensure her documentation accurately reflects the course of events and actions taken in all emergencies associated with childbirth. If notes are written retrospectively, this fact should be recorded when documenting the date and time of the events.

Any emergency associated with childbirth can be a terrifying experience for the woman and her family as well as the midwife involved. Prompt recognition and management requires experience and a calm sense of purpose on the part of the midwife in both the home and hospital setting. Having a thorough knowledge of protocols and participating in multidisciplinary emergency drills in the clinical setting can assist in developing the midwife's confidence and competence to deal with future emergencies associated with childbirth.

## Maternal collapse

When an emergency occurs, the midwife's management must always begin with an assessment of the maternal and then, when appropriate, the fetal condition. Although the most common causes of cardiopulmonary arrest are hypovolaemia and eclampsia, in the majority of emergencies associated with childbirth, respiratory or cardiac arrest may not have occurred when management begins, as complete or partial loss of consciousness is rare in pregnancy.

### Causes of loss of consciousness

Loss of consciousness may be caused by:
- simple faint;
- epileptic fit;
- hypoglycaemia;
- hypoxia;
- amniotic fluid embolism;
- pulmonary embolism;
- eclampsia;
- cerebrovascular accident/stroke;
- myocardial infarction;
- anaphylaxis;
- major haemorrhage;
- uterine inversion;
- septic shock;
- drug/anaesthetic toxicity.

It is, therefore, important that the midwife assesses the situation quickly, including the need to undertake basic life support.

## Basic life support

In situations where an individual has collapsed, standards have been agreed for health professionals and lay people throughout Europe. This involves the three principles of assessing and maintaining the *airway*, *breathing* and *circulation* of the collapsed patient (ABC), without any specialist equipment other than a pharyngeal airway. The midwife first establishes the level of consciousness by gently shaking the woman's shoulders and enquiring whether she can hear. Assistance is called for by pulling the emergency cord/ ringing the emergency bell, if in hospital/health centre, or by asking the partner to telephone for help, if in the home environment. The midwife should always remain with the woman.

The pregnant woman is laid flat, removing any pillows and is then positioned in a left lateral tilt to prevent aortocaval compression. This can be achieved by the use of pillows or a wedge under the right side. Tilting the head back and lifting the chin is effective in maintaining the airway. The airway is cleared of any mucus or vomit. If dentures are well fitting, they should be left in place. The chest is observed for signs of respiratory effort. The midwife listens for breathing sounds and feels for breath being exhaled from the mouth and nose. An oropharyngeal airway may then be inserted, if available.

If there is no spontaneous respiration, the midwife should pinch the nose closed, take a deep breath and exhale into the woman's mouth so that the chest can be seen to rise. The air is allowed to escape and the chest observed to fall. This is repeated to achieve two effective breaths. If after five attempts the woman remains unresponsive, the carotid pulse is felt in order to assess for signs of circulation.

Should there be an absence of a carotid pulse, external chest compression should be commenced at a rate of 100 compressions per minute with a ratio of 15 chest compressions to every two breaths. The midwife locates the xiphisternum and places her hands palm downwards one on top of the other with the fingers interlinked. The heel of the lower hand is placed on the lower two-thirds of the sternum. With arms straight the midwife leans on the sternum depressing it 4–5 cm and releases it slowly at the same rate as compression. The midwife may need to kneel over the woman or find something to stand on to ensure she is suitably positioned to carry out resuscitation. It is also essential that the woman is on a firm surface for the manoeuvre to be successful.

It is important to obtain as much help as is possible immediately. Within the hospital environment, it would be usual to summon the cardiac arrest team and, in most labour wards, an obstetric anaesthetist may also be available. However, if the emergency occurs in the home, the midwife would be expected to call for an emergency ambulance stressing the exact nature of the call to ensure the appropriate personnel attend (i.e. trained paramedics). If competent in the skill and in the absence of any medical support, a second midwife may proceed to insert an intravenous cannula in order to replace any fluid the woman may have lost. Oxygen therapy may also be commenced. Once the woman's condition has been stabilized, medical interventions, including venepuncture for haematological and biochemical analysis and for cross-matching, will ultimately aim to determine the likely cause of the collapse and determine the most appropriate treatment.

---

### Basic adult life support actions

**Actions**
- Check conscious state (shake and shout)
- Call for help
- Clear airway (head tilt, chin lift)
- Check breathing (look and listen)
- Two effective breaths (watch chest for movement)
- Check circulation (carotid pulse for 10 seconds or spontaneous movement)
- No circulation: commence chest compression at 100 per minute
- Check circulation again
- Use two breaths for every 15 compressions
- Continue until help arrives

---

### Pulmonary embolism

Pulmonary embolism (PE) occurs in association with approximately 3:1000 pregnancies. Two-thirds of cases occur in the puerperium. In the UK, it is the commonest cause of maternal death directly associated with pregnancy. In the latest triennial report (2000–2002), 25 deaths were associated with or caused by pulmonary embolism and a further five deaths from cerebral thrombosis (Lewis and Drife 2004). This is a reduction

from previous years, probably as a consequence of improvements in the early detection of high-risk pregnancies and the implementation of the Royal College of Obstetricians and Gynaecologists (RCOG) guidelines on thromboprophylaxis.

The clinical signs of PE are related to the size of the clot that is obstructing the pulmonary circulation but, such is the risk of the condition, it is important for the midwife to recognize such signs so that appropriate treatment can be sought and implemented immediately.

---

### Clinical manifestations of pulmonary embolism and subsequent investigations

| Common signs and symptoms | Associated signs and symptoms | Investigations |
| --- | --- | --- |
| • Acute breathlessness | Haemoptysis | Chest X ray |
| • Pleuritic chest pain | Tachypnoea | Electrocardiogram |
| • Cough | Tachycardia | Clotting studies (thrombophilias and lupus anticoagulant) |
| • Peripheral oedema | Cyanosis | Oxygen levels (saturation and blood gases) |
| • Crackles on listening to the chest | Hypotension | Ventilation perfusion scan (V/Q scan) |
| • Distended neck veins | | |
| • Tricuspid flow murmur | | |
| • Acute cor pulmonale | | |
| • Pyrexia | | |
| • Anxiety | | |
| • Confusion (hypoxia) | | |

---

The aetiology, diagnosis and management of thromboembolic disorders are discussed in detail in Chapter 12. However, although rare, a massive PE may present with sudden cardiorespiratory collapse, and the midwife would be expected to undertake immediate resuscitation (ABC) and administer oxygen until medical assistance arrives. The responsibilities that the midwife would be expected to fulfil are highlighted (see box), a number of which can be instigated in the home while awaiting emergency transfer to hospital.

## The midwife's responsibilities in a pulmonary embolism emergency

- Summon appropriate emergency assistance (obstetrician, anaesthetist, physician, haematologist, radiologist/arrange emergency transfer to hospital ICU/HDU in maternity unit)
- Undertake cardiac massage as necessary
- Administer oxygen via mask/nasal prongs
- Initiate IV access
- If appropriate, sit the woman up to maximize respiratory effort
- Assist with endotracheal intubation as necessary
- Assess and record cardiovascular and respiratory vital signs
- Attach oximeter and record electrocardiogram
- Administer heparin and other drugs (e.g. opiate to relieve discomfort and anxiety) according to medical instructions
- Maintain accurate fluid balance (urinary catheter/CVP line)
- Observe for signs of excessive bleeding
- Monitor fetal well-being (if appropriate)/arrange care of the baby
- Provide psychological support to the woman and her family

CVP, central venous pressure; HDU, high dependency unit; ICU, intensive care unit; IV, intravenous.

## Amniotic fluid embolism

Amniotic fluid embolism occurs when amniotic fluid enters the maternal circulation. It is an emergency that is impossible to predict and offers few, if any, warning signs, with often a tragic outcome. The incidence of this rare condition is approximately 1:30 000 pregnancies. There were five maternal deaths attributed to amniotic fluid embolism in the UK during 2000–2002 (Lewis and Drife 2004).

Traditionally diagnosis of amniotic fluid embolism has only been made on postmortem examination when, during histological examination, fetal cells and debris have been found in the maternal lungs. It has been associated with rupture of the membranes, rapid labour, precipitate vaginal birth and Caesarean sections. The mechanism appears to be the access of amniotic fluid at a higher pressure than usual, directly into the maternal circulation through a defect somewhere near the placental site. This consequently causes acute cardiorespiratory compromise and severe disseminated intravascular coagulation. In some cases, there is evidence to suggest that an abnormal maternal reaction to amniotic fluid may also cause an amniotic fluid embolism.

As these women are critically ill, there is no time to undertake any investigations. Prognosis is generally poor, with around 30 per cent of women dying in the first hour and an overall mortality rate of up to 90 per cent. It has been suggested that diagnosis should be made on the basis of clinical signs and symptoms (see box). The sudden onset of a triad of symptoms – hypotension, hypoxia and coagulopathy – are highly

## Clinical presentation and treatment of amniotic fluid embolism

| Signs and symptoms | Treatment |
|---|---|
| - Sudden severe chest pain | - Call for emergency help |
| - Dyspnoea | - Intravenous access and fluids |
| - Hypotension | - Urgent resuscitation/ intubation/IPPV |
| - Tachycardia | - Cardiac massage, as necessary |
| - Pulmonary oedema | - Monitor condition with CVP/arterial lines |
| - Cyanosis | - Monitor clotting and correct coagulopathy |
| - Coagulopathy and consequent haemorrhage | - Careful fluid balance and renal assessment |
| - Convulsions due to hypoxia or cardiac arrest | - Administer drugs as necessary: |
| | – dopamine (increases cardiac output) |
| | – hydrocortisone (reduces inflammatory response) |
| | – sodium bicarbonate (to correct acidosis) |
| | – syntocinon (uterine atony) |
| - Fetal distress | - Transfer to ICU/HDU |
| | - Support partner and family members |
| | - Psychological care to woman regarding self/ fetal/neonatal outcome |

CVP, central venous pressure; HDU, high dependency unit; ICU, intensive care unit; IPPV, intermittent positive pressure ventilation.

suspicious of amniotic fluid embolism. It is, therefore, important that the midwife always suspects an amniotic fluid embolism should a previously asymptomatic healthy woman suddenly develop cardiac or respiratory failure during labour, Caesarean section or immediately following the birth of her baby. Amniotic fluid embolism may also occur during termination of pregnancy.

These symptoms can appear in any order, alone or in combination. It is worth noting that, in 10–15 per cent of cases, the first sign of amniotic fluid embolism is a convulsion that has the potential for the initial diagnosis to be confused with that of eclampsia.

## Pre-eclampsia and eclampsia

In the latest triennial report of maternal deaths in the UK, hypertensive disorders were identified as being the second most common cause of maternal death (direct) in the UK. Of the 14 deaths in this category, 8 deaths were attributed to pre-eclampsia and 6 deaths associated with eclampsia (Lewis and Drife 2004).

## Definitions

Pre-eclampsia is a disease of pregnancy characterized by a blood pressure of 140/90 mmHg or more on two separate occasions after the 20th week of pregnancy in a previously normotensive woman. This is accompanied by significant proteinuria (more than 0.3 g in 24 hours). Pre-eclampsia is discussed in detail in Chapter 10.

Severe or fulminating pre-eclampsia (sometimes known as impending eclampsia) is the transitional condition that is characterized by increasing signs and symptoms, and a consequential worsening in the woman's condition. Such a severe medical condition should be treated as an emergency so that timely intervention and appropriate treatment may prevent an eclamptic seizure.

Eclampsia (a Greek word meaning *lightening*) often strikes with random ferocity causing devastating consequences. It is defined as the new onset of convulsions during pregnancy or after the baby's birth unrelated to other cerebral pathological conditions, in a woman with pre-eclampsia. It is thought to be due to intense vasospasm of the cerebral arteries, oedema secondary to ischaemic damage of vascular endothelium and intravascular clot formation. The

following sections discuss the management of severe or fulminating pre-eclampsia, and eclampsia.

## Incidence and epidemiology

Although eclampsia is relatively rare in the UK, occurring in approximately 1:2000 pregnancies, 40 per cent of which occur during the antenatal period, 20 per cent during labour and a further 40 per cent in the postnatal period, severe pre-eclampsia is much more common.

## Severe/fulminating pre-eclamspia

Characteristic signs and symptoms (see box) will signal the onset of eclampsia. It is of importance that the midwife is alert to any of these signs and symptoms, and summons medical assistance immediately. In the absence of proteinuria, pre-eclampsia is suspected when hypertension is accompanied by symptoms including headaches, blurred vision, abdominal/epigastric pain or altered biochemistry, for example, low platelet counts, abnormal liver enzyme levels [alanine aminotransferease (ALT), aspartate aminotransferase (AST) and gamma glutamyl transpeptidase (GGT)]. These signs and symptoms, together with a blood pressure of 160/110 mmHg or more, and proteinuria of 2+ or 3+ on a dipstick, demonstrate the more severe form of the disease. On abdominal examination, the fetus may appear smaller than its gestational age, and

### Signs and symptoms associated with severe/fulminating pre-eclampsia

- A sharp rise in blood pressure
- Diminished urinary output: owing to acute vasospasm
- Increase in proteinuria
- Headache: usually severe, persistent and frontal in location
- Drowsiness or confusion: owing to cerebral oedema
- Visual disturbances (blurring of vision, flashing lights): owing to retinal oedema
- Facial and peripheral oedema
- Epigastric pain: owing to liver oedema and infarctions impairing function
- Hyper-reflexia
- Presence of clonus
- General malaise, nausea and vomiting
- Intrauterine growth restriction, oligohydramnios and reduced fetal movements

there may be oligohydramnios and diminished fetal movements.

A multidisciplinary approach involving an obstetrician and anaesthetist (at consultant level), haematologist, paediatrician and appropriately experienced midwife should be involved in the planning and provision of care. The aim of the care and management is to preclude death of the woman and fetus by controlling the hypertension, inhibiting convulsions and preventing coma. This involves providing one-to-one midwifery care with drugs and equipment for managing an eclamptic fit, monitoring the fetal condition and supporting adequate ventilation and oxygen therapy.

---

### Midwifery care relating to severe/fulminating pre-eclampsia

- Monitor and record blood pressure, vital signs and level of consciousness every 15 minutes
- Monitor and record intravenous intake, urinary output, level of proteinuria and CVP
- Administer oral hygiene as the woman is usually nil by mouth
- Administer drugs as prescribed and titrate according to blood pressure response
- Monitor daily biochemical blood results for detection of changes reflecting deterioration (full blood count, electrolytes, uric acid, liver enzymes, fibrinogen, platelets, clotting studies and blood urea nitrogen)
- Monitor fetal well-being electronically and administer steroids as prescribed to hasten fetal lung maturity
- Observe for signs of the onset of labour/assess progress in labour
- Maintain a calm quiet environment
- Assess for symptoms of worsening condition
- Provide psychological care for the woman and her family
- Notify any significant changes in the woman's condition to the obstetrician and/or anaesthetist

---

### Treatment

The initial aim is not for the blood pressure to return to normal but to a considerably safer level. This may be achieved using either hydralazine to relax arteriolar smooth muscle, or the alpha- and beta-blocker, labetalol. A bolus dose is first given followed by a continuous infusion, titrated against the blood pressure. Even if the blood pressure returns to near normal, this does not mean that the disease process has been stopped, but merely that one manifestation of it has been temporarily pharmacologically corrected. However, nine of the 14 deaths associated with pre-eclampsia and eclampsia in the last triennial report were due to intracranial haemorrhage, suggesting a failure of effective antihypertensive therapy.

Anticonvulsants are also prescribed to prevent an eclamptic fit or further convulsions, and magnesium sulphate is the drug of choice. This acts as a cerebral vasodilator and membrane stabilizer, and has been demonstrated to be very effective. A loading dose of 4 g is given over 5–10 minutes intravenously followed by a maintenance dose of 5 g/500 mL normal saline given as an intravenous infusion at the rate of 1–2 g/hour. Although magnesium sulphate is generally a safe drug, respiratory depression and even cardiac arrest may supervene, should toxicity occur. A maximum serum magnesium level of 4 mmol/L is therapeutic, but around 7 mmol/L is associated with respiratory distress and levels around 12 mmol/L can trigger cardiac arrest. If necessary, the effects can be reversed with calcium gluconate, which should always be readily available.

Management of fluid balance can be problematic. In pre-eclampsia, there is intense peripheral vasoconstriction accompanied by a decrease in the plasma volume, together with redistribution of the extracellular fluid. The urine output falls, and overenthusiastic efforts to maintain a fluid balance may cause pulmonary and cerebral oedema. Intravenous gelatin solutions, such as Haemaccel and Gelofusine, may be used to increase the colloid osmotic pressure and pull fluid back into the circulation, thereby attempting to reduce the oedema and increase the blood volume. The administration of diuretics, therefore, should be avoided if possible.

In severe pre-eclampsia, a central venous pressure (CVP) line may be considered in order to monitor the fluid balance more effectively. This is inserted and supervised by an anaesthetist. Measurements should be taken hourly and maintained at around 4–6 mmHg. Intravenous fluids are administered using infusion pumps and, in the absence of bleeding, no more than 100 mL per hour of fluids (oral and intravenous) should be given. Urine output and urinalysis should be monitored every hour. In severe pre-eclampsia, a urinary catheter should be *in situ*: a level of 30 mL urine per hour indicates adequate renal function.

When it is clear that the early birth of the fetus is most likely, if the gestation is less than 34 weeks, steroids are usually given to improve lung maturity and decrease neonatal complications. Steroid administration, however, must not delay delivery if this is necessary for control of severe maternal problems. In fulminating pre-eclampsia or eclampsia, the birth of the baby should take place as soon as possible once the woman's condition has been stabilized. Oxytocin should be given to assist with the delivery of the placenta and membranes as ergometrine and syntometrine cause vasoconstriction with a consequential increase in blood pressure.

## Eclampsia

Eclampsia is obvious as a grand mal convulsion. However, other causes of seizures, such as epilepsy, have to be considered. Any convulsion in pregnancy should be considered to be eclamptic until proved otherwise.

### Immediate care and treatment of the eclamptic woman

- Summon an obstetrician and anaesthetist.
- Protect the woman from injury during the tonoclonic phase.
- Maintain the woman's airway using suction, if necessary.
- Administer oxygen and prevent severe hypoxia.
- Turn the woman on to her side with her head down (recovery position).
- Obtain intravenous access and monitor fluid balance.
- Treat the convulsion: magnesium sulphate intravenously.
- Possibly sedate to prevent hyperstimulation.
- Monitor and record vital signs.
- Assess fetal well-being risk/fetal distress from hypoxia/abruption.
- Stabilize the woman's condition.
- Plan the mode of delivering the baby.
- Implement the plan without further delay.

If the woman's condition stabilizes to enable labour to be induced, and should the clotting studies be satisfactory, epidural analgesia is often selected for pain relief. This has the additional benefits of lowering the blood pressure as well as eliminating painful stimuli that may trigger convulsions. If labour is well established, then a vaginal birth may be possible; however,

the most frequent mode of delivering the baby is by Caesarean section. Wherever possible, any clotting disorders must be corrected before any mode of delivery is attempted.

Timing of delivery depends upon the gestation, the presence of other complicating factors, the severity of the disease and the stability of the woman's condition. In general, if the woman has disease severe enough to warrant antihypertensive and anticonvulsant therapy, the birth of the baby should follow once her condition has been stabilized.

### Indications for urgent delivery
Indications for urgent delivery are as follows:

- blood pressure persistently at 160/100 mmHg or more with significant proteinuria;
- elevated liver enzymes;
- low platelet count;
- eclamptic fit;
- anuria;
- significant fetal distress.

Once the woman's condition has stabilized and the baby has been born, the aggressive approach to the management of pre-eclampsia needs to be maintained as there is still risk to the mother of eclampsia occurring during the first 24 hours of the postnatal period.

## HELLP syndrome

HELLP syndrome (haemolysis, elevated liver enzymes and low platelets) is a serious complication usually associated with women who have pre-eclampsia, and manifests between 32 and 34 weeks of pregnancy. However, around 30 per cent of cases may also occur during the postnatal period. Eight deaths in the last triennial report were associated with HELLP syndrome.

Serious maternal morbidity and mortality may consequently result from the development of disseminated intravascular coagulation, acute renal failure, pulmonary oedema, and subcapsular liver haematoma or rupture of the liver, with the latter creating a combined medical, surgical and obstetric emergency. Babies whose mothers have HELLP syndrome are often small for gestational age and are at risk from perinatal asphyxia, placental abruption and fetal death. Diagnosis is based on a combination of laboratory and clinical signs and symptoms with which the midwife should be familiar (see box).

## HELLP syndrome

| Possible signs and symptoms | Laboratory findings | Treatment |
| --- | --- | --- |
| • Malaise/ fatigue | • Haemolysis | • Immediate hospitalization to consultant unit/ICU/HDU |
| • Epigastric pain | • Anaemia | • Under 34 weeks: conservative management (plasma expanders/ antihyper- tensives and steroids) |
| • Nausea and vomiting | • Low/falling platelets | • In term pregnancies or deterioration in maternal/ fetal condition: expedite delivery |
| • Non-specific viral syndrome- like symptoms | • Elevated liver transaminases (AST, ALT and GGT) | |
| • Headache | • Elevated lactate dehydrogenase and raised bilirubin levels | |
| • Gastrointestinal bleed | | |
| • Hypertension | | |
| • Proteinuria | | |

ALT, alanine aminotransferease; AST, aspartate aminotransferase; GGT, gamma glutamyl transpeptidase; HDU, high dependency unit; HELLP, haemolysis, elevated liver enzymes and low platelets; ICU, intensive care unit.

## Haemorrhage during childbirth

### Definition

Any blood loss from the vagina during pregnancy that is greater than a show or an excessive blood loss after the birth of the baby. According to the last triennial report, there were 17 maternal deaths attributed to haemorrhage: three as a result of placental abruption, four due to placenta praevia and ten to postpartum haemorrhage (PPH) (Lewis and Drife 2004). This is a significant increase from one death (1997–1999) to ten deaths attributed to PPH where the number of deaths from placental abruption and placenta praevia remain unchanged.

## Understanding the pathophysiology

The haemochorial nature of the human placenta places the pregnant women at particular risk of haemorrhage. The placental cotyledons are directly bathed in maternal blood. Any disruption of this interface may lead to blood loss that may occur behind (retro) or around (peri) the placental site. The blood loss will often be concealed and may extend. Extension to the edge of the placenta leads to revealed blood loss. There are important differences in clinical presentation depending on whether the placenta is normally sited or low-lying. Controlling the haemorrhage depends upon haemostasis in the placental bed, achieved by myometrial contraction (living ligatures). Coagulation factors and platelets are secondary to this process. If placental bleeding occurs during the antenatal period, it can only be stopped by emptying the uterus of the baby and placenta. Effective management of major haemorrhage requires aggressive supportive measures at the same time as measures to resolve the bleeding, and prevent maternal shock and any sequelae from developing. Whatever the cause, the need for resuscitation and subsequent management will depend upon the maternal condition, the fetal condition, the cause of the bleeding and the gestation of the pregnancy.

Blood loss during childbirth is almost always maternal. As a result, the fetus may be affected by maternal hypoxia, hypotension or by the secondary effects of placental separation reducing the available interface for oxygen delivery. An unusual exception is vasa praevia where blood vessels on the fetal surface of the placenta are ruptured causing direct blood loss from the fetus. Losing even a small quantity of blood can be catastrophic for the well-being of the fetus.

## Antepartum haemorrhage

### Definition

Bleeding from the genital tract after 24 weeks' gestation and before the birth of the baby.

## Action plan for managing severe haemorrhage

- Arrange emergency transfer to hospital (if at home)/ transfer to ICU/HDU in maternity unit
- Summon appropriate emergency assistance (paramedics/senior obstetrician, anaesthetist)
- Position woman to avoid supine hypotension
- Undertake venepuncture for full blood count, clotting studies and cross-matching
- Notify blood bank and consult haematologist: cross-match at least 6 units urgently
- Obtain intravenous access and commence fluid replacement: plasma expander
- Administer oxygen via mask/nasal prongs
- Observe blood loss
- Monitor fetal well-being (if appropriate)
- Transfuse blood as soon as possible: if not cross-matched, it must be the same blood group as the mother or, in extreme cases, O rhesus negative
- May need fresh-frozen plasma, platelets and cryoprecipitate (consult haematologist)
- Maintain and record accurate fluid balance using urinary catheter and CVP line
- Test for renal function and liver function tests
- Eliminate the cause: deliver the baby and placenta (hysterectomy in extreme cases)
- Observe for signs of postpartum haemorrhage

CVP, central venous pressure; HDU, high dependency unit; ICU, intensive care unit.

### Epidemiology and aetiology

Antepartum haemorrhage (APH) complicates 2–5 per cent of pregnancies. Most cases involve relatively small quantities of blood loss, but may still have sequelae relating to poor placental function, intrauterine growth restriction and premature birth (see also Chapter 11). Some cases are also life threatening.

There are three classifications of APH:

- *accidental* – placental abruption;
- *inevitable* – placenta praevia;
- *incidental* – from local lesions in the genital tract.

In addition to taking a detailed history from the woman as to the nature and extent of vaginal bleeding, the midwife should also recognize the clinical differences between placental abruption and placenta praevia as defined in Table 16.1, as well the possibility of any local cause, in order to aid diagnosis and effect appropriate management. Until the location of the placenta is confirmed, a vaginal examination should *never* be performed. However, in the majority of cases in UK practice, the placental site will probably have been established by routine ultrasound scan before major bleeding occurs.

## Placental abruption

A placental abruption is separation of a normally situated placenta from the uterine wall. In more than two-thirds of cases, the separation reaches the edge of the placenta, tracks down to the cervix and is revealed as vaginal bleeding. The remaining cases present with uterine pain without any obvious bleeding (concealed). The woman is at risk of hypovolaemic shock, clotting disorders and consequentially more widespread organ damage, while the fetus is at risk of hypoxia as a result of placental separation and premature birth. The aetiology and pathophysiological consequences of

**Table 16.1** – Comparison of haemorrhage from placenta abruption with that from placental praevia

| Placental abruption | Placenta praevia |
| --- | --- |
| Painful | Painless |
| Woman is distressed | Woman is less distressed |
| Tender tense abdomen | Soft abdomen |
| Normal lie and presentation | Abnormal lie and presentation |
| Abnormal cardiotocograph (CTG) likely | CTG usually normal |
| May be associated with pre-eclampsia | No particular association with pre-eclampsia |
| Coagulation defect may occur early | No coagulation defect initially |

placental abruption are discussed in further detail in Chapter 10.

The midwife's management depends upon recognition of the problem, acknowledging that the true blood loss may be far greater than the blood loss seen, and immediate implementation of the action plan for severe haemorrhage (see earlier). In very severe cases, the fetus may be dead and vaginal birth can be accelerated by artificial rupture of the membranes and oxytocics once the woman's condition is reasonably stable. If the fetus is alive, a Caesarean section will be undertaken as a matter of urgency, providing the resuscitation of the woman is not compromised.

## Placenta praevia

A placenta that is praevia is partially, or wholly, implanted in the lower uterine segment on either the anterior or posterior wall. The incidence in the UK is 5:1000. As the lower segment grows and stretches, the placenta praevia may separate causing bleeding to occur on more than one occasion. A vaginal birth may be possible with the lesser degrees of placenta praevia, providing the condition of the woman and fetus are satisfactory and any blood loss is not life threatening. However, with major degrees of placenta praevia, it is usual for a Caesarean section to be undertaken by a senior obstetrician at around 37–38 weeks' gestation before the cervix begins to dilate. Delivery would also be indicated if the woman presents with a massive antepartum haemorrhage of >1500 mL or continues to experience significant bleeding of lesser severity.

The risk to the fetus is mainly prematurity owing to early Caesarean section. However, should the cervix begin to dilate and bleeding ensue, there is also the risk of severe hypoxia to the fetus owing to placental separation and also maternal shock as a result of torrential haemorrhage. Severe bleeding usually occurs after the 34th week of pregnancy and about 50 per cent of women with placenta praevia will give birth before 35 weeks.

A woman who has placenta praevia is also at risk of major bleeding during the Caesarean section. The risk of excessive bleeding is particularly great when the placenta is situated anteriorly or is morbidly adhered to an old Caesarean section scar. The placental bed in the lower segment does not contract as efficiently as those in the upper uterine segment once the placenta

has been removed. The midwife should also closely observe the woman for signs of excessive postpartum haemorrhage.

## Vasa praevia

Vasa praevia is an extremely rare condition in which the umbilical cord vessels pass through the placental membranes and lie across the cervical os. Predisposing factors include placenta praevia and multiple pregnancy. The fetal blood vessels, therefore, are at risk of rupturing at spontaneous rupture of membranes or can be damaged as artificial rupture of membranes is undertaken, resulting in fetal blood loss. Although only slight bleeding may be seen, major fetal heart rate changes soon become apparent as a consequence of acute fetal exsanguination. Fetal tachycardia develops, followed by deep decelerations. Although tests for fetal haemoglobin are possible, by the time they are completed, the fetus may be dead. Faced with this situation, the midwife should be highly suspicious of the cause of the antepartum haemorrhage and alert medical colleagues into undertaking a Caesarean section with the utmost speed.

## Uterine rupture

Rupture, or tearing of the uterus, occurs most commonly in association with a previous scar on the uterus, such as a previous classical longitudinal Caesarean section scar. However, it may also occur in the absence of a scar. Almost all cases occur during labour and particular caution should be taken when labour is induced in women who have a uterine scar.

The midwife's vigilance in recognizing cases that are at risk and the potential signs by which uterine rupture may present is vital. Instigating prompt management will help to avert a major maternal haemorrhage. This will involve summoning assistance from senior colleagues, resuscitating the woman according to the degree of shock apparent, and assisting in preparing her for surgical delivery or laparotomy.

The woman complains of continuous abdominal pain with some vaginal blood loss, which may be slight. Contractions cease, the fetal heart rate pattern becomes abnormal and, without immediate laparotomy and delivery, the fetus will usually die. If rupture occurs in

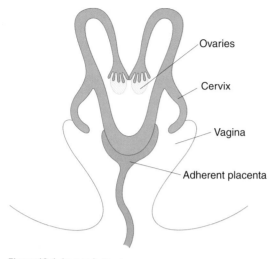

**Figure 16.1** Inverted uterus.

the second stage of labour, it is frequently not recognized. In this situation, the fetus may be delivered by ventouse extraction or forceps. Owing to the internal bleeding, the woman will begin to show signs of circulatory collapse while complaining of abdominal discomfort. It may be possible to repair the uterus following the baby's birth but, in most cases of uterine rupture, the only way to control the bleeding is for the obstetrician to perform a hysterectomy. During the postnatal period, the midwife has an important role to play by offering the woman and her family the opportunity to discuss the outcome of the uterine rupture and the long-term significance it has for them.

## Uterine inversion

Uterine inversion is a very rare but life-threatening complication associated with the third stage of labour (Figure 16.1). It is described when the uterine fundus has prolapsed into the body of the uterus, through the cervix or even through the vulva. The inverted uterus may be seen at the vulva, felt in the vagina or, in lesser cases, identified as a dimpling of the uterine fundus on abdominal examination. It can be caused by mismanagement of the third stage of labour, such as early and excessive controlled cord traction, and after rapid decompression of the uterus following the birth of a large baby or multiple pregnancy. All midwives should be familiar with both the active and expectant management of the third stage of labour.

The woman experiences sudden and profound shock that may be disproportionate to the blood loss visible and degree of inversion. The extent of bleeding will depend on whether the placenta is still attached. The attached placenta prevents bleeding as the uterine sinuses are not exposed and should, therefore, be left alone. Should manual removal of the placenta be necessary, this should be done in theatre under general anaesthesia because of the risk of postpartum haemorrhage.

As with all acute emergencies, the midwife must summon help from a senior obstetrician and anaesthetist. An assisting midwife may undertake appropriate resuscitation measures and treat the shock while the midwife who has assisted the woman give birth attempts to replace the uterus by manual compression (Johnson's manoeuvre). The midwife inserts her hand into the vagina and cups the fundus in the palm of her hand. Pressure is exerted back up and along the long axis of the vagina towards the posterior fornix of the vagina. This position needs to be held for at least 5 minutes or until a firm contraction occurs, to ensure the uterus remains in the pelvis. Intravenous oxytocics should then be given to maintain uterine contraction and enable the cervix to reform.

If manual replacement fails, then medical or surgical intervention will be necessary. This can be achieved by O'Sullivan's hydrostatic method. Warm saline is infused through a giving set into the vagina. As several litres are run into the vagina, the pressure of the fluid builds up restoring the uterus to the normal position, while the operator seals off the introitus by one hand inserted in the vagina. Alternatively, tocolytic agents, such as ritodrine or salbutamol, can be used to relax the cervical contraction ring before an attempt to return the uterus manually is made. If manual replacement continues to fail, a laparotomy will be required.

Throughout all these procedures, the midwife should keep the woman and her partner informed of what is happening. The midwife's assessment and recording of vital signs, including the level of consciousness, is vitally important.

## Postpartum haemorrhage

### Definitions

Excessive bleeding from the genital tract at any time following birth of the baby up to 6 weeks after the birth is defined as postpartum haemorrhage (PPH).

If it occurs during the third stage of labour or within the first 24 hours of the birth, it is classed as *primary postpartum haemorrhage*. If it occurs after the first 24 hours and up until 6 weeks postpartum, the bleeding is defined as *secondary postpartum haemorrhage*. Although traditionally excess loss is described as >500 mL, as blood loss is extremely difficult to measure, the midwife should consider any blood loss, however small, that adversely affects the woman's condition, as constituting a postpartum haemorrhage. A loss of >1000 mL occurs in 1 per cent of cases. However, it is the speed with which it may be lost that is so problematic.

### Aetiology and management

There are several reasons why a primary PPH may occur, including atonic uterus, retained placenta, trauma and blood coagulation disorders. Uterine atony, when the uterus is not contracted, accounts for 90 per cent of all PPH. In these cases, after summoning assistance, the midwife should ensure the bladder is emptied and then attempt to stop the bleeding, by massaging the uterus with a smooth circular motion to cause it to contract. There should be no undue pressure applied to the uterus and, when a contraction is felt, the hand is held still. An intravenous oxytocic infusion is commenced to sustain the contraction. If the woman is able to put the baby to the breast, this may also assist with promoting uterine muscle contraction by the further release of oxytocin. Should other oxytocics prove ineffective, prostaglandin F2 alpha (Haemabate) may also be injected systemically or directly into the myometrium through the anterior abdominal wall by the obstetrician.

The initial action of rubbing up a contraction is always the same regardless of whether bleeding occurs with the placenta *in situ* or later. Once the uterus is contracted, the midwife should then carefully ensure it is emptied, by delivering the placenta (if necessary) or gently expressing any clots with firm but gentle pressure on the fundus. If the placenta is retained, once the woman's condition is stable and she has adequate analgesia, a manual removal is performed by an experienced obstetrician under aseptic conditions. If this situation arises in the home following a home birth, the midwife should make prompt arrangements to transfer the woman and her baby to hospital. The midwife is responsible for ensuring an intravenous infusion is sited and that the woman's condition is stable before she and her baby are transferred.

She is also responsible for examining the placenta and membranes when they are finally delivered to ensure they appear complete.

If bleeding persists following the delivery of the placenta, and is becoming potentially life threatening, the midwife should perform internal bimanual compression. This involves placing one clenched fist in the anterior fornix of the vagina, while the other hand massages the fundus via the abdominal wall, thereby pressing the walls of the uterus together. As this procedure is extremely painful for the woman, the midwife should only attempt it when other measures have not been effective and while awaiting medical assistance. Alternatively, bimanual compression may be attempted externally when the uterus is grasped with both hands and squashed between them. It may be necessary to maintain bimanual compression until clotting disorders have been corrected, as fibrin degradation products, increased in disseminated intravascular coagulation, may themselves cause the uterus to relax.

Should bleeding persist despite uterine contraction, it may be due to other causes, such as genital tract trauma requiring repairing. Clotting disorders must be excluded before exploration of the vagina and uterus is performed under a general anaesthetic. If the woman's haemodynamic status does not improve or deteriorates despite apparent control of revealed bleeding, the cause may be as a consequence of broad ligament or paravaginal bleeding, or even uterine rupture.

Where a PPH persists, the midwife may be called upon to assist the obstetrician with other measures, such as uterine packing and the insertion of intrauterine balloons (e.g. a Rusch catheter). In rare cases, bilateral internal iliac artery ligation or hysterectomy may be necessary.

### Secondary postpartum haemorrhage

This is most likely to occur between 10 and 14 days following the baby's birth. The cause is usually due to a fragment of placenta or membranes, the presence of a large uterine blood clot and/or uterine infection. The lochia is heavier than normal and appears bright red in colour, and may be offensive in smell. Pyrexia and tachycardia usually present if the cause is due to infection. As this is an event that is likely to occur at home, the midwife should advise all women of the possible signs of secondary PPH prior to discharge from midwifery care.

### Action points for secondary postpartum haemorrhage

- Summon medical assistance/paramedic team depending on environment
- Reassure the woman and her partner/family
- Rub up a contraction by massaging the uterus, if it is still palpable
- Express any clots
- Encourage the woman to empty her bladder
- Administer an oxytocic drug intramuscularly/intravenously
- Keep all soiled pads and linen to assess the volume of blood loss
- Commence an intravenous infusion
- Resuscitate as appropriate
- Transfer to hospital once condition is stable, if bleeding severe
- If bleeding persists, discuss the range of treatment options: conservative antibiotics, oxytocin and iron/operative intervention in theatre

## Fetal emergencies

The fetus may be severely affected by any of the maternal emergencies that occur before it is born. However, there are some intrapartum emergencies that directly affect the fetus without any immediate major physical compromise to the mother. Major abnormalities of the fetal heart rate, in particular prolonged fetal bradycardia, warrant immediate delivery. Acute fetal distress is discussed in Chapter 15.

## Umbilical cord accidents

### Definitions and diagnosis

*Cord presentation* exists when a loop or loops of umbilical cord lie below the presenting part of the fetus with the membranes intact. When the membranes rupture, the cord may prolapse through the cervix and eventually the vulva, giving rise to a *cord prolapse*. Both cord presentation and cord prolapse are associated with prematurity, malpresentations of the fetus and polyhydramnios. Although it is impossible to diagnose cord presentation from abdominal examination, the midwife should be suspicious of those pregnancies that carry a higher risk.

The incidence of cord prolapse is around 1:500 births. The umbilical vein is compressed between the presenting part and the maternal pelvis, reducing or stopping flow of oxygenated blood to the fetus, which can result in severe fetal hypoxia and death. If continuous fetal heart rate monitoring is in progress, deep variable decelerations will be seen, leading to severe bradycardia.

### Management

Although cord presentation may be suspected when the midwife detects abnormalities in the fetal heart rate, it is usual to make the diagnosis on vaginal examination. The midwife should summon medical assistance immediately and communicate her findings and the need for emergency measures to the woman and her partner. The membranes should always be left intact and the woman helped into a position that will relieve cord compression: either a knee–chest or an exaggerated Sims' position (Figures 16.2 and 16.3). The foot of the bed may also be raised. The well-being of the fetus and the stage of labour will determine the mode of birth and the speed at which it should be undertaken.

Cord prolapse may be seen externally or palpated in the vagina by the midwife. Once diagnosed, the objective is to maintain the fetal circulation by preventing cord compression and immediate delivery of the fetus. If the incident occurs during a home birth and the fetus is still alive, then transfer to hospital should be without delay with the maternity unit staff fully aware and prepared to deal with the fetal emergency upon arrival. If the cord has prolapsed through the vulva, it should be replaced in the vagina to keep it warmer, otherwise it should not be handled in order to avoid vasospasm.

While arranging for Caesarean section to be performed, manual elevation of the presenting part above the pelvic outlet, to relieve pressure on the umbilical vein and allow oxygen to reach the fetus, is achieved by the midwife inserting two fingers on to the presenting part and applying pressure. The woman should adopt an all-fours position or an exaggerated Sims' position to elevate her buttocks and relieve pressure off the umbilical cord. The latter position is more appropriate when transferring the woman by ambulance. Manual elevation should be maintained until the fetus is about to be born either vaginally or by Caesarean section, and can be both tiring and uncomfortable for the midwife involved.

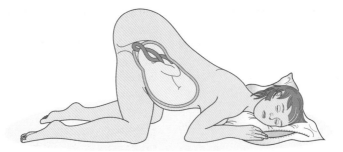

**Figure 16.2** All-fours position: pressure on the umbilical cord is relieved as the fetus gravitates to the uterine fundus. (© Boyle 2002: *Emergencies around childbirth: a handbook for midwives.* Oxford: Radcliffe Medical Press Ltd. Reproduced with permission of the copyright holder.)

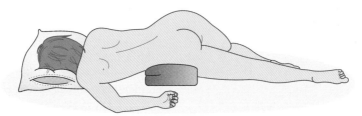

**Figure 16.3** Exaggerated Sims' position. Pillows or wedges are used to elevate the woman's buttocks to relieve pressure on the umbilical cord. (© Boyle 2002: *Emergencies around childbirth: a handbook for midwives.* Oxford: Radcliffe Medical Press Ltd. Reproduced with permission of the copyright holder.)

A less intrusive approach that avoids handling the cord is to fill the woman's bladder with 500 mL of normal saline to displace the fetal presenting part upwards and inhibit uterine contractions.

Intravenous access and venepuncture for full blood count and cross-matching are undertaken and the woman given oral ranitidine should a Caesarean section be justified. A second midwife should make every effort to monitor the fetal heart continuously, particularly through contractions. These findings should be accurately documented in the woman's records along with details of the care and management decisions that are made in conjunction with the medical team.

An urgent Caesarean section is required in the majority of cases. However, if the cervix is fully dilated and the presenting part is engaged, a vaginal birth may be appropriate through maternal effort or with forceps or ventouse extraction. Even when the cervix is fully dilated, if the head is high or there are other factors that may suggest attempting a vaginal birth would be difficult, a Caesarean section should be the performed as soon as possible with prior empty-ing of the maternal bladder. Before commencing Caesarean section, the second midwife should listen to the fetal heart to ensure that the fetus is alive.

*Prognosis*

The outcome of a prolapse of the umbilical cord will depend upon the gestation, other complicating factors, such as intrauterine growth restriction, and the length of time that the cord has been compressed. Should the diagnosis and subsequent action be made promptly in hospital and the fetus is at term, the prognosis is usually good. However, if the cord prolapse occurs in the home setting, there is a greater risk of fetal death occurring by the time the woman is admitted to hospital. It is worth noting that total cord compression for longer than 10 minutes will cause cerebral damage and, if it continues for around 20 minutes, death is usual. These time parameters may be further reduced should the fetus be already compromised.

## Shoulder dystocia

*Definition and aetiology*

There are many variations regarding the definition of shoulder dystocia. One simple definition that is commonly used is when the shoulders fail to traverse the pelvis spontaneously after the fetal head is born.

The incidence varies from 0.2 per cent to 1.2 per cent depending on the definition used. A universally accepted definition of shoulder dystocia is yet to be produced.

In passing through the pelvis, the fetal head and shoulders rotate to make use of the widest pelvic diameters. After the fetal head is born, it is usual for restitution to occur and the shoulders rotate into the anterior–posterior diameter of the pelvis, making use of the widest diameter of the pelvic outlet. However, if the shoulders have not entered the pelvic brim then the anterior shoulder may become caught above the maternal symphysis pubis and cause dystocia. Occasionally, both shoulders may remain above the pelvic brim. In cases of shoulder dystocia, although the birth may have initially been uncomplicated, the head may have advanced slowly with the chin having difficulty sweeping over the perineum. Once the head has been born, it may look as though it is trying to return into the vagina due to reverse traction. This is commonly known as the 'turtle sign'.

Vessels in the fetal neck are occluded after the head is born causing asphyxia. Cerebral damage will occur if the delay in the baby being born exceeds 5 minutes. If labour has been prolonged, the fetus may already be compromised. However, inappropriate traction, particularly downward traction on the head causing lateral flexion of the head on the neck, will cause stretching of the brachial plexus and nerve damage, increasing the likelihood of Erb's palsy. In some cases, fractures of the clavicle and humerus may also result. It is, therefore, important that the baby is carefully examined by an experienced paediatrician for signs of any birth trauma as soon as it has been born.

### Management

Although it would be useful for the midwife to identify those women at risk from a birthing complication associated with shoulder dystocia, only in a minority of cases will it be recognized before the baby's birth. Even combinations of risk factors have poor predictive value. However, if the baby is known to be very large (>4.5 kg) and shoulder dystocia has complicated a previous pregnancy, particularly in a diabetic mother, an elective Caesarean section would be appropriate in order to prevent shoulder dystocia from occurring. In the majority of cases, in recognizing any risk factors the midwife should then ensure that experienced colleagues are present at the birth of

the baby to help manage the problem. Should shoulder dystocia be suspected or diagnosed during a home birth, the midwife has a responsibility to inform the woman and her partner of her findings and subsequent concerns and make arrangements for emergency transfer to the hospital maternity unit.

---

**Risk factors for shoulder dystocia**

- Fetal macrosomia (over 4000 g)
- Diabetes mellitus
- Maternal obesity
- Postmaturity
- Excessive maternal weight gain
- Previous large baby
- Previous shoulder dystocia
- Multiparity
- Prolongation of late first stage of labour (dilatation of the cervix 7–10 cm)
- Prolonged second stage of labour
- Arrest or failure of descent of presenting part
- Need for assisted vaginal delivery

---

Shoulder dystocia is managed by a sequence of manoeuvres designed to facilitate the birth of the baby without fetal damage. This sequence must be part of a prepared plan of action that all midwifery and obstetric staff are familiar with and have practiced in labour ward drills.

The midwife should make an accurate record of the time the head and body were born, the manoeuvres that were used and the personnel who were present during the birth. The number of attempts of traction on the head and the relationship of these attempts to the other manoeuvres should also be recorded. As the complication of the Erb's palsy may lead to subsequent litigation up to 25 years after the birth, it is vital that records are made contemporaneously and accurately reflect the events that have taken place.

There are various manoeuvres that may be used to attempt resolving shoulder dystocia. No single manoeuvre has been proven to be superior to any other in disimpacting the shoulder and none is entirely free from potential injury to the fetus or woman. A mnemonic (HELPERR) has been designed to assist midwives and obstetricians involved with a birth complicated with shoulder dystocia (see box).

### Shoulder dystocia drill (HELPERR)

- Help: call for help and activate protocol
- Episiotomy: improves access to the fetus and for internal manoeuvres
- Legs: McRoberts manoeuvre (30–60 seconds)
- Pressure: external suprapubic (30–60 seconds)
- Enter the vagina:/Rubin's/Woods' screw manoeuvre (30–60 seconds)
- Remove the posterior arm
- Roll the woman over on to all fours
- Zavanelli manoeuvre (not strictly part of the mnemonic)
- Symphysiotomy (not strictly part of the mnemonic).

## Non-invasive procedures

The *McRoberts position* involves assisting the woman to lie flat and to bring her knees up to her chest as far as possible. It is recommended as the first manoeuvre to attempt as it does not involve manipulation of the fetus and appears to be relatively safe. In this position, the angle of the symphysis pubis is rotated superiorly and the weight of the woman's hyperflexed legs, creating gentle pressure on her abdomen, releases the impaction of the anterior shoulder.

Applying *suprapubic pressure* on the side of the fetal back towards the fetal chest may help to adduct the shoulders, reduce the bisacromial diameter and push the shoulders into the oblique position and off the symphysis pubis. This manoeuvre may also be used in conjunction with the McRoberts' manoeuvre.

The *all-fours* position may also be useful in alleviating shoulder impaction. The actual movement of the woman turning on to her hands and knees may help dislodge the shoulder, particularly if it is the posterior shoulder that is impacted behind the sacral promontory. However, the anterior shoulder may remain impacted against the symphysis pubis.

## Manipulative procedures

Although the problem is a bony one, performing a *large episiotomy* or extending an existing one may be considered to provide more space at the outlet. The majority of cases will resolve with non-invasive management. However, if such procedures prove unsuccessful, the midwife should consider techniques involving direct manipulation of the fetus.

*Rubin's manoeuvre* requires the midwife to identify the posterior shoulder on vaginal examination and then to push the posterior shoulder in the direction of the fetal chest, thus adducting the shoulders and rotating the anterior shoulder away from the symphysis pubis.

An alternative would be for the midwife to use the *Woods' screw rotational manoeuvre*. This involves the midwife inserting her hand into the vagina to identify the fetal chest. Then by exerting gentle pressure on to the posterior fetal shoulder, it is pushed backwards through 180°. Although this manoeuvre abducts the shoulders, it does rotate the shoulders into a more favourable diameter to allow the baby to be born.

Should rotational manoeuvres be unsuccessful, the midwife may attempt to *deliver the posterior arm*. The midwife inserts her hand into the vagina and places two fingers under the posterior shoulder. Applying pressure in the antecubital fossa will help the forearm to flex so that it can be swept over the chest. Delivery of the arm may facilitate rotation of the fetus through a 180° arc, bringing the posterior shoulder under the symphysis pubis to enable the rest of the birth to be completed normally. Should there be further difficulty when delivering the second arm, and if time permits, positioning the woman in an all-fours position and either using Rubin's or the Woods' screw manoeuvres should be considered by the midwife. In some instances, the obstetrician may decide to break the fetal clavicle as a means of ensuring the fetus is born alive.

If all of these manoeuvres fail as a last resort to deliver a live fetus, the obstetrician may consider the *Zavanelli manoeuvre*. This involves the reversal of the mechanism of birth where the fetal head is returned to its pre-restitution position and, with pressure exerted on the occiput, the head is then replaced in the vagina. A Caesarean section is then promptly undertaken. In rare cases, a *symphysiotomy* is performed. This is where the maternal symphysis pubis is surgically separated to enlarge the pelvis so the fetus may be born. It is common in developing countries where there may be cephalopelvic disproportion.

Shoulder dystocia is a most alarming fetal emergency for the midwife and obstetrician. Furthermore, it can be very frightening for the woman and her partner. Without delaying matters unduly, every opportunity should be taken to explain what is happening and to give a full explanation to the woman and her partner after the baby is born.

## Key Points

The role that midwives play in any childbirth emergency is fundamental to ensuring that the well-being of mother and fetus remains optimal. This involves the following.

- Being aware of any risk factors in order to avoid untoward childbirth events
- Making an appropriate diagnosis and taking prompt action, involving summoning appropriate assistance and ensuring that the woman is in the most appropriate environment
- Undertaking basic life support measures until further assistance arrives
- Recognizing their duty of care to inform women and their partners/families of the significance and subsequent management of the emergency
- Assisting with procedures undertaken by medical colleagues
- Maintaining clear lines of communication both verbally, and through accurate and contemporaneous record keeping
- Being responsible for keeping up to date with local emergency procedures/protocols, including taking part in multidisciplinary emergency practice drills
- Engaging in the review of practice to ensure that policies and procedures are regularly reviewed in the light of best possible evidence

## References and additional reading

Boyle M (ed.). *Emergencies around childbirth: a handbook for midwives*. Oxford Radcliffe Medical Press, 2002.

Lewis G, Drife J (eds). *Confidential Enquiry into Maternal and Child Health; why mothers die 2000–2002*. Sixth report of the confidential enquiry into maternal deaths in the United Kingdom. London: RCOG Press, 2004.

Woodward V, Bates, K, Young N. *Managing childbirth emergencies in community settings*. Basingstoke: Palgrave Macmillan, 2005.

# The puerperium

## OVERVIEW

The puerperium is the 6-week period following the birth of the baby when considerable physiological changes occur as the mother's body returns to its pre-pregnant state. This is the time when the mother learns how to care for her baby and begins to adapt to motherhood. The mother experiences many emotions and is also vulnerable to psychological disturbances that may be affected by her social circumstances. It is important that the mother receives understanding and support from her partner and family. Appropriate care and support from the midwife, general practitioner and health visitor is also vital. In the UK, birth may take place at home or in the hospital from where the mother may be transferred home within 6 hours of an uncomplicated birth. The mother and baby may stay longer in hospital according to their individual needs and well-being. The midwife has a statutory responsibility to support and care for the mother and baby for at least 10 days and any longer period that the midwife considers necessary [Nursing and Midwifery Council (NMC) 2004a]. Thereafter, the health visitor takes on responsibility for continuing care, particularly of the infant.

## Physiological changes

The physiological changes that occur following childbirth take place without complication for most mothers. The midwife must assess maternal well-being with regard to these physiological changes and identify any potential or actual complications, making referral to other health professionals or agencies as appropriate. The assessment includes observing the mother, talking with and listening to her, and physical examination. This may be done on a daily basis or according to individual needs and risk assessment.

## Genital tract changes

Following delivery of the placenta and membranes, the lower segment of the uterus and cervix appear flabby and there may be small cervical lacerations. In the first few days, the cervix remains slightly open but, by the end of the second week, the cervix has regained its tone and the internal os should be closed. The external os can remain open permanently, giving a characteristic slit like appearance to the parous cervix. In the first few days, the stretched vagina is smooth and oedematous but, by the third week, rugae begin to reappear.

## Uterine involution

Involution is the process by which the postpartum uterus, weighing about 1 kg, returns to its pre-pregnancy state of less than 100 g. Immediately after the birth, the uterus should be well contracted with the fundus about 4 cm below the umbilicus or 12 cm above the symphysis pubis. Within 2 weeks, the uterus is no longer palpable above the symphysis. Involution occurs by a process of ischaemia and autolysis of the myometrium whereby muscle cells diminish in size as a result of enzymatic digestion of cytoplasm. This has virtually no effect on the number of muscle cells and the excess protein produced from autolysis is absorbed into the bloodstream and excreted in the urine. Involution appears to be accelerated by the release of oxytocin in women who breast feed.

The midwife will assess the process of involution by asking the mother about her physical health, palpating the uterus abdominally to ensure it is contracted and assessing the height of the uterine fundus. In the event of any delay in involution (see box), the midwife will decide whether referral to the doctor is required. A delay in involution in the absence of any other signs or symptoms (e.g. vaginal bleeding) is unlikely to be of clinical significance.

---

### Causes of delayed involution

- Full bladder
- Loaded rectum
- Uterine infection
- Retained products of conception
- Fibroids
- Broad ligament haematoma

---

## Lochia

Lochia is the bloodstained uterine discharge comprised of blood and necrotic decidua. Only the superficial layer of decidua becomes necrotic and sloughs off. The basal layer adjacent to the myometrium is involved in the regeneration of new endometrium, which is complete by the third week. Initially, the lochia is red; this gradually changes to pink as the endometrium is formed and becomes serous by the second week. The midwife should ask the mother about the amount and colour of the lochia and, if necessary, inspect the sanitary pad. It is important that any abnormalities in relation to the lochia are recognized so that appropriate referral to a doctor can be made and relevant treatment prescribed. Persistent red lochia suggests delayed involution that is usually associated with infection or a retained piece of placental tissue. Offensive lochia, which may be accompanied by pyrexia and a tender uterus, suggests infection and should be treated with a broad-spectrum antibiotic. Retained placental tissue is associated with increased red blood cell loss and clots, and this may be suspected if the placenta and membranes were incomplete at delivery. Antibiotics and evacuation of retained products under regional or general anaesthesia may be required.

---

### Puerperal disorders

## Perineal complications

Perineal pain can be a significant problem for mothers in the initial days after birth, often continuing after 10 days. Perineal oedema and lacerations can cause discomfort, although discomfort is greatest in women who sustain spontaneous tears or have an episiotomy, and especially following instrumental delivery. The midwife should advise the mother about hygiene, bathing or showering and appropriate analgesia. A number of non-pharmacological and pharmacological therapies have been used empirically with varying degrees of success. However, local cooling (with crushed ice, witch hazel or tap water) and topical anaesthetics such as 5 per cent lignocaine gel provide short-term symptomatic relief (Grant and Sleep 1989). Effective analgesia following perineal trauma can be achieved with paracetamol, although anti-inflammatory preparations may be more effective. Codeine derivatives have a tendency to cause constipation.

Infections of the perineum are generally uncommon considering the risk of bacterial contamination during birth; therefore, when signs of infection (redness, pain, swelling and heat) occur, especially when associated with pyrexia, these must be taken seriously and the midwife should refer to a doctor. Swabs for microbiological culture must be taken from the infected perineum and broad-spectrum antibiotics and analgesia should be prescribed. Drainage of pus should be encouraged by removal of any skin sutures, otherwise infection would spread with increasing morbidity and a poor anatomical result. Spontaneous opening of repaired perineal tears and episiotomy is usually the result of secondary infection. Surgical repair would not be attempted in the presence of infection. The wound should be irrigated twice daily and healing should be allowed to occur by secondary intention. If there is a large gaping wound, secondary repair should only be performed when the infection has cleared, there is no cellulitis or exudate present and healthy granulation tissue can be seen.

## Bladder function

Voiding difficulty and overdistension of the bladder are not uncommon after childbirth, especially if regional anaesthesia (epidural/spinal) has been used. After epidural anaesthesia, the bladder may take up to 8 hours to regain normal sensation and about 1 L of urine may be produced. Therefore, urinary retention can cause considerable damage to the detrusor muscle. Overstretching of the detrusor muscle can dampen bladder sensation and make the bladder hypocon-tractile, particularly with fibrous replacement of smooth muscle. In this situation, overflow incontinence of small amounts of urine may be mistaken for normal voiding. Fluid overloading prior to epidural anal-gesia, the antidiuretic effect of high concentrations of oxytocin during labour, increased postpartum diur-esis, particularly in the presence of oedema, and increased fluid intake by breast-feeding mothers all contribute to the increased urine production in the puerperium.

Women who have undergone a traumatic delivery, such as a difficult instrumental birth, or who have suffered multiple/extended lacerations or a vulvovagi-nal haematoma, may find it difficult to void because of pain or periurethral oedema. Other causes of pain, such as prolapsed haemorrhoids, anal fissures, abdom-inal wound haematoma or even stool impaction of the rectum may interfere with voiding. The midwife needs to be particularly vigilant to avoid bladder dis-tension after an epidural or spinal anaesthetic. The distended bladder may be palpable as a suprapubic cystic mass or it may displace the uterus laterally or upwards, thereby increasing the height of the uterine fundus.

To minimize the risk of overdistension of the blad-der in women undergoing a Caesarean section under regional anaesthesia, a urinary catheter may be left in the bladder for the first 12–24 hours. The benefit of leaving a catheter *in situ* for about 12 hours after epidural insertion should be evaluated against encour-aging normal voiding and the small risk of urinary tract infection. Any woman who has not passed urine within 4 hours of giving birth should be encouraged to do so before resorting to catheterization. In gen-eral, a clean catch specimen of urine should be sent for microscopy, culture and sensitivity and, if the residual urine in the bladder is greater than 300 mL, a catheter may need to be left in to allow free drainage for 48 hours.

Although vaginal delivery is strongly implicated in the development of urinary stress incontinence, it rarely poses a problem in the early puerperium. There-fore, any incontinence should be investigated to exclude a vesicovaginal, urethrovaginal or rarely an ureterovagi-nal fistula. Pressure necrosis of the bladder or urethra may occur following prolonged obstructed labour and incontinence usually occurs in the second week when the slough separates. Small fistulae may close spontaneously after a few weeks of free bladder drainage; large fistulae will require surgical repair by a specialist.

## Bowel function

Constipation is common in the puerperium. This may be due to an interruption in the normal diet and pos-sible dehydration during labour. Advice on adequate fluid intake from the midwife and increase in fibre intake may be all that is necessary. However, constipa-tion may also be the result of fear of evacuation owing to pain from a sutured perineum, prolapsed haemor-rhoids or anal fissures. Avoidance of constipation and straining is of utmost importance in women who have sustained a third or fourth degree tear. A large hard bolus of stool may disrupt the repaired anal sphincter and cause anal incontinence. It is important that these women are prescribed lactulose and ispaghula husk (Fybogel, Regulan) or methylcellulose immediately after the repair, for a period of 2 weeks.

The high prevalence of anal incontinence and fae-cal urgency affecting primiparous and parous women following childbirth has only recently been recog-nized. Long-term anal incontinence following pri-mary repair of a third or fourth degree tear occurs in 5 per cent of women and anovaginal/rectovaginal fistulae occur in 2–4 per cent of these women. It is important to consider a fistula as a cause of anal incontinence in the postpartum period, particularly if the woman complains of passing wind or stool per vaginam. Small anovaginal fistulae will close spontaneously over a period of 6 months but larger fistulae will require formal repair frequently with a covering colostomy.

## Secondary postpartum haemorrhage

This is defined as fresh bleeding from the genital tract between 24 hours and 6 weeks after birth. The most common time for secondary postpartum haemorrhage (PPH) is between 7 and 14 days, so it is most likely that it will occur at home. The cause is most commonly attributed to retained placental tissue. Associated features include crampy abdominal pain, a uterus larger than appropriate, passage of pieces of placental tissue or tissue within the cervix, and signs of infection. The midwife must seek medical assistance while supporting and reassuring the mother. The management of heavy bleeding includes an intravenous infusion, cross-match of blood, syntocinon, and an examination under anaesthesia and evacuation of the uterus. Antibiotics should be given if placental tissue is found, even without evidence of overt infection. The doctor may consider pelvic ultrasound to exclude retained products, although, if blood loss is not excessive, its use is contentious; distinction between retained products and blood clot can be extremely difficult.

Other causes of secondary postpartum haemorrhage include endometritis, hormonal contraception, bleeding disorders (e.g. von Willebrand's disease) and choriocarcinoma.

## Obstetric palsy

Obstetric palsy, or traumatic neuritis, is a maternal condition where one or both lower limbs may develop signs of a motor and/or sensory neuropathy following birth. Presenting features include sciatic pain, foot drop, parasthesia, hypoaesthesia and muscle wasting, and may result from exaggerated lithotomy position and instrumental delivery. The midwife should take appropriate preventative action during labour and birth. If it occurs, an obstetric and orthopaedic opinion is needed. Management includes bedrest with a firm board beneath the mattress, analgesia and physiotherapy.

## Symphysis pubis diastasis

Separation of the symphysis pubis can occur spontaneously in at least 1 in 800 vaginal births. Deliberate surgical separation of the pubis in labour (symphysiotomy) is no longer practised in the UK. Spontaneous separation may be noticed after birth and has been associated with forceps delivery, rapid second stage of labour or severe abduction of the thighs during labour. Common signs and symptoms include, symphyseal pain aggravated by weight-bearing and walking, a waddling gait, pubic tenderness and a palpable interpubic gap. Treatment includes bedrest, anti-inflammatory agents, physiotherapy and a pelvic corset to provide support and stability.

## Thromboembolism

The risk of thromboembolic disease rises five-fold during pregnancy and the puerperium in part due to the normal physiology. The latest *Confidential Enquiry into Maternal Deaths* (Lewis and Drife 2004) identifies seven deaths following vaginal birth and 10 deaths following Caesarean section. If deep vein thrombosis or pulmonary embolism is suspected by the midwife, medical aid must be sought. The obstetrician will commence full anticoagulant therapy and a bilateral venogram and/or lung scan should be carried out within 24–48 hours (Ch. 12).

## Puerperal pyrexia

The risk of puerperal infection is important. Significant puerperal pyrexia is defined as a temperature of 38°C (100.4°F) or higher on any two of the first 10 days postpartum, exclusive of the first 24 hours. A mildly elevated temperature is not uncommon in the first 24 hours, but any pyrexia associated with tachycardia should be referred for a medical opinion and investigation. In about 80 per cent of women who develop a pyrexia in the first 24 hours following a vaginal delivery, no obvious evidence of infection can be identified. However, a wound infection should be considered for women delivering by Caesarean section. Common sites associated with puerperal pyrexia include chest, throat, breasts, urinary tract, pelvic organs, abdominal or perineal wounds and legs.

## Chest complications

Chest complications are most likely to appear in the first 24 hours following birth, particularly after general anaesthesia. Atelectasis may be associated with fever and can be prevented by early and regular chest physiotherapy. Aspiration pneumonia (Mendelson's syndrome) must be suspected if there is wheezing, dyspnoea, a spiking temperature and evidence of hypoxia.

## Genital tract infection

Until 1937, puerperal sepsis was the major cause of maternal mortality but gradually declined (Lewis and Drife 2004). The discovery of sulphonamides in 1935 and the simultaneous reduction in the virulence of the haemolytic streptococcus helped towards a dramatic fall in maternal mortality. There were no deaths due to puerperal sepsis in 1984, but it accounted for eight maternal deaths between 2000 and 2002 (Lewis and Drife 2004). Five deaths were following vaginal birth, two home births and three hospital births, and three following Caesarean section. The risk factors for puerperal sepsis are listed (see box). The possible signs and symptoms of sepsis (see boxes) must be considered. Referral to the obstetrician is necessary for prompt, appropriate treatment, including antibiotic therapy, can be started to prevent mortality or morbidity.

---

### Common risk factors for puerperal infection

- Antenatal intrauterine infection
- Caesarean section
- Cervical cerclage for cervical incompetence
- Prolonged rupture of membranes
- Prolonged labour
- Multiple vaginal examinations
- Internal fetal monitoring
- Instrumental delivery
- Manual removal of the placenta
- Retained products of conception
- Non-obstetric, e.g. obesity, diabetes, human immunodeficiency virus (HIV)

---

### Signs of puerperal pelvic infection

- Pyrexia and tachycardia
- Uterus – poorly contracted, tender and larger
- Infected wounds – Caesarean/perineal
- Peritonism
- Paralytic ileus
- Indurated adnexae (parametritis)
- Bogginess in pelvis (abscess)

---

### Symptoms of puerperal pelvic infection

- Malaise, headache, fever, rigors
- Abdominal discomfort, vomiting and diarrhoea
- Offensive lochia
- Secondary postpartum haemorrhage

---

### Aetiology

A mixed flora normally colonizes the vagina with low virulence. Puerperal infection is usually polymicrobial and involves contaminants from the bowel that colonize the perineum and lower genital tract. Following birth, natural barriers to infection are temporarily removed and, therefore, organisms with a pathogenic potential can ascend from the lower genital tract into the uterine cavity. Placental separation exposes a large raw area, and retained products of conception and blood clots within the uterus provide an excellent culture medium for infection. Vaginal birth may be associated with lacerations of the genital tract. Although these lacerations may not need surgical repair, they can become a focus for infection similar to iatrogenic wounds, such as Caesarean section and episiotomy.

Transmission can occur by droplet infection, infected dust or by direct skin contact. The toxins produced by these organisms can result in a rapid deterioration into septicaemic shock and yet produce minimal local signs. With the advent of penicillin, serious infection is now rare, although penicillin-resistant staphylococcus now poses a new threat.

The midwife must ensure that hygiene and universal precautions in relation to hand-washing and prevention and control of infection are strictly adhered to by all midwives and health professionals. She must also advise the mother and her family in relation to hygiene.

**Table 17.1** – Investigations for puerperal genital infections

| Investigations | Abnormalities |
|---|---|
| Full blood count | Anaemia, leucocytosis, thrombocytopenia |
| Urea and electrolytes | Fluid and electrolyte imbalance |
| High vaginal swabs and blood culture | Infection screen |
| Pelvic ultrasound | Retained products, pelvic abscess |
| Clotting screen (haemorrhage or shock) | Disseminated intravascular coagulation |
| Arterial blood gas (shock) | Acidosis and hypoxia |

Investigations for puerperal genital infections are shown in Table 17.1.

A number of factors determine the clinical course and severity of the infection: the general health and resistance of the woman; the virulence of the offending organism; presence of haematoma or retained products of conception; and timing of antibiotic therapy and associated risk factors. The common methods of spread of puerperal infection are outlined below.

- An ascending infection from the lower genital tract or primary infection of the placental site may spread via the Fallopian tubes to the ovaries giving rise to a salpingo-oophoritis and pelvic peritonitis. This could progress to a generalized peritonitis and pelvic abscesses.
- Infection may spread by contiguity directly into the myometrium and the parametrium giving rise to a metritis or parametritis, also referred to as pelvic cellulitis. Pelvic peritonitis and abscesses may occur.
- Infection may spread to distant sites via lymphatics and blood vessels. Infection from the uterus can be carried by uterine vessels into the inferior vena cava via the iliac vessels or, directly, via the ovarian vessels. This could give rise to a septic thrombophlebitis, pulmonary infections or a generalized septicaemia and endotoxic shock.

Mild to moderate infections can be treated with a broad-spectrum antibiotic (e.g. Co-amoxiclav) or a cephalosporin, such as Cephalexin plus Metronidazole. Depending on severity, the first few doses should be given intravenously.

With severe infections, there is a release of inflammatory and vasoactive mediators in response to the endotoxins produced during bacteriolysis. The resultant local vasodilation causes circulatory embarrassment and poor tissue perfusion. This phenomenon is known as septicaemic/septic/endotoxic shock and delay in appropriate management could be fatal.

Necrotizing fasciitis is a rare but frequently fatal infection of skin, fascia and muscle. It can originate in perineal tears, episiotomies and Caesarean section wounds. Perineal infections can extend rapidly to involve the buttocks, thighs and lower abdominal wall. In addition to measures taken in the management of septic shock, wide debridement of necrotic tissue under general anaesthesia is absolutely essential to avoid mortality.

## Prevention of puerperal sepsis

Increased awareness of the principles in general hygiene, use of aseptic techniques and good surgical approach have contributed to the decline in severe puerperal sepsis. However, the risk of sepsis is higher following Caesarean section, particularly when performed after the onset of labour. There is evidence that prophylactic antibiotics during emergency Caesarean section reduce the risk of postoperative infection (Lewis and Drife 2004), namely wound infection, metritis, pelvic abscess, pelvic thrombophlebitis and septic shock. Antibiotics should be given after clamping of the umbilical cord to avoid unnecessary exposure of the baby. The benefit of prophylaxis for elective Caesarean sections would be of greater significance in units where the background infectious morbidity is high.

**Table 17.2** – Diagnosis and management of puerperal pyrexia

| Symptoms | Diagnosis | Special investigations | Management |
|---|---|---|---|
| Cough | Chest infection | Sputum M, C&S | Physiotherapy |
| Purulent sputum<br>Dyspnoea | Pneumonia | Chest X-ray | Antibiotics |
| Sore throat<br>Cervical lymphadenopathy | Tonsillitis | Throat swab | Antibiotics |
| Headaches<br>Neck stiffness (epidural/<br>spinal anaesthetic) | Meningitis | Lumbar puncture | Antibiotics |
| Dysuria<br>Loin pain and tenderness | Pyelonephritis | Urine M, C&S | Antibiotics |
| Secondary PPH | Metritis | Pelvic ultrasound | Antibiotics |
| Tender bulky uterus | Retained placental tissue | | Uterine evacuation |
| Pelvic/calf pain/tenderness | Deep vein thrombosis<br>Pulmonary embolism | Dopplers/venogram of legs<br>Lung perfusion scan<br>angiogram<br>Chest X-ray and blood gases | Heparin |
| Painful engorged breasts | Mastitis<br><br>Abscess | Milk M, C&S | Express milk<br>Antibiotics<br>Incision and drainage |

## The breasts

### Anatomy

The breasts consist of glandular, adipose and connective tissue (Figure 17.1). They lie superficial to the pectoralis major, external oblique and serratus anterior muscles extending between the second and sixth rib from the sternum to the axilla. A pigmented area called the areola, containing sebaceous glands, surrounds the nipple. During pregnancy, the areola becomes darker and the sebaceous glands become prominent (Montgomery's tubercles). The breast comprises 15–25 functional units arranged radially from the nipple, and each unit is made up of a lactiferous duct, a mammary gland lobule and alveoli. The lactiferous ducts dilate to

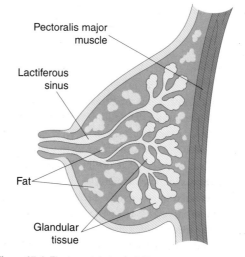

**Figure 17.1** The breast during lactation.

form a lactiferous sinus before converging to open in the nipple. Contractile myoepithelial cells surround the ducts as well as the alveoli.

## Physiology

Breast development occurs at puberty and can produce milk within 2 weeks of hormonal stimulation. The control of mammary growth and development is not fully understood, and many hormones may contribute to this process. In general, oestrogens stimulate proliferation of the lactiferous ducts (possibly with adrenal steroids and growth hormones) while progesterone is responsible for the development of the mammary lobules. During early pregnancy, lactiferous ducts and alveoli proliferate, while in later pregnancy, the alveoli hypertrophy in preparation of secretory activity. The lactogenic hormones, prolactin and human placental lactogen probably modulate these changes during pregnancy.

## Colostrum

Colostrum is a yellowish fluid secreted by the breast that can be expressed as early as the 16th week of pregnancy and is replaced by milk during the second/third postpartum day. Colostrum has a high concentration of proteins, but contains less sugar and fat than breast milk, although it contains large fat globules. The proteins are mainly in the form of globulins, particularly immunoglobulin (Ig) A, which plays an important role in protection against infection. Colostrum is believed to have a laxative effect, which may help empty the baby's bowel of meconium.

## Breast milk

The major constituents of breast milk are lactose, protein, fat and water (Table 17.3). The composition of breast milk is not constant; early lactation differs from late lactation, one feed differs from the next and the composition can change during a feed. Artificial infant formulas cannot, therefore, be identical to breast milk. Compared to cow's milk, breast milk provides slightly more energy, has less protein but more fat and lactose. The major protein fractions are lactalbumin, lactoglobulin and caseinogen. Lactalbumin is the major protein in breast milk, whereas caseinogen

**Table 17.3** – Comparison between human and cow's milk

|  | Human breast milk | Cow's milk |
| --- | --- | --- |
| Energy (kcal/mL) | 75 | 66 |
| Lactose (g/100 mL) | 6.8 | 4.9 |
| Protein (g/100 mL) | 1.1 | 3.5 |
| Fat (g/100 mL) | 4.5 | 3.7 |
| Sodium (mmol/L) | 7 | 22 |
| Water (mL/1000 mL) | 87.1 | 87.3 |

forms 90 per cent of the protein in cow's milk. The mineral content is much higher in cow's milk, particularly sodium and can, therefore, be dangerous if given to a baby who is dehydrated from gastroenteritis. In addition to IgA, breast milk contains small amounts of IgM and IgG, and other factors, such as lactoferrin, macrophages, complement and lysozymes. Although breast milk contains a lower concentration of iron, its absorption is better than from cow's milk or iron-supplemented infant formula. The improved bioavailability may be related to lactoferrin, an iron-binding glycoprotein, which also inhibits bacterial growth. With the exception of vitamin K, all other vitamins are found in breast milk and, therefore, vitamin K is offered to the baby to minimize the risk of haemorrhagic disease.

## Prolactin

Prolactin is a long-chain polypeptide produced from the anterior pituitary, and levels rise up to 20-fold during pregnancy and lactation. Peak levels of prolactin are reached within 45 minutes of suckling but return to normal immediately after weaning and in non-breast feeding mothers. The exact mechanism of action is not fully understood but prolactin appears to have a direct action on the secretory cells to synthesize milk proteins. Prolactin is essential for lactation and it is hypothesized that nipple stimulation prevents release of prolactin-inhibiting factor from the hypothalamus, thereby initiating the production of prolactin by the anterior pituitary.

## Oxytocin

Milk produced under the influence of prolactin has to be delivered to the baby. The milk-ejection or let-down reflex is initiated by suckling, which stimulates the pulsatile release of oxytocin from the posterior pituitary. Oxytocin contracts the myoepithelial cells surrounding the alveoli and the myoepithelial cells lying longitudinally along the lactiferous ducts, thereby aiding expulsion of milk. Oxytocin release can be stimulated by visual, olfactory or auditory stimuli (e.g. hearing the baby cry), but can be inhibited by stress. Oxytocin also stimulates uterine contractions giving rise to the 'after pains' of childbirth.

## Breast feeding

An important aspect of the role of the midwife is to promote breast feeding and to help women to make an informed choice as to feeding. Women who choose to bottle feed also need advice and support. Women who opt to breast feed often decide before or very early in pregnancy. This decision is usually based on previous experience, influence of family or friends, culture and custom. The Baby Friendly Initiative [World Health Organisation (WHO)/UNICEF 1991] identifies that women be given information about breast feeding during pregnancy, need support from the midwife as breast feeding is being established, and ongoing support when the mother is discharged from the care of the midwife.

The most common reasons mothers give for abandoning breast feeding are inadequate milk production or sore and cracked nipples. These problems can be overcome by correct positioning of the baby on the breast (Figure 17.2). The mouth should be placed over the nipple and areola so that suction created within the baby's mouth draws the breast tissue into a teat which extends as far back as the junction of the soft and hard palate. The tongue applies peristaltic force to the underside of the teat against the support of the hard palate. In this way there should be no to and fro movement of the teat in and out of the baby's mouth, thus minimizing friction. The mother should be shown how to implement the rooting reflex. When the skin around the baby's mouth is touched the mouth begins to gape. The mother should reposition the baby so the lower rim of the baby's mouth fits well below the nipple allowing a liberal mouthful of breast

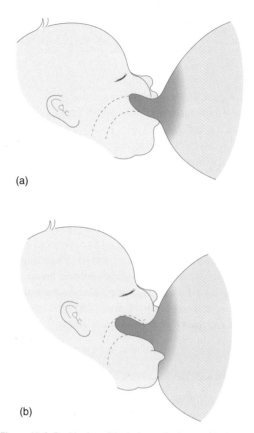

(a)

(b)

**Figure 17.2** Positioning of the baby on the breast: (a) poor positioning; (b) good positioning.

tissue. When the baby is properly attached, breast feeding should be pain free.

Early suckling appears to be beneficial and the mother should be helped to initiate breast feeding within half an hour of birth. The midwife should ensure that the mother is comfortable and fully supported. The mother should be advised to feed her baby on demand (WHO/UNICEF 1991) and the baby left on the breast until feeding finishes spontaneously. Supplementary feeds of formula, glucose or water should not be given to the breast feeding baby and dummies/pacifiers are not recommended.

### Advantages of breast feeding

- Readily available at the right temperature and ideal nutritional value
- Cheaper than formula feed

- Associated with a reduction in:
  - childhood infective illnesses, especially gastroenteritis
  - fertility with amenorrhoea
  - atopic illnesses (e.g. eczema and asthma)
  - necrotizing enterocolitis in preterm babies
  - juvenile diabetes
  - childhood cancer, especially lymphoma
  - pre-menopausal breast cancer

### *Non-breast feeding mothers*

There are various reasons as to why a woman may choose not to breast feed, ranging from personal choice to stillbirth and infections, such as HIV. These mothers may suffer considerable engorgement and breast pain, and the midwife must provide advice and support in such circumstances. Suppression of lactation may need to be facilitated by pharmacological means.

## Breast disorders

### Painful nipples

The nipple can become very painful if the covering epithelium is denuded or if a fissure develops giving rise to 'cracked nipples'. As this is most likely to be caused by poor positioning of the baby on the breast, it can be prevented. However, thrush (candidiasis) may also cause soreness. Cracked nipples are associated with an increased risk of a breast abscess developing. While the mother can be guided to continue breast feeding, 'cracked nipples' may require resting the affected nipple and manually expressing milk. Breast feeding should then be reintroduced gradually.

### Breast engorgement

Engorgement of the breasts usually begins by the second or third postpartum day and, if breast feeding has not been effectively established, the overdistended and engorged breasts can be very uncomfortable. The midwife should support and encourage the mother during what can be a very distressing time, helping the mother to have confidence in her ability to breast feed.

Breast engorgement may cause puerperal fever. Although the fever rarely lasts more than 16 hours, other infective causes must be excluded. A number of remedies for treatment of breast engorgement, such as manual expression, firm support, applying an ice bag and an electric breast pump, have all been recommended in the past, but allowing the baby easy access to the breast is the most effective method of treatment and prevention.

## Mastitis

Inflammation of the breast is not always due to an infective process. Mastitis can occur when a blocked duct obstructs the flow of milk and distends the alveoli. If this pressure persists, the milk extravasates into the perilobular tissue initiating an inflammatory process. The affected segment of the breast is painful, and appears red and oedematous (Figure 17.3). Flu-like symptoms develop associated with a tachycardia and pyrexia. In general, suppurative mastitis usually presents at the third to fourth postpartum week and is usually unilateral. Symptoms include rigors, fever, pain and reddened swollen breasts. The most common infecting organism is *Staphylococcus aureus*. The most frequent source of infection is from the baby's nose or throat and, second, from an infected umbilical cord. Management may include isolation of mother and baby, ceasing breast feeding from the affected breast, expression of milk either manually or by electric pump, and microbiological culture and sensitivity of a sample of milk. Flucloxacillin can be prescribed while awaiting sensitivity results.

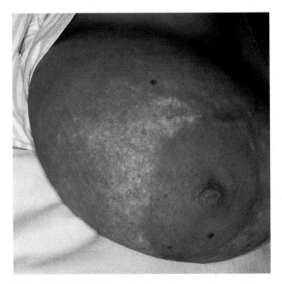

**Figure 17.3** Mastitis demonstrating redness, oedema and engorged veins.

About 10 per cent of women with mastitis develop a breast abscess. Treatment is by a radial surgical incision and drainage under general anaesthesia.

## Contraception

The exact mechanism of lactational amenorrhoea is poorly understood but the most plausible hypothesis is that, during lactation, there is inhibition of the normal pulsatile release of luteinizing hormone from the anterior pituitary. Breast feeding, therefore, provides a contraceptive effect, but it is not totally reliable. However, a mother who is still in the phase of postpartum amenorrhoea while *fully* breast feeding her baby has a less than 2 per cent chance of conceiving in the first 6 months (Kennedy et al. 1989). Although this is comparable to some other methods of contraception, it is likely that the mother will use additional contraception, such as a barrier method. If an intrauterine contraceptive device or intrauterine system is preferred, it is usual to wait until about 6 weeks postpartum after vaginal birth, particularly if the mother is breast feeding, and 8 weeks after Caesarean section. The combined oral contraceptive pill increases the risk of thrombosis in the early puerperium but can be started at anytime from 3 weeks after giving birth. It should be avoided by breast feeding mothers as it can have an adverse effect on the quality and constituents of breast milk. Women who are not breast feeding should commence the pill within 4 weeks of the birth as ovulation can occur by 6 weeks postpartum.

The progesterone-only pill is suitable when breast feeding and should be commenced about day 21 following birth, prior to which there may be puerperal breakthrough bleeding. Injectable contraception, such as depot medroxyprogesterone acetate (Depo provera) given 3-monthly is very effective. It is preferable to be given at 6 weeks postpartum, as it can cause heavy or prolonged bleeding in the early puerperium. Sterilization can be offered to mothers who are certain that they have completed their family. Tubal ligation can be performed during Caesarean section or by the open method (mini-laparotomy) in the first few postpartum days. However, it is better delayed until after 6 weeks postpartum, when it can be done by laparoscopy. This allows the mother to spend more time in comfort with her newborn baby and laparoscopic clip sterilization is less traumatic and associated with a lower failure rate.

## Pelvic floor exercises

It is a widespread belief that pelvic floor exercises tone up muscles of the pelvic floor and should be advocated in the postpartum period. Studies to evaluate their benefit in preventing genital prolapse, urinary incontinence or anal incontinence are lacking. There is also no evidence that antenatal exercises prevent incontinence or prolapse. However, as general exercise is known to strengthen striated muscle and pelvic floor exercises are unlikely to be harmful, women are taught postnatal exercise. Pelvic floor awareness is vital, so that women with pelvic floor dysfunction may seek help sooner.

## Perinatal death

Definitions used are as follows:
- *stillbirth*: a baby born after the 24th week of pregnancy that has not breathed or shown any sign of life [Stillbirth (Definition) Act 1992];
- *perinatal death*: stillbirth at or after 24 weeks' gestation or death within 7 days of birth;
- *live birth*: any baby which shows sign of life irrespective of gestation.

The parents and family needed to be cared for empathetically and sensitively throughout this very distressing time. The midwife may be the ideal person to provide emotional support and comfort, information and advice. Effective communication and support are crucial and women should be encouraged to make contact with organizations such as SANDS (Stillbirth and Neonatal Death Society). The grieving process can be facilitated by practices such as seeing and holding the dead baby, naming the baby, and taking hand/foot prints and photographs.

In many hospitals, bereavement counsellors, often a midwife, can provide specialist counselling and support. Support may be required for some time; the mother will need to have her physical well-being monitored and will need much emotional support. Every mother who has lost a baby should have the 6-week postnatal visit at hospital or in an environment most suited to her needs. The midwife must notify her supervisor of midwives in the event of a stillbirth and the supervisor can provide support for the midwife.

The midwife or doctor in attendance or who examines the body after a stillbirth can sign and issue the stillbirth certificate (NMC 2004a). The certificate should be given to the parents to register the death with Registrar of Births and Deaths. The parents can make private funeral arrangements or may prefer the hospital to arrange this.

## The postnatal examination

This is carried out at about 6 weeks postnatal by the general practitioner or the obstetrician, if the birth was complicated. With the flexibility regarding the definition of the postnatal period (NMC 2004a), the midwife may become increasingly involved in the 6-week postnatal examination and discussion with the mother. In doing so, the midwife must ensure that she is practising within her sphere of competence, and that she has the education and skills to extend such care provision.

The examination includes an assessment of the woman's emotional, mental and physical health, and progress of the baby. Direct questions should be asked about urinary, bowel and sexual function. Weight, urine analysis and blood pressure are checked, and a complete general, abdominal and pelvic examination is performed. A cervical smear may be taken, although it is best taken after 3 months postpartum. Advice can be given about sexual activity and pelvic floor exercises are discussed.

### CASE HISTORY

During the antenatal period, Mary, a primigravida, was unsure about how she would feed her baby; her preference appeared to be to bottle feed. As her midwife, you discussed both breast and bottle feeding with Mary. Mary has just had a planned birth at home of a healthy baby at term and she has decided to breast feed.

**What are the main issues you as the midwife should consider as you help Mary to breast feed?**

- Mary's comfort and privacy
- The involvement of Mary's partner
- Encouraging Mary by giving her information and helping her to understand the physiology of lactation and the needs of her baby

- Advising Mary on the advantages of breast feeding for her baby and herself
- Application of the Baby Friendly Initiative ten steps as they apply to Mary (WHO/UNICEF 1991)
- Support and encouragement for Mary, initially during the first feed and ongoing support as she requires it
- Correct positioning of the baby at the breast
- Advising Mary on nutrition and fluid intake, hygiene, rest and sleep
- Identification of Mary's needs regarding breast feeding and planning your postnatal visits to her appropriately
- Information about postnatal and/or breast feeding support groups

### Key Points

- The puerperium refers to the 6-week period following childbirth.
- Midwifery care and support for at least 10 days is crucial as the woman physically returns to her pre-pregnancy state and adjusts to motherhood.

- Support and education for the mother and her partner relating to parenting, feeding and caring for the baby are vital aspects of the midwife's role.
- Disorders include perineal pain, puerperal sepsis, thromboembolism, bowel and bladder dysfunction.

## References and additional reading

Bick D, MacArthur C, Knowles H, Winter H. *Postnatal care: evidence and guidelines for management.* Edinburgh: Churchill Livingstone, 2002.

Grant A, Sleep J. Relief of perineal pain and discomfort after childbirth. In: Chalmers I, Enkin M, Keirse M (eds). *Effective care in pregnancy and childbirth.* Oxford: Oxford Medical, 1989.

Kennedy KI, Rivera R, McNeilly AS. Consensus statement on the use of breast feeding as a family planning method (Bellagio 1988). *Contraception* 1989; **39**:477–96.

Lewis G, Drife J (eds). *Confidential Enquiry into Maternal and Child Health; why mothers die 2000–2002.* Sixth report of the confidential enquiry into maternal deaths in the United Kingdom. London: RCOG Press, 2004.

Nursing and Midwifery Council. *Midwives' rules and standards.* London: NMC, 2004a.

Nursing and Midwifery Council. *Standards of proficiency for pre-registration midwifery education.* London: NMC, 2004b.

World Health Organisation/UNICEF. *Protecting, promoting and supporting breast feeding: the special role of the maternity services.* Geneva: WHO, 1991.

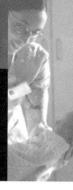

# Mental health in pregnancy and the puerperium

## OVERVIEW

Pregnancy affects mental health in a complex way but equally mental health has an important bearing on the outcome of pregnancy both from the maternal viewpoint as well as the development of the child. During recent years, it has been recognized that mental health is as important as physical health both during pregnancy and in the postpartum period.

## The importance of psychiatry in obstetrics

Pregnancy is one of the greatest risk factors for mental illness in a woman's life and it is thus incumbent on midwives, obstetricians and other health care professionals to be aware of the issues surrounding diagnosis and treatment both during pregnancy and the puerperium.

The impact of mental health problems has been highlighted in successive Confidential Enquiries into Maternal Deaths (1994–1996, 1997–1999 and 2000–2002, Lewis and Drife 2004). Twelve per cent of all direct, indirect and late indirect maternal deaths were the fatal consequence of psychiatric illness, with the majority of these accounted by suicide. These suicides are notably unusually violent (shootings, jumpings, hangings) in contrast with suicide attempts in other younger women, which commonly take the form of overdoses and are frequently less successful.

Recommendations have been made from these Enquiries that management protocols should be in place in every Trust to enable the identification of pregnant women with a history of mental health problems to ensure that care plans are in place to reduce risk during this vulnerable time.

### Antenatal aspects

The antenatal period is a particularly high-risk time for the onset of new psychiatric disease. Epidemiological studies have shown that the incidence/prevalence of psychiatric morbidity is around 10 per cent of all expectant mothers (Golding et al. 2001). Research studies of the effect of stress, from whatever cause, have confirmed a detrimental impact both on the outcome of pregnancy from the maternal viewpoint, and on the development of the fetus. Effects include early onset of labour (Wadhwa et al. 1991, Sandman 1997) increased incidence of pre-eclampsia (Kurki et al. 2000), and intrauterine growth restriction (Feldman et al. 2000) and increased incidence of abnormality (Hansen et al. 2000). It is of importance to recognize this during antenatal consultation and treat the symptoms and underlying cause appropriately. This includes adequate treatment of any mental illness.

Women suffering from longstanding recurrent and enduring mental illness can present a challenge to maternity services. Pregnancy, childbirth and the stresses of life as a new parent may destabilize conditions that had previously been under control. Treatment should not be stopped but certain pharmacological treatments are known to be contraindicated during different phases of pregnancy and suitable alternatives may need to be found. Optimizing the relationship between mother and baby may require specialist intervention.

## Postnatal aspects

In the year following childbirth, women have a greatly increased risk of suffering from a serious mental illness, including a psychotic or a depressive illness, and being referred to a psychiatrist or being admitted to a psychiatric hospital (see box).

### Incidence of postpartum mental disorders

- 15–30 per cent    'Depression'
- 10 per cent    Major depressive illness
- 3–5 per cent    Moderate/severe depressive illness
- 1.7 per cent    Referred to a psychiatrist
- 4/1000    Admitted to a psychiatric unit
- 2/1000    Admitted with puerperal psychosis

While over 80 per cent of women with postpartum psychiatric illness may suffer a milder form of depressive/anxiety disorder that is managed quite effectively in primary care, it is important that this is recognized and treated, especially in view of the detrimental effect this might have on the mother–infant interaction and subsequent infant development.

## The role of the midwife

The responsibility of the midwife is clearly defined in Rule number 6, *Midwives' rules and standards* [Nursing and Midwifery Council (NMC) 2004]. The rule stipulates that:

*where a deviation from the norm which is outside her current sphere of practice becomes apparent in a woman or baby during the antenatal, intranatal or postnatal period, a practising midwife shall call such qualified health professional as may reasonably be expected to have the necessary skills and experience to assist her in the provision of care.*

Historically, midwives have not received mental health training and, in accordance with the rules, both in previous years with the United Kingdom Central Council for Nursing, Midwifery and Health Visiting (UKCC) and, more recently, the NMC (2004), the midwife is entitled to refuse to provide such care to pregnant women. However, the midwife still has a responsibility to ensure that the woman receives the necessary care from an appropriately qualified professional. The pattern has been for the midwife to fulfil her responsibility by referring women with mental health problems to their general practitioners, who might then refer them to their local community mental health team or to their local psychiatric unit. This leads to a patchy, inconsistent and fragmented pattern of care.

### 'Normal' emotional and psychological changes during pregnancy

Diagnosing mental illness in pregnancy may be complicated by the wide variety of 'normal' emotional and behavioural changes that can occur, and it can be difficult to determine when a normal and understandable response to a challenging situation becomes abnormal.

Common antenatal patterns include:
- mixed feelings about being pregnant;
- fears of being unable to cope;
- increased emotional lability;
- minor depressive symptoms (most marked in first trimester);
- anxiety and fears regarding delivery;
- obsessional thoughts regarding the safety of the baby (more common in the third trimester,

particularly in women who have specific pregnancy complications).

Common postnatal patterns include:

- *The 'pinks'.* For the first 24–48 hours following delivery, it is very common for women to experience an elevation of mood, a feeling of excitement, some overactivity and difficulty sleeping.
- *The 'blues'.* As many as 80 per cent of women may experience the 'postnatal blues' in the first 2 weeks after delivery. Fatigue, short-temperedness, difficulty sleeping, depressed mood and tearfulness are common, but are usually mild and resolve spontaneously in the majority of cases.

The following psychological disruptions should not be considered normal during pregnancy and require further assessment:

- panic attacks;
- episodes of low mood of prolonged duration (>2 weeks);
- low self-esteem;
- guilt or hopelessness;
- thoughts of self-harm or suicide;
- any mood changes that disrupt normal social functioning;
- 'biological' symptoms (e.g. poor appetite, early wakening);
- change in 'affect'.

## Management of pregnancy in women with pre-existing psychiatric disease

Women with pre-existing mental health issues should come to the attention of maternity services at booking, but they are sometimes reluctant to admit this. Often women, particularly those with more serious mental health problems, are under the care of a community mental health team but this is not often disclosed. Appropriate screening questions should form part of all routine booking histories and good communication between all health care professionals is paramount. It is essential that optimum treatment for the illness is continued during pregnancy and the knee-jerk response of discontinuing all medication is resisted. These women are at risk of relapse during pregnancy and post delivery, if incorrectly treated. The mental health services should be involved at an early point in the pregnancies of women who have

either ongoing disease or a past history of significant mental illness and to formulate a robust care plan to optimize health care during the pregnancy. This care plan might include the possibility of conjoined admission of the mother and infant to a mother and baby mental health unit. There might also be potential child protection issues and early involvement of the local authority in care planning would be helpful.

## Schizophrenia

Women suffering from schizophrenia still have strong maternal instincts and many do want to have children. Ideally, these women should receive counselling related to their treatment from their psychiatrist prior to conception, but there is often a reluctance to discuss this with their mental health team for fear of censure and a concern that their babies will be removed from their care as a matter of course without proper debate. Instead, these women may discontinue medication secretly, suddenly and abruptly in order to conceive, risking serious relapse during the later stages of pregnancy. While older antipsychotic medications impair fertility, this is not the case with newer drugs, and thus the risk of unplanned pregnancies in this group of women is increased.

There is no evidence that any of the antipsychotic agents have teratogenic effects and this includes the newer atypical agents. As the safety database grows, the newer agents are to be preferred to the older drugs, which have a plethora of side effects, such as anticholinergic effects causing constipation, retention of urine and hesitancy of micturition, which add to the discomfort of pregnancy. After the first trimester, during mid-pregnancy and the period of fetal growth, there is also an increased volume of distribution, which leads to a dilutional effect of any drugs administered. While conventional wisdom supports the concept of administration of the lowest effective dose, given this physiological phenomenum, dosage sometimes needs to be adjusted upwards at this stage in pregnancy to achieve the same therapeutic benefit and to be adjusted down again towards the end of pregnancy. The later stages of pregnancy and the immediate postpartum period are the times of most risk, and it is important that the woman is monitored carefully and frequently during this time so that early warning signs of destabilization are treated promptly and effectively.

Schizophrenia is an illness that causes considerable disruption to lifestyle. Sufferers may lead a chaotic existence and lack a network of social support. This may seriously limit parenting skills. Issues to discuss, as well as the effects of pregnancy and the postpartum period on mental health, include the capacity to be a successful parent in the long term, and there is a significant risk that an affected mother will not ultimately remain the primary carer of her own child. Extra social support and surveillance will usually be necessary but this is often tolerated poorly by the mother suffering from schizophrenia. The local authority responsible for the welfare of the child often institute child protection proceedings. Attitudes between different teams vary: some are helpful and nurturing, facilitating the mother and infant interaction; others are more punitive, confirming the often unspoken fears of the woman even before pregnancy.

Postnatally, the woman and her baby may benefit from an in-patient stay in a specialized mother and baby unit, especially when the risk of relapse and deterioration in mental state is adjudged particularly high, under the review and encouragement of a perinatal mental health team. Breast feeding is to be encouraged to promote bonding with the newborn, unless there is deterioration in mental state, and antipsychotic drugs in moderate doses are not a contraindication to this.

Schizophrenia demonstrates multifactorial inheritance and the offspring of affected parents are at increased risk themselves of developing the condition.

## Bipolar affective disorder

This condition, also known as 'manic depression', is usually controlled with a combination of mood-stabilizing drugs (lithium, carbamazepine and sodium valproate), antidepressants and neuroleptics.

The mood-stabilizing drugs are all recognized teratogens, particularly carbamazepine and sodium valproate, which are associated with a 50 per cent incidence of congenital abnormality. Lithium increases the risk of Ebstein's anomaly, an abnormality of the tricuspid valve of the heart, although recently there has been some debate about the risk in real terms, as the numbers involved are relatively small. If a mother is known to have taken lithium in early pregnancy, a series of specialized ultrasound scans can detect the presence of the defect at an early stage. Used in the third trimester,

lithium has been known to cause fetal hypothyroidism, polyhydramnios and diabetes insipidus.

Management of a woman suffering from bipolar disorder who wishes to become pregnant can be problematic. For this reason, some women do not disclose their illness, preferring instead to stop medication of their own volition, risking a relapse, which may be very harmful. If the illness is stable, then the mood stabilizers may be reduced and replaced by antidepressants and/or neuroleptics depending on whether the pattern of illness is predominantly hypomanic or depressive. Ideally, this is done following pre-pregnancy counselling, when the decision to stop contraception has been made.

Women should be monitored closely during pregnancy and especially after delivery. Postpartum relapse occurs in approximately 50 per cent of women with bipolar illness and it is important that treatment is commenced promptly should the need arise. There is no clear consensus regarding prophylaxis. There is probably the best evidence to support the use of lithium but this is contraindicated in breastfeeding. It may be best to treat with one of the newer antipsychotics and olanzapine has been shown to be very helpful.

## Depression

Depression is the most common of the mood disorders and varies considerably in severity. At least one in ten women will suffer some form of depression throughout their lifetime. There is no evidence that pregnancy reduces the risk of a relapse or improves the mood of women with active depression. Milder forms of this illness are common and it may be difficult for a midwife to assess risk. If a woman has had a past history of depression and has needed care from a community mental health team, or even a hospital admission, this is indicative of a higher degree of risk than if she had merely suffered episodes of tearfulness following a relationship break-up some years previously.

Women may be receiving treatment for depression when they become pregnant. Currently, the automatic response is to stop all medication suddenly and immediately, and while this may be the right way forward, careful risk assessment needs to be undertaken. Depression untreated during pregnancy carries its own hazards and this includes increased incidence of minor congenital abnormality, maternal malnutrition, premature onset of labour, impaired intrauterine growth and babies being born early and small-for-dates. Sufferers also self-medicate with alcohol and cigarettes, agents known to be potentially harmful.

There is now ample experience with the use of antidepressant drugs during pregnancy and women can be reassured that they carry no teratogenic risk. There is still a tendency, especially amongst older practitioners, to recommend the use of tricyclic antidepressant drugs, as they have been around for longer, but they have their own problems regarding their side-effect profile with the wide-range of anticholinergic effects and are toxic in overdose. The situation with SSRIs (selective serotonin reuptake inhibitors) is becoming increasingly clear regarding safety, as more evidence accumulates. No causative association with fetal harm has been demonstrated and their use in younger women is increasing. It is difficult to evaluate reports of increase in preterm labour risk and low birth weight, as this is a known consequence of untreated depressive illness itself.

Dosage of medication during pregnancy needs careful monitoring. The dilution effect due to increased volume of distribution during mid-pregnancy means that dosage may have to be adjusted upwards at this time. Both tricyclic antidepressants and the SSRIs have been associated with a withdrawal syndrome in the neonate. The tricyclic drugs occasionally lead to the emergence of anticholinergic and/extrapyramidal symptoms in the newborn, and SSRIs have been associated with a withdrawal syndrome comprising increased irritability and restlessness. In the case of the SSRIs, the phenomenum is seen more frequently in the drugs with a short half-life, such as paroxetine and venlafaxine. In all instances, the effects are transient, mild and resolve without the need for treatment. There is no evidence of any longer term difficulties. The risk may be minimized by reduction of dosage prior to delivery. In all cases, risks and benefits should be weighed carefully. Untreated depression carries a significant morbidity.

Women with a history of depression not related to pregnancy carry between a one in three and one in five risk of a major postpartum depression. If the previous depressive illness occurred in the postpartum period, the recurrence risk is as high as 50 per cent. At the very least, skilled monitoring should be planned for the postnatal period. Treatment should be given promptly, when needed. There is no evidence that antidepressants given prophylactically are effective.

Antidepressants are safe in breast feeding. Special care should be taken if fluoxetine is chosen. It is known to be excreted into breast milk in measurable amounts. There have been reports that, in the short term, the infant suffers increased colic, restlessness and goes to sleep less readily. There is no evidence of long-term problems. In one follow-up study, infants have been monitored over a 36-month period and there have been no findings of developmental problems, either physically or emotionally.

## Generalized anxiety states

It is important to make a distinction between anxiety and depression, although there is often comorbidity. The treatment for anxiety states has a stronger emphasis on the use of psychological techniques and aid in the reduction of stress levels from whatever cause.

Pregnancy and the anticipation of labour and the arrival of a new baby may exacerbate an existing anxiety disorder. Benzodiazepine use during the first trimester may be associated with an increased risk of cleft lip and/or palate. Benzodiazepines should be avoided in late pregnancy. Neonatal withdrawal effects are evident in the babies. Immediate effects include respiratory depression and hypotonia, and there may be more protracted withdrawal symptoms. Benzodiazepines are excreted into breast milk. It has been reported that, because of this, breast feeding by mothers who continue to take benzodiazepines may help to reduce the severity of the neonatal withdrawal (neonatal abstinence syndrome) but this practice should not be generally encouraged.

## Obsessive compulsive disorder

Women with a history of this condition often suffer exacerbations during pregnancy or the postpartum period. Vulnerability factors include 'perfectionist' personality traits, a certain inflexibility of personality and a liking of routine. Having a baby is neither conducive to the maintenance of routines nor to keeping to high internal standards. There is often more mess for the woman to deal with than previously (babies are not the tidiest of people!), and this is a powerful precipitant in the exacerbation of any relapse.

## Eating disorder

Women with a history of an eating disorder, although recovered at the time they become pregnant, frequently run into difficulty during pregnancy as weight gain and change of body shape is inevitable. It is also recognized that babies born to women with a history of eating disorder are known to be lighter than might be anticipated and a certain number of such women have some difficulties with infant feeding. A syndrome of 'anorexia by proxy' has been reported. The new mother is fearful that her baby will put on too much weight. She makes up feeds that are inadequate in amount and also in content, making up three-quarter or half-strength feeds for fear that full-strength feeds are 'too rich' for her baby. Changes happen insidiously. The infant fails to thrive and gradually falls down the percentile growth charts.

## Personality disorder

It is important to differentiate between mental illness and personality disorder, although this may be difficult for the midwife. Personality disorder is characterized by longstanding dysfunctional patterns of behaviour that are outside accepted social norms, and cause suffering and distress to the persons themselves as well as others. Many types are recognized, but two in particular, dissocial personality disorder and emotionally unstable personality disorder, cause the woman to have difficulties adjusting to pregnancy and the demands of motherhood. These women look for immediate gratification of their needs and have difficulty prioritizing the needs of anyone, let alone a baby above their own. Women with emotionally unstable personality disorder frequently have suffered abusive early-life experiences, have a low tolerance to stress and respond to stressful situations by destructive means, including self-harm. It is important not to label such women as suffering from mental illness (although they may be more vulnerable to a formal psychiatric illness), as personality disorders are difficult to treat, do not respond to medication and only long-term psychotherapy has been shown to be of any benefit.

## Substance misuse

Women who misuse prescribed drugs, alcohol and illicit substances pose a threat to themselves and their babies. This may have arisen as recreational practice or as a form of coping strategy when overcome by life stresses. The habit may be deeply entrenched and may be a practice the woman is reluctant or unable to stop.

Pregnancies are fraught. The newborn often suffers withdrawal symptoms and may require intensive and protracted support in a neonatal intensive care unit. The practice of substance misuse is frequently associated with personality disorder, and chaotic and hazardous lifestyles.

## Domestic violence

Domestic violence may occur for the first time in a relationship when a woman is pregnant. If it already exists within a relationship, it may escalate. The frequency with which this occurs is becoming better known and it is now generally accepted that 1 in 12 women are victims of domestic violence when pregnant. The impact upon the mental health of the woman is complex and domestic violence may coexist with major mental health problems, such as depression, psychosis and substance misuse. Child protection issues may well result from this. The subject should be sensitively approached in the antenatal period.

## Specific syndromes of the puerperium

The postnatal period represents perhaps the highest risk period in a woman's life for the development of a psychiatric disorder. There is debate as to whether these syndromes are diagnostic entities in their own right or whether they are part of a continuum of illness, sometimes with the first episode occurring in the puerperium.

## Puerperal psychosis

This very severe disorder affects between 1 in 500 and 1 in 1000 women after delivery. It rarely presents before the third postpartum day (most commonly the fifth) and usually before 4 weeks. The onset is characteristically abrupt with a rapidly changing clinical picture.

The aetiology of postpartum psychosis is discussed below but remains unclear. Powerful risk factors are recognized, however, and these include the following:

- previous history of puerperal psychosis;
- previous history of bipolar affective disorder;

- previous history of severe non-postpartum depressive illness;
- family history (first/second-degree relative) of bipolar disorder/affective psychosis.

### Characteristic symptoms of puerperal psychosis

- Restless agitation
- Insomnia
- Perplexity
- Confusion
- Fear and suspicion
- Delusions (often involving the baby)
- Hallucinations
- Failure to eat and drink
- Thoughts of self-harm
- Depressive symptoms (guilt, worthlessness, hopelessness)

## Management

The patient should be referred urgently to a psychiatrist and will usually require admission to a psychiatric unit. The mother may be so acutely disturbed that admission under the Mental Heath Act may be necessary. Although it is a recommendation from the Confidential Enquiry into Maternal Deaths that, if admission is deemed necessary, if possible, this should be a mother and baby unit under the supervision of a specialized perinatal mental health care team, it should also be recognized that initially the mother may be too unwell for this to be safe procedure. Conjoined admission should follow as quickly as is safely appropriate once the mother's mental health is stabilized to prevent separation of the baby from its mother, and to facilitate bonding and the future relationship.

Immediate treatments include the following.

- Acute treatment with neuroleptics. The atypical antipsychotics are preferred and olanzapine is the treatment of choice. Chlorpromazine and haloperidol should be avoided unless absolutely necessary because of their side-effect profile.
- Benzodiazepines can be useful in this situation with their tranquilizing effect. It is unlikely that the mother will be able to sustain breast feeding during such an acute illness.

- Acute treatment of mania with lithium carbonate.
- Electroconvulsive therapy, for both a manic and a depressive type of presentation.
- Antidepressants may be indicated in a depressive presentation.

Recovery usually occurs over 4–6 weeks. Treatment will need to be continued for at least 6–12 months. These women remain at high risk of pregnancy-related and non-pregnancy-related recurrences. The risk of recurrence in a future pregnancy is approximately 1:2, particularly if the next pregnancy occurs within 2 years of the one complicated by puerperal psychosis. Women with a previous history of puerperal psychosis should be considered for prophylactic lithium, started on the first postpartum day, but this means that breast feeding should not be attempted.

### Postnatal depression – postpartum (non-psychotic) depression

Depression has already been discussed. There is a similar debate as to whether postnatal depression is an illness in its own right. It is useful term, as it is probably less stigmatizing to be labelled as suffering from postnatal depression (PND) rather than a major depressive disorder and the use of the term heightens awareness of the possibility of mental health problems postpartum. It is a term that includes a heterogeneous group of conditions and it is important that it is not used as a blanket term, as each episode of illness in each person needs to be assessed in its own right. The majority of cases will fulfil diagnostic criteria for a mixed anxiety/depressive disorder and are probably best managed within primary care. It is important to distinguish postpartum depression of any degree from the postpartum 'blues'.

Between 10 and 15 per cent of women will suffer with some form of depression in the first year after the delivery of their baby. At least 7 per cent will satisfy the criteria for mild major depressive illness (see symptoms box). Three–five per cent will suffer a severe major depressive disorder with symptoms of depression that are indistinguishable from depressive illness occurring at any other time. Without treatment, most women will recover from mild episodes spontaneously within 3 to 6 months. One in 10 however will remain depressed at one year.

### Adverse sequelae of postnatal depression

**Immediate**
- Physical morbidity
- Suicide/infanticide
- Prolonged psychiatric morbidity
- Damaged social attachments to infant
- Disrupted emotional development of infant

**Later**
- Social/cognitive effects on the child
- Psychiatric morbidity in the child
- Marital breakdown
- Future mental health problems

### S Symptoms of severe postnatal depression

- Early morning wakening
- Poor appetite
- Diurnal mood variation (worse in the mornings)
- Low energy and libido
- Loss of enjoyment
- Lack of interest
- Impaired concentration
- Tearfulness
- Feelings of guilt and failure
- Anxiety
- Thoughts of self-harm/suicide
- Thoughts of harm to the baby

Risk factors for postnatal depression include:
- past history of psychiatric illness;
- depression during pregnancy;
- obstetric factors (e.g. Caesarean section/fetal or neonatal loss);
- social isolation and deprivation;
- poor relationships;
- recent adverse life events (bereavement/illness);
- severe postnatal 'blues'.

## Clinical features

In contrast to puerperal psychosis, non-psychotic postpartum depression usually presents later in the postnatal period, most commonly around 6 weeks, with a more gradual onset. The 6-week postnatal check is an ideal opportunity to detect early postnatal depression but the signs are often missed. The Edinburgh Postnatal Depression Scale is a screening questionnaire that all women should be asked to perform at their postnatal check. Particular interest should be exercised in the assessment of women with risk factors for postnatal depression. The questionnaire should only be regarded as a screening tool to heighten awareness that the mother might be depressed. Although a score above 12 correlates well with a diagnosis of depressive illness, the questionnaire was never intended as a diagnostic tool and should not supersede clinical assessment. Mothers may have difficulty disclosing any negative feelings to a health visitor in an interview. Equally they may not disclose their true feelings on a sheet of paper.

It is probably helpful to divide depressive illness into two classes depending on severity. Severe postnatal depression may present earlier than milder forms and, in this group, biological risk factors are more important than psychosocial factors. It is this group that is more associated with maternal mortality and which should be referred for formal psychiatric intervention.

## Treatment

Treatment options for mild/moderate postnatal depression of the mixed depressive/anxiety kind include:
- remedy of social factors;
- non-directive counselling;
- cognitive behavioural therapy;
- drug therapy (when the depressive component is more than mild).

Randomized trials, however, have demonstrated the benefits of non-directive counselling from specially trained midwives and health visitors. Even simple encouragement to join a local postnatal group may prevent social isolation and limit the chances of mild postnatal depression.

If pharmacotherapy is deemed necessary, then tricyclic antidepressants or preferably SSRIs are appropriate. There is good evidence to support the safety of both in breast feeding with the reservation that fluoxetine is excreted into breast milk. This has been associated with the emergence of short-term side effects in the baby but there is no evidence for any longer term effect.

There has been a vogue in the past for treating postnatal depression with progestogens in the erroneous belief that the fall in progesterone levels postpartum is the cause of postnatal depression. There is no good evidence to support this and it may even be harmful, if the use of other effective treatments is delayed because of it. This practice should, therefore, be avoided. High-dose oestrogen regimes have been tried in research trials but the evidence regarding their effectiveness remains limited, and they are not used routinely.

## Aetiology

There have always been attempts to try to determine a unitary basis for the onset of puerperal illnesses and, given the temporal relationship to the major life event of childbirth, the temptation to link these illnesses to hormonal factors is understandable. However, this is to ignore the heterogeneous nature of the illnesses described, and the multiplicity of vulnerability factors and stressors operating at this time.

### Pathophysiology of puerperal illnesses

Although psychosocial factors are clearly of importance in the aetiology of milder forms of postnatal depression, this is not so clearly the case for severe postnatal depression nor puerperal psychosis, where biological risk factors, such as family history, predominate. The constancy of incidence across cultures and the temporal relationship with childbirth might suggest a neuroendocrine basis for the more severe conditions. Changes in cortisol, oxytocin, endorphins, thyroxin, progesterone and oestrogen have all been implicated in the causation, and all have been investigated. Comparable dramatic changes in steroidal hormones outside of the postpartum period have a well-known association with affective psychoses and mood disorders.

A plausible recent theory is that the sudden fall in oestrogen postpartum triggers a hypersensitivity of certain dopamine receptors in a predisposed group of women and may be responsible for the severe mood disturbance that follows. The occurrence and the severity of the postnatal blues, therefore, could possibly be related to both the absolute level of progesterone and the relative drop from a pre-partum level.

However, there is no clear association between the postpartum blues and affective psychoses and no evidence as yet to implicate progesterone in the severe conditions. The occurrence and the severity of the postnatal blues are thought to be related to both the absolute level of progesterone and the relative drop from a pre-partum level. However, there is no clear association between the postpartum blues and affective psychoses, and no evidence as yet to implicate progesterone in the aetiology of puerperal psychosis or severe postnatal depression.

## The role of the midwife

Presently, the type of care received is often dependent on the individual midwife and local access to mental health services for childbearing women. Specialist midwives can have a positive impact on resourcing care for women and supporting midwives in practice. Recognized care pathways for women with mental health problems will provide appropriate individualized care.

Antenatal mental health clinics have been of benefit in providing effective care for vulnerable women. A multiagency approach to care is important involving midwives, obstetricians, psychiatrists and nurses specializing in perinatal psychiatry, neonatal nurses, paediatricians, drug workers or substance misuse midwives, social services and hospital child protection teams. Interpreters and local support agencies specializing in mental health are also utilized. Domestic violence support is also important to give advice and a confidential service of referral, if requested.

Training regarding mental health issues during pregnancy for midwives to assist detection and referral is given from a specialist perinatal psychiatry team. Midwives refer women to the specialist midwife who acts in a central role, directing the woman to the appropriate available service. Arrangements can then be made for the woman to be seen and assessed in the mental health clinic, where an appropriate care plan can be formulated. This referral requires the consent of the woman. If there is a reluctance to give consent, the case can be discussed in detail between the midwifery staff and the psychiatric team concerning the level of risk. Even in the absence of consent, the midwife has a professional duty to ensure that any dangers posed to the mother or the newborn are addressed, and steps taken to attempt to reduce the risk. These steps may involve alerting the general practitioner and health visitor and may also require input from child protection services.

## CASE HISTORY

The following two case histories illustrate the various problems that are encountered, the function of the assessment process, the care plan that was formulated and the outcome. The reports are not a complete representation of any one particular woman but a composite of salient features of several women within each of the categories described.

### Case AA

AA is a 40-year-old primigravida who caused concern to her booking midwife because of her unusual demeanour. Although she was living alone and unsupported by any family and was expecting twins, she appeared unduly untroubled and brushed away any discussion about the practicalities of how she would manage two babies. Her mood appeared overbright and she said she was feeing 'on top of the world'. She denied any past psychiatric history, although she did say she had taken some medication from time to time but was 'all right' now.

Her presentation was discussed with the specialist midwife who made arrangements for her to be seen in the mental health liaison clinic by the consultant psychiatrist. Assessment, including tactful questioning, elicited that this lady had a lengthy psychiatric history, that she was currently attending a day centre and that she saw a doctor from time to time. After identifying the day centre and communicating with the consultant psychiatrist who attended and who was her responsible medical officer, a diagnosis of longstanding bipolar affective disorder was confirmed.

As her mental state during the pregnancy was euphoric and elated, advice was given by the consultant perinatal psychiatrist as to the best medication to continue during her pregnancy, and in conjunction with the midwives and her treating psychiatrist, a care plan was formulated to ensure that she remained well during her pregnancy. In view of the high risk of destabilization after delivery, this plan included conjoined admission with her twins after delivery to monitor her mental state to ensure optimum treatment and also to assess her parenting abilities. As it was recognized at this early stage that she would undoubtedly need support in this

latter respect, the local authority were alerted and child protection measures started through a prebirth conference. The local authority was involved throughout the care planning process and were in agreement with the care plan proposed.

In the event, the care plan worked well and she was admitted together with her twins. Her mental state, as predicted, proved somewhat fragile and adjustments to her medication were made quickly and effectively. In spite of this, concerns about her ability to parent her daughters remained and the local authority gave more support and enlisted help from family members.

It is probable that, had this situation not been identified at an early stage during the pregnancy, crises would have arisen to the detriment of mother and children.

### Case BB

BB is a 27-year-old married lady expecting her first child and was identified by her booking midwife as having a past history of depression, sufficiently severe to need treatment with antidepressant medication. Her mood appeared low and flat during the booking procedure. After discussion, an appointment was made for her to be seen in the mental health clinic. During the assessment, it became apparent that her main symptoms related to an anxiety state and this had its origins in her early life experiences. She had been subject to sexual abuse during her childhood and the memories of this were reawakened as she was expecting her own child. Additionally, she expressed a particularly intense fear of handling a newborn baby. She disclosed an incident when she had with some reluctance agreed to bathe her sister's baby and described how, slippery with soap, the baby had slid through her hands. Although the baby had not come to any harm, the memory of this had stayed with her and she had associated it in her mind with her own abusive experiences.

Although her mood appeared somewhat flat, there was no other indication of depressive disorder and it was felt there was no need to continue with antidepressant medication. Instead she was offered psychological therapy in the form of cognitive behavioural therapy to help her manage her anxiety from within her own resources. Having identified her specific fear of handling newborn babies, she was encouraged to engage with the specially trained nursery nurses working in the mother and baby psychiatric unit and, with their help, this fear resolved before her baby was born.

Follow-up continued after delivery. Her mental state remained stable and she enjoyed motherhood. She is contemplating starting longer-term psychotherapy to help her come to terms with her past abuse, probably when her daughter is 1 year old.

This case illustrates the principle that an initial report of depression may not be indicative of a depressive illness, and further and specific enquiry is essential to determine all the factors operational for one particular person. Furthermore, an automatic prescription of antidepressants, while helpful for some, is not a universal panacea. In this particular instance, intervention during the antenatal period led to a reduction of stress levels during the pregnancy and the mother enjoying the company of her daughter when she was born.

## Conclusion

The successive Confidential Enquiries into Maternal Deaths (CEMD) have rightly drawn attention to importance of mental health issues by highlighting the psychiatric causes of maternal mortality. Their strong recommendations have been to establish management protocols for pregnant women with mental health problems. Compliance with these recommendations can achieved through good multidisciplinary working across a number of agencies and an example of good practice may be seen in a mental liaison clinic located within an antenatal department. As well as fulfilling the original remit of the CEMD recommendations, the joint working between midwifery and mental health professionals has resulted in a generally higher level of care given to each pregnant woman in a more holistic way.

## 🔑 Key Points

- Midwives should ask all women at booking about previous psychiatric history – personal or family.
- Close collaboration is recommended between midwives, obstetricians and psychiatrists for women with mental illness, a previous history of severe mental ill-health, or a strong family history of bipolar affective disorder.
- Recognized care pathways with close multiagency working can ensure the provision of appropriate individualized care and reduce the risk to mental health morbidity.
- Women with previous serious mental illness should be appropriately counselled regarding the recurrence risks associated with pregnancy.
- Prescribing of psychoactive drugs in pregnancy and breast feeding should be done with care under the guidance of a psychiatrist with a particular interest in pregnancy-related mental illness.
- Specialist perinatal psychiatric services should be available to all women.

## References

Feldman PJ, Dunkel-Schetter C, Sandman CA, Wadhwa PD. Maternal social support predicts birthweight and fetal growth in human pregnancy. *Psychosomatic Medicine* 2000; **62**:715–25.

Golding J, Pembrey M, Jones R, et al. ALPSAC – The Avon longitudinal study of parents and children. *Paediatric and Perinatal Epidemiology* 2001; **15**:74–87.

Hansen D, Lou HC, Olsen J. Serious life events and congenital malformations: a national study with complete follow-up. *Lancet* 2000; **356**:875–80.

Kurki T, Hilesmaa V, Raitasalo R. Depression and anxiety in early pregnancy and risk for pre eclampsia. *Journal of Obstetrics and Gynaecology* 2000; **92**:487–90.

Lewis G, Drife J (eds). *Confidential Enquiry into Maternal and Child Health; why mothers die 2000–2002*. Sixth report of the confidential enquiry into maternal deaths in the United Kingdom. London: RCOG Press, 2004.

Nursing and Midwifery Council. *Midwives' rules and standards*. London: NMC, 2004.

Sandman CA, Wadhwa P, Chicz-Demet C, et al. Maternal stress, HPA activity and fetal/infant outcome. *Annals of the New York Academy of Science* 1997; **814**:266–75.

Wadhwa P, Culhane JF, Rauh V, et al. Stress, infection and pre-term birth: a behavioural perspective. *Paediatric and Perinatal Epidemiology Supplement* 2001; **15**(Suppl 2): 17–29.

## Key additional reading

Crandon AJ. Maternal anxiety and neonatal well being. *Journal of Psychosomatic Research* 2002; **23**:113–15.

Mulder EJH, Robles de Medina PG, Van den Burgh J. Prenatal maternal stress: effects on pregnancy and the (unborn) child. *Early Human Development* 2002; **70**(1–2):3–14.

Scottish Intercollegiate Guidelines Network. *Postnatal depression and puerperal psychosis.* Publication no. 60. Edinburgh: Scottish Intercollegiate Guidelines Network, 2002 (www.sign.ac.uk).

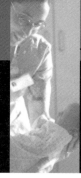

# Neonatal care

## OVERVIEW

More than half a million babies are born every year in the UK and over 200 million are born worldwide. In industrialized countries, the majority of babies are born normally at term, healthy, cared for by their parents, and grow and develop without complications. A small proportion of babies will be born preterm and/or will suffer complications, and a very small proportion of the babies will die. The earlier the gestation the baby is born, the lower the birth weight and the sicker the baby is, the higher the mortality. Sophisticated, highly technical neonatal units are available to provide the skilled nursing and medical care to any baby who is preterm or sick. In less developed countries, maternal health is poorer generally and in pregnancy, there are fewer facilities to care for preterm and sick babies, and the mortality rate is very much higher than in industrialized countries. However, the reasons babies die are similar regardless of where they are born, with preterm birth and its consequences, infections, congenital malformations, and hypoxia or trauma acquired intrapartum being the most common. The midwife has an important role in the prenatal period, along with obstetricians, to try to prevent such complications. In the postnatal period, the midwife has a continuing role in trying to prevent complications but also in working in partnership with parents to give appropriate care to meet the needs of the baby. If any other complications occur, the midwife must quickly detect them, refer to the neonatologist or family doctor, and assist in the investigation and treatment, including caring for the dying baby and supporting the family.

## Neonatal care by the midwife

Midwives in the UK are responsible for overseeing the care of the healthy term baby and his mother principally in the first 10 days of life, but this can extend to the full neonatal period in hospital and in the community. However, some midwives have specialized in neonatal care as part of their role and, along with nurses, have developed the specialty of neonatal nursing. Working mainly in hospital-based neonatal units with other health care professionals, neonatal nurses provide highly specialized care for preterm and sick babies from birth to discharge, which usually extends longer than the neonatal period. If required, many neonatal services offer continuing care after the baby has gone home until care is transferred to the paediatric services.

## Organization of neonatal care and provision of services

The care of neonates in the UK is organized around guidelines produced by the British Association of

Perinatal Medicine (BAPM) (2001). Healthy term babies require normal care, usually given by their mother in the postnatal ward and at home. About 10 per cent of all babies born in the UK require admission to a neonatal unit, with a wide range between hospitals of 4 to 35 per cent. Most of these admissions are for special care, while about 2 per cent of babies need full intensive care. Examples of what is defined as special care, high-dependency care and intensive care (BAPM 2001) are given (see box).

---

## Categories of babies requiring neonatal care (BAPM 2001)

### Level 1 intensive care (maximal intensive care)
Care given in an intensive care nursery that provides continuous supervision by a suitably trained nurse, ideally 1:1, with immediate medical aid available.

Examples of babies who need intensive care are those:
- receiving any respiratory support via a tracheal tube
- who are <29 weeks' gestation and <48 hours old

### Level 2 intensive care (high-dependency intensive care)
Care given in an intensive care nursery that provides care by specially trained nursing staff, who may care for two babies at a time.

Examples of babies who need level 2 intensive care are those:
- requiring parenteral nutrition
- having convulsions
- having frequent apnoeic attacks
- requiring oxygen treatment and weighing <1500 g

### Special care
Care given in a special care nursery that provides care and treatment exceeding normal routine care. Nurses may care for four babies at a time. Some aspects of special care may be undertaken by a mother supervised by qualified nursing staff.

Examples of babies who need special care are those:
- being tube fed
- undergoing phototherapy
- receiving special monitoring (e.g. frequent glucose or bilirubin estimations)

---

Neonatal units vary with some offering only special care, some special care and high-dependency care, some just intensive care and others all three levels of care. Neonatal surgery is usually provided in separate units. Units can be known by a variety of titles, such as special care baby unit or intensive care unit. The term neonatal unit (NNU) is used in this chapter to include all types of unit.

Many health care professionals are involved in neonatal care apart from midwives, such as doctors, neonatal nurses, physiotherapists, pharmacists, dieticians and occupational therapists. They have specific yet complementary roles as part of a neonatal team.

## Principles of neonatal care

The needs of all babies are very similar but the level of care varies. In this chapter, an overview is given of the midwife's role in the care of the healthy term baby. Part of that role is to be alert for deviations, to work with doctors to investigate and treat complications, and to recognize when high dependency or intensive care is required.

Midwives have a responsibility to ensure that the mother is fully able to provide normal care for her baby (BAPM 2001). However, if the baby is admitted to the NNU, the neonatal team will provide much of the care, but will involve the parents in decision-making and the delivery of as much care as the parents feel they want to give.

Midwives should understand the definitions that apply to the categorization of all babies. These include the following:
- term, preterm, post-term/postmature;
- low birth weight, very low birth weight, extremely low birth weight;
- appropriate for gestational age, small for gestational age, large for gestational age, intrauterine growth restriction.

The midwife has a responsibility to examine the baby from top to toe in the first hours after birth to establish weight, length, head circumference, vital signs, and to exclude or identify external congenital abnormalities. If any deviations from normal are identified, the midwife must give any emergency care, refer to a doctor, give basic information to the parents and provide care to meet the baby's needs. Further involvement in care depends on the extent and nature of the deviation.

In the UK, all babies are routinely examined by a doctor or other suitably qualified practitioner within the first 7 days of life (Baston and Durward 2001), who may be a midwife with an additional qualification in examination of the newborn. The purposes of the examination are:

- diagnosis of congenital malformations;
- diagnosis of common minor problems, with advice about management or appropriate reassurance, if no intervention is indicated (e.g. Mongolian blue spots, naevi);
- continuing screening, which began antenatally, to identify those babies who should be offered specific intervention (e.g. hepatitis vaccination);
- health education advice (e.g. regarding breast feeding, cot death prevention, immunization, safe transport in cars);
- general parental reassurance

The midwife must have a working knowledge of the most common congenital abnormalities that can be diagnosed *in utero*, those that are obvious at birth, those that are incompatible with life, those that require immediate midwifery interventions to sustain life, those that present in the first weeks of life, the signs exhibited and their management. For many abnormalities, the sooner the treatment is instituted, the better the outcome for the baby and parents. The midwife should also be aware of the common minor problems, their presentation and treatment, so that she can augment any discussion between the doctor and the parents, if required.

Any model of neonatal care is likely to address the baby's physical and social/emotional needs, and the parents' educational needs.

Physical needs include the following:

- airway and respiratory;
- temperature regulation;
- cardiovascular and haematological;
- nutrition and elimination;
- infection, skin care and hygiene;
- neurological and pain;
- sleep, rest and self-regulation.

These also include care of the dying baby and his family.

Social/emotional needs include developing positive interaction with parents. The parents' educational needs will vary depending on their parenting experience, but may include learning how to care for the baby's physical needs and learning how to nurture the baby.

## Physical needs

### Airway and respiratory

The vast majority of babies achieve a smooth transition from intrauterine to extrauterine life, making their first respiratory efforts within 10 seconds of birth. Fetal lungs are filled with 'lung liquid', a fluid that is important for normal lung development and growth. During labour, production of lung liquid ceases and reabsorption begins. Lung liquid is squeezed out during normal birth. When the baby takes his first gasp and then establishes and sustains respirations, the remaining lung liquid is gradually absorbed by the lymphatics and the pulmonary capillaries. At the same time as the airways fill with air, the pulmonary vascular resistance begins to fall and blood supply to the alveoli increases dramatically. Gas exchange between alveoli and capillaries occurs and the increased arterial oxygen tension sustains the transition to extrauterine life in the respiratory system but also stimulates necessary adaptations in the cardiovascular system.

Normal care of the baby who establishes spontaneous respirations at birth is to dry him immediately to prevent heat loss, facilitate skin-to-skin contact with his mother and cover him with warm blankets. If the mother prefers, the baby can be dried, wrapped in warm blankets and given to her to cuddle in her arms. The father can also be offered his baby to hold, especially if the mother is unable to do so. The midwife should continue to monitor the baby's condition to ensure that these initial adaptations are sustained.

Babies who fail to breathe after birth may do so as a result of deprivation of oxygen and blood supply to the brain before birth, or because they are unable to make respiratory movements at birth due to extreme preterm birth, a central nervous system or muscle disease, or because they are systemically ill with infection, with resultant increasing hypoxaemia/hypoxia. The responses to hypoxia/anoxia are illustrated in Figure 19.1.

Most babies who fail to breathe spontaneously at birth will respond to basic resuscitation; therefore, all professionals who attend births must be able to recognize when a baby is not establishing normal extrauterine respirations and circulation, and be able to initiate resuscitation. Certain situations are clearly high risk

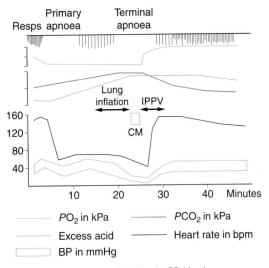

**Figure 19.1** The response to asphyxia. BP, blood pressure; bpm, beats per minute; CM, cardiac massage; IPPV, intermittent positive pressure ventilation. (Reproduced with permission from the Northern Region handbook.)

---

### Situations in which advanced resuscitation skills may be required

- Preterm deliveries
- Vaginal breech deliveries
- Thick meconium staining of the amniotic fluid
- Significant fetal distress
- Significant antepartum haemorrhage
- Serious fetal abnormality (e.g. hydrops, diaphragmatic hernia)
- Rotational forceps or vacuum deliveries
- Caesarean section – unless elective and under regional anaesthesia
- Multiple deliveries

---

and, in these cases, a person with advanced resuscitation skills should be present at the birth (see box).

However, about 20–30 per cent of babies who require resuscitation do not fall into high-risk categories. The inability to predict which babies will fail to make a successful transition to extrauterine life is the reason why all those who attend births have a responsibility to maintain their neonatal resuscitation skills. As in many countries, in the UK, standardized resuscitation courses and updates are available. The Resuscitation Council-UK (2005) web site is a valuable resource and the current guidelines also include an excellent algorithm for resuscitation.

## The Apgar score

The Apgar score is a tool that was designed to help identify a baby who is making a successful transition to extrauterine life or not (Table 19.1). A normal score is between 7 and 10. The reason for a low Apgar score (less than 7) may not be asphyxia, but the baby certainly has a problem and the sooner it is recognized and treated the better. The item 'grimace' reports the baby's response and originally this was a response to a suction catheter. Suction catheters are rarely required in neonatal resuscitation and inappropriate, poorly performed or frequent deep suction of the oropharynx can cause bradycardia; therefore, this item is no longer assessed as a response to a suction catheter. The baby may respond to other acceptable forms of tactile stimulation or intervention and a score given.

The Apgar score is usually awarded at 1 and 5 minutes. If the Apgar score is still low at 5 minutes, further observations should be made at intervals. Recording the Apgar score is helpful because it has become an internationally recognized shorthand way of summarizing a baby's condition at birth. However, resuscitative efforts should not be delayed by any necessity to calculate an Apgar score and the Apgar score can never replace the required detailed narrative describing the baby's condition, the resuscitative efforts and the response to resuscitation.

## Resuscitation

If the baby is healthy, no active resuscitation is required and care is given as above. However, babies who require resuscitation at birth usually fall into one of the two following categories within a minute of birth.

1. Not breathing/not breathing adequately, but with a heart rate of more than 100 beats per minute (bpm) and centrally cyanosed. The baby should be dried and placed under a radiant heat source wrapped in a warm dry towel. Drying often provides enough stimulation to induce adequate breathing. More vigorous tactile stimulation is unhelpful. If there is no response, begin active resuscitation using five 'inflation breaths' via a self-inflating bag, valve and mask apparatus or a T-piece resuscitation system. If inflation is successful, the chest wall will rise and fall in time with inflations by the fourth of fifth inflation breath. Regular breaths of 30–40 per minute should continue until the baby makes spontaneous breaths. Help should be called in case the baby does not respond.

**Table 19.1** – The Apgar score

| | | Score | | |
|---|---|---|---|---|
| | | 0 | 1 | 2 |
| A | Appearance: central trunk colour | White or blue all over | Pink with blue extremities | Pink all over |
| P | Pulse rate[a] | Absent | <100 bpm | >100 bpm |
| G | Grimace (response to stimulation) | Nil | Grimace | Cry or cough |
| A | Activity | Limp | Some flexion | Well flexed, active movement |
| R | Respiratory effort | Absent | Gasping or irregular | Regular or strong cry |

[a]Best to record the actual rate.
bpm, beats per minute.

2. Not breathing, or with a heart rate of less than 100 bpm or is pale. This baby is usually completely floppy. Prompt resuscitation is required and the baby will not recover without it. Dry him quickly, place him on the resuscitation surface in a warm dry blanket and call for help. Initiate basic resuscitation as above. If the heart rate remains less than 60 bpm, commence chest compressions. If the response is not rapid, proceed to intubation as soon as a person with the necessary skill arrives. Very occasionally, drugs may be required to augment ventilation and compressions.

While time is of the essence in neonatal resuscitation, this is no excuse for rough handling or sloppy thermal care. The parents will be extremely anxious and every action or verbal utterance is likely to be imprinted on the parents' memory. Therefore, team members must always act in a professional manner, be mindful of the parents' presence, and one member should take time to talk to them as soon as possible to inform them of treatment and progress.

It is essential that the knowledge and skills of the midwife in relation to resuscitation are up to date. Some may have undertaken additional education to become an advanced resuscitator. Midwives must ensure that the resuscitation equipment is readily available, in good working order and is restocked after any resuscitation event. They must be able to assess the needs of the baby for resuscitation and intervene appropriately to initiate basic resuscitation, obtain help as necessary, assist with advanced resuscitation, ensure care of the baby after resuscitation and ensure care of the parents throughout.

It is important that the midwife can recognize specific problems that alter the usual resuscitation process. Two of the more common problems are extreme preterm birth and meconium aspiration.

### Extreme preterm birth

For babies born before 34 weeks' gestation, there is an increased risk of respiratory distress syndrome/surfactant deficiency disease (RDS/SDD). Current BAPM (1998) best practice guidelines recommend that, in threatened preterm birth before 34 weeks, the mother is given steroid injections to stimulate the fetal lungs to mature, particularly maturation of surfactant. Evidence suggests that, should the baby subsequently be born preterm, the severity of RDS/SDD will be less than expected for his gestation. As an adjunct to prenatal steroids, it is recommended that prophylactic surfactant replacement therapy is given before the baby takes a breath. Therefore, as soon as the baby is born, he is wrapped in warm towels, brought to the resuscitation area, placed under a radiant warmer and has his vocal cords visualized using a laryngoscope. The surfactant is then instilled into the trachea and the baby is given assisted ventilation via bag, valve and mask/ tube, or T-piece apparatus to distribute the surfactant through the airways.

Another factor that severely compromises extremely preterm babies is the heat loss they endure during the resuscitative efforts, resulting in hypothermia that increases the risks of morbidity and mortality. Recently, these vulnerable babies have been born and immediately put feet first in a plastic bag/polyethylene bag to their neck while still wet. They are placed under a radiant warmer and the head is dried and covered with a hat. The baby remains in the bag until transfer to a humidified incubator in the NNU. The bag is then removed and the baby thoroughly dried and then covered/clothed as much as his condition will allow. The evidence indicates that these babies maintain a body temperature within the normal range.

## Meconium aspiration

The meconium expelled by term and post-term fetuses in response to intrauterine/intrapartum hypoxia can result in inhalation of meconium into the airways. If the baby cries/breathes spontaneously when born, is active, has a heart rate of more than 100 bpm, no active resuscitation is required, and the baby receives normal care. However, if the baby is severely asphyxiated with no respiratory movements, floppy tone, little response, pale or cyanosed and a heart rate of less than 100 bpm, advanced resuscitation is required but with the following caveats.

When the baby is born, he is gently wrapped in warm towels and taken to the resuscitation area. An advanced resuscitator should visualize the vocal cords using a laryngoscope. Using a large-bore suction catheter, any meconium is then aspirated from above the cords, the catheter is renewed and meconium is aspirated from below the cords. The baby is then quickly dried and rewrapped in warm blankets, and resuscitation proceeds as usual, depending on the baby's needs. This baby will require intensive care in the NNU.

In the past, babies born through meconium were suctioned more often and more vigorously. However, evidence suggests that suctioning the mouth and nose when they appear at the perineum during birth, and subsequent deep suctioning of the oropharynx are not helpful, and may cause more meconium to be aspirated. Trying to stop the baby breathing by splinting the chest wall, saline lavage and repeated blind suctioning are also now outlawed.

However, if the person present at the birth of a severely asphyxiated baby born through meconium does not have advanced resuscitation skills and immediate assistance by an advanced resuscitator is not available, after birth the mouth and nose should be gently suctioned to clear any obvious meconium and basic resuscitation begun. The consequences of meconium in the airways are serious, but the consequences of permanent brain damage due to prolonged hypoxia are potentially worse.

## Failure to respond to resuscitation

Most babies who are respiratorily depressed at birth respond readily to resuscitative efforts; however, very occasionally, a baby will not respond. If advanced resuscitation including drug administration has been ineffective, consideration has to be given to other conditions that can influence response to resuscitation. A pneumothorax should be excluded or given emergency treatment, if diagnosed. If the baby looks pale, the possibility of a massive fetomaternal haemorrhage, blood loss at delivery or a failure of an adequate placental transfusion owing to extreme cord compression must be considered and the baby should be given O-negative blood (not cross-matched) immediately via an umbilical venous catheter.

However, if there is no cardiac output after about 20 minutes of adequate cardiopulmonary resuscitation, the prognosis for intact survival is very poor, and the most senior person present should consider discontinuing resuscitation in consultation with the neonatal team and possibly the parents, if they are available.

## Ethical issues surrounding resuscitation

This is an area that generates a great deal of anxiety. A doctor or midwife suddenly faced with a very preterm or abnormal baby is insufficiently experienced to make a value judgement about resuscitation. Ideally, this situation should be avoided by prior warning, so that a discussion can be held between the most senior paediatrician available, a senior obstetrician and the parents. If the parents, after being informed of the chances of intact survival, do not wish active resuscitation of their baby who will be born at 23 or 24 weeks' gestation, or of a severely malformed baby, most neonatologists would support their decision and offer 'comfort care' only. Experience teaches that is wise to warn the parents beforehand that sometimes there is a surprise and the baby is bigger and more mature than expected, in which case it may be appropriate to offer intensive care on a 'wait and see' approach.

If there is not time to consult with the parents beforehand, or there is any conflict or doubt, then full resuscitation should be offered (Mifflin 2003). Most tiny babies who die do so very quickly, within 24 hours, and a period of intensive care allows time for the parents to take in the situation and to grieve afterwards because they are certain that 'everything has been done'. This course of action avoids the possibility of anger developing because of doubt about viability remaining in the parent's minds.

### Care after resuscitation

Effective resuscitation does not necessarily mean the baby is pink and crying lustily. Some babies will be and the parents should be informed of the situation and that the baby will be monitored carefully over the subsequent days to ensure there are no further problems. The baby will then be transferred with the mother to the postnatal ward.

### Postnatal respiratory problems

In the postnatal ward and at home, midwives assess babies' respiratory efforts during the daily baby examination they conduct. If there are no complications, the baby will be discharged as healthy. If complications develop, the baby will require investigation and specific care, usually requiring transfer to the NNU.

For the babies who have complex resuscitation and those who develop complications, NNU admission will be required for observation, further investigation and treatment. Babies who are admitted immediately after birth should be stabilized and then transferred in a transport incubator to the NNU.

The baby's respiratory needs are further assessed. Negative signs indicating respiratory distress include a rate of more than 60 breaths per minute, increased inspiratory effort (nasal flaring and intercostal or sternal recession/indrawing), poor colour (pale, dusky, grey, cyanosed) and expiratory grunting. Newborns usually have irregular/periodic breathing except when they are in a deep sleep.

If respiratory distress is diagnosed, the baby should be transferred to a NNU for further assessments that would include blood gas analysis, monitoring arterial oxygen saturation and possibly a chest X-ray. Depending on the diagnosis, respiratory support would be given and might include the following:

- supplemental oxygen administration;
- continuous positive airways pressure, usually via nasal prongs/catheters;
- positive pressure mechanical ventilation;
- respiratory stimulants, such as caffeine citrate;
- antibiotics;

- chest physiotherapy and suction of secretions;
- inspired nitric oxide.

There are numerous respiratory conditions that can affect the baby, such as respiratory distress syndrome, meconium aspiration syndrome, transient tachypnoea of the newborn, apnoea of prematurity and pneumonia.

## Temperature regulation

The normal core body temperature is considered to be 36.7–37.2°C, with variations of no more than 1°C to the periphery. Continuous temperature readings from skin probes are used with babies requiring intensive care; otherwise the temperature is measured intermittently under the axilla with an electronic infrared device that may be unreliable. Mothers can choose from a variety of non-invasive techniques to measure temperature in the home situation. Mercury thermometers and rectal temperature measurements are no longer considered safe.

Babies are at risk for disruptions of temperature regulation because they cannot compensate for the heat they lose. A baby cannot generate heat via voluntary or involuntary muscle movement; therefore, the main generation of heat is via non-shivering thermogenesis, the burning of brown fat deposits.

Heat loss from the body core to the periphery is usually impeded by subcutaneous fat insulation and by vasoconstriction. Babies, especially preterm babies and those that are small for gestational age, have little subcutaneous fat, so heat loss is increased.

Heat loss from the skin surface to the environment is by conduction, convection, radiation and evaporation. The baby is predisposed to lose heat easily via all these mechanisms. Therefore, it is essential that the midwife understands the mechanism for heat loss via these routes and takes steps to prevent or reduce such loss. Caring for the baby on warm surfaces, avoiding draughts, positioning cots away from windows and outside walls, drying babies after birth, not bathing babies, using humidification in incubators and to deliver respiratory gases, changing wet nappies, and dressing the baby are all important strategies. If the baby does become hypothermic, measures to reverse the condition must be implemented immediately to prevent further heat loss and deterioration of the baby's overall condition.

Babies are prone to hyperthermia owing to their inability to sweat. The main cause is usually a high environmental temperature, so prevention is possible. However, if the baby does develop hyperthermia, adjusting the environmental temperature should be carefully undertaken so that the baby's temperature returns to within normal limits.

## Cardiovascular and haematological

The changes that occur in the respiratory system at birth are the primary stimulus for the transition from a fetal circulation pattern to an adult one. The loss of the placental flow that occurs when the vessels in the umbilical cord constrict and/or when the cord is clamped and cut is a secondary, although important, stimulus, as the lack of flow through the umbilical vein, ductus venosus and the hypogastric arteries results in their closure. The reversal of pressure relationships in the pulmonary artery and the aorta increases the flow of blood to the lungs, increases the volume returning to the left atrium, forces the foramen ovale flap to close, and thus halts the flow across this temporary structure from the right atrium. The flow of blood through the ductus arteriosus also reverses, allowing blood to leave the aorta and shunt into the pulmonary artery, thus exposing the ductal cells to increased oxygen tensions. This stimulates constriction of the ductus arteriosus, and stops all shunting between the right and left sides of the circulation. The transition to the adult circulation pattern should persist if the baby establishes normal respirations.

### Vitamin K deficiency bleeding
Previously known as haemorrhagic disease of the newborn, vitamin K deficiency bleeding (VKDB) occurs in three forms as follows.
1. *Very early VKDB* is limited to babies whose mothers have taken drugs that interfere with the manufacture of vitamin K-dependent clotting factors, such as antituberculous or anticonvulsant drugs. These mothers should be given extra vitamin K (5 mg daily) in the last month of pregnancy and the babies must be given intramuscular vitamin K (1 mg) prophylaxis.
2. *Classical VKDB* presents on days 2–7 of life, with bleeding from the umbilical stump, bruising or melaena. The mortality of classical VKDB is low and the disorder can be prevented by a single dose of vitamin K given to the baby by any route.

3. *Late VKDB* occurs virtually exclusively in babies who are breast fed, unless they have liver disease. Small warning bleeds from the gums are a common feature but the worst problems are associated with the high (50 per cent) chance of intracranial haemorrhage that can cause permanent neurological handicap. It can be prevented by a single intramuscular dose of vitamin K (1 mg) given at birth but a single oral dose is ineffective. For healthy babies of 36 weeks' gestation and older a single dose of intramuscular (IM) vitamin K (1 mg) shortly after birth should be given. Alternatively, oral doses of vitamin K (2 mg) should be given on the first day and between days 4–7. If the baby is exclusively breast fed, he should receive a further 2 mg dose at one month and monthly doses thereafter until solid food and/or formula feeding is introduced. Term babies who are at special risk and babies of less than 36 weeks' gestation should receive intravenous or IM vitamin K shortly after birth, but the dose vaires depending on their weight. Local guidelines should be consulted.

Any abnormal bleeding must be investigated. Confirmation of the diagnosis of VKDB is obtained from coagulation tests, which show a normal platelet count and prolonged thrombin and prothrombin times. Treatment is with intravenous vitamin K and fresh-frozen plasma.

## Fluids, nutrition and elimination

The gastrointestinal (GI) tract of the term baby is developed sufficiently to enable breast feeding. The younger the gestation of the baby and the sicker he is, the less able he is to suck feeds, or digest or absorb them.

The method chosen by the mother to feed her baby should be respected by all concerned and she should be supported in her efforts to feed her baby. However, the benefits of breast milk for all babies, especially preterm and sick babies are well known and, if the baby requires NNU care, the mother may express breast milk, even if she chooses to feed her baby using milk formula by bottle.

All babies should have some fluids and nutrition within the first hour of life, whether enteral or parenteral. Healthy term babies will gradually develop a variable demand feeding pattern. Regardless of the method of feeding chosen, mothers usually require supervision and support to ensure their technique is correct.

To assist the mother and to ensure accurate information is given, the midwife must understand the physiology of the breast and the process of lactation and milk ejection, how these can differ if the baby is born preterm, the options for comfortable positions for breast feeding, the position of the baby at the breast, attachment/latching, the usual feeding behaviour during the feed and how the baby usually finishes a feed. Much of this understanding can also be used if the mother is expressing breast milk, but the midwife should also understand the methods of hand expression, use of mechanical pumps, breast stimulation and massage, collection, storage and use of expressed milk in order to help the mother express milk efficiently (Lang 2002).

Breast feeding should not be painful and, if pain is experienced, the midwife should explore with the mother the possible reasons. Damaged nipples, engorgement, blocked ducts, mastitis and breast abscess are examples of problems that may occur. Most are a result of poor breast feeding technique and, if this is corrected, many of the problems will resolve. Symptomatic relief, antibiotics and aspiration of an abscess may be required, depending on the diagnosis, and the midwife must ensure that the required treatment is prescribed.

There are many lay and official groups worldwide to promote breast feeding. This is especially important in developing countries, where access to clean water is limited and GI infections are life threatening. However, in industrialized countries, many women who are breast feeding rely on the support and encouragement given by these groups to sustain breast feeding.

If the mother chooses to bottle feed her baby, she should have information, supervision and support from the midwife about the following: techniques; the formulae available; suitable sources of water; preparing, storing and using feeds; feeding equipment, and its cleaning and sterilization.

Usually, calculation of fluid and calorie requirements is unnecessary in healthy term babies, especially for those who are breast feeding. The assessment of whether the baby is receiving sufficient for his needs is estimated by how well he tolerates the volume, how often he feeds, whether his urine and faecal outputs are normal, if he settles to sleep after a feed and wakes for the next feed.

However, in some industrialized countries, where breast feeding support is less than ideal, some babies are failing to feed efficiently or effectively, and are developing severe dehydration, usually complicated by hypernatraemia, requiring NNU intensive care. This potentially fatal condition is easily prevented if breast feeding mothers can ensure the baby is correctly positioned, correctly attached and feeds using the correct technique. However, she needs to learn these skills, and it is the midwife's responsibility to teach and supervise these (p. 281).

If the baby is preterm or sick, fluid and calorie requirements will be calculated, and guidelines are available to ensure the baby receives sufficient for his needs. This usually involves working up to an intake of 150–175 mL/kg per 24 hours by 5–7 days of life. These babies are unlikely to be able to breast or bottle feed. The alternatives are parental nutrition using dextrose solutions followed by inclusion of an amino-acid solution and lipid emulsion, delivered as total parenteral nutrition. As soon as possible, babies receive milk into their GI tract. If the baby is very preterm, nutritive milk volumes would exceed tolerance; therefore, a non-nutritive regime is commenced. This involves administering a small unchanging volume of preferably breast milk at regular intervals via a gastric tube. Such minimal enteral feeding/trophic feeding/gut priming is not expected to nourish or contribute to the baby's fluid requirements, but does help stimulate further development and colonization. It has also been shown to improve tolerance of nutritional feeds once they commence.

Babies unable to feed by mouth usually receive enteral nutrition by nasogastric or orogastric tube. Feeds are usually given intermittently by bolus or by gravity. Continuous feeds are less often used because of the complications that can occur with the equipment, contamination of the milk and in the baby.

### Hypoglycaemia

Healthy term babies of appropriate weight who are breast fed have lower blood glucose concentrations than those of formula-fed babies in the first 2–3 days of life. They also have raised ketone body concentrations and the neonatal brain can use ketone bodies as an alternative fuel. Healthy, normally grown term babies who are breast feeding well do not need to have their blood glucose concentrations measured for screening purposes. There is no agreement on the lower limit of the normal range in this situation; bedside testing with reagent strips is notoriously inaccurate and there is no evidence that a lower limit exists below which asymptomatic 'hypoglycaemia' is damaging. Recognition of these facts makes the use of supplementary feeding less likely and encourages breast feeding (Rennie and Roberton 2002). However, there are undoubtedly babies who are at high risk of developing symptomatic hypoglycaemia and for whom screening is appropriate (see box).

---

### Babies at risk of developing symptomatic hypoglycaemia

- Babies with intrauterine growth restriction
- Babies of diabetic mothers
- Preterm babies
- Babies who have suffered fetal distress in labour
- Babies who are 'large for dates' – possibility of undiagnosed maternal gestational diabetes

---

Babies who are at the highest risk are those whose growth has been restricted *in utero* and those born to diabetic mothers. Occasionally an apparently healthy term baby has a rare condition, such as idiopathic hyperinsulinaemic hypoglycaemia of infancy (formerly called neisidioblastosis), which will manifest as symptomatic hypoglycaemia in the first days of life. Very rarely, a healthy baby becomes hypoglycaemic from breast milk insufficiency. In these situations, prolonged symptomatic hypoglycaemia can occur and this can be brain damaging. A balance needs to be struck between screening for and prevention of symptomatic hypoglycaemia in at-risk babies, with recognition of symptomatic hypoglycaemia in babies who are ill, whilst avoiding overinvestigation and overtreatment in the normal term baby whose mother is trying to establish breast feeding.

Signs of hypoglycaemia in the newborn are vague and include lethargy/floppiness, apnoea and excessive jitteriness. These non-specific signs can also be due to sepsis. If a term baby of normal weight is sleepy, he needs help to feed directly from the breast or to be given expressed breast milk or formula from a cup, syringe or bottle. However, if the signs are more than just sleepiness, worsen or persist, the baby must be examined fully by a doctor and investigations to exclude sepsis and/or hypoglycaemia should be considered. Checking a glucose level in this situation is not an excuse for omitting a proper examination.

If a low serum glucose is confirmed, then the diagnosis is symptomatic hypoglycaemia until proven otherwise. This is an emergency and intravenous glucose must be given without delay. Blood samples for true blood glucose, insulin and ketone body levels should be collected at the same time as commencing an intravenous infusion of 10 per cent dextrose. To avoid rebound hypoglycaemia, boluses of dextrose should be avoided if possible or restricted to 'miniboluses' of 3 mL/kg of 10 per cent dextrose.

Hypoglycaemia in at-risk babies should be prevented by screening and supplementary feeding. Small for gestational age babies can require as much glucose as 12 mg/kg per minute to maintain glucose levels. Asymptomatic hypoglycaemia is managed with an increase in feeds in the first instance, with recourse to intravenous treatment only if the baby cannot tolerate feeds, symptoms develop or the hypoglycaemia persists (Rennie and Roberton 2002).

### Inborn errors of metabolism

There are many such conditions but the ones of immediate importance to the midwife are those that are screened for in the first week of life. Screening procedures have changed over time in response to other changes in neonatal care and society. Parental consent now has to be gained before the screening can be done. Midwives should check their local policies.

#### Phenylketonuria:

Screening for phenylketonuria (1 in 13 000 babies) using dried blood spots collected on to filter paper (the Guthrie test) was introduced in 1969. Milk feeds need to be established first, and midwives collect blood by heel stab on the fifth to ninth day of life, posting the cards to the laboratory. If the test is positive, an alteration in diet can successfully control the condition without complications.

#### Hypothyroidism

The same system was expanded to include a screen for congenital hypothyroidism (1 in 3000) from 1981. Audit of the programme shows that it has been extremely successful, and that it detects far more cases than were suspected clinically at a much earlier stage in life. Virtually all babies with congenital hypothyroidism now start treatment by 28 days of age and have a better IQ as a result.

#### Cystic fibrosis and other conditions

Certain areas of the UK use the dried blood spot to screen for cystic fibrosis (usually by measuring immunoreactive trypsin) and haemoglobinopathies, such as sickle cell haemoglobin or thalassaemia. Tests are also available for a host of other rare conditions including maple syrup urine disease, Duchenne muscular dystrophy, fragile X syndrome and congenital adrenal hyperplasia, but none have been implemented in the UK. Screening for neonatal neuroblastoma using vanillylmandelic acid (VMA) levels in urine is implemented only in Japan where the incidence is peculiarly high.

# Elimination

The baby should urinate within the first 12 hours of life and, if being fed appropriately, should have at least six large and forceful urinations in each 24 hours of clear, straw coloured urine. A reduced urine output or abnormalities in the characteristics of the urine or the flow associated with a baby who is lethargic, feeding poorly, has increased jaundice or vomits must be investigated, as urinary tract infections and congenital abnormalities of the genitourinary tract are common.

Meconium should be passed within the first 24 hours of life and may continue for 48 hours. Assuming the baby is being fed appropriately, the colour and consistency of the faeces will change, becoming lighter, more green–yellow and less sticky than meconium. This 'changing stool' may continue for 48 hours and then the faeces become yellow, seedy and looser in consistency, a 'normal stool'. Any disruptions to this pattern or in the characteristics of the faeces must be investigated and the cause treated. Congenital abnormalities of the GI tract, such as stenosis or atresia, malrotation, volvulus or imperforate anus, will require surgical intervention.

## Necrotizing enterocolitis

This is an acquired condition of the small and large intestine thought to be due to bowel ischaemia and superimposed infection. It is more common in preterm and small for gestational babies who required resuscitation at birth and/or have serious medical or surgical problems. The baby may present with bile-stained vomiting, abdominal distension, diarrhoea and then constipation with melaena, and non-specific signs of infection. Parenteral nutrition, nil by mouth, decompression of the GI tract and antibiotic treatment can be effective, although to prevent bowel perforation, some babies have surgical removal of the affected bowel with possible stoma formation on a temporary or permanent basis.

## Jaundice

All babies develop hyperbilirubinaemia in the first days of life owing to excess haemolysis of red blood cells, the limited ability of the liver to process (conjugate) bilirubin, the waste product from the haemolysis, and the sterility of the bowel and reabsorption of bilirubin from the bowel that has not undergone its final conversion before elimination. The reabsorbed bilirubin is recycled to the liver, where it overloads the already overloaded system. Storage of the unprocessed (unconjugated) bilirubin in fatty tissue, particularly in subcutaneous fat is common. When this occurs, a visible skin colour change is detected – jaundice. The midwife must detect and monitor the baby's condition and bilirubin level carefully.

Usually this is a physiological process that has the following characteristics:

- the appearance of jaundice after 24 hours of life;
- peak serum bilirubin levels on day 4–5 of life;
- bilirubin levels do not rise above the agreed threshold levels for the baby's gestation and days of life;
- the jaundice resolves by day 7–10 of life;
- the baby is generally well throughout.

If these criteria are met, the jaundice is considered physiological and the baby requires no treatment, but specific aspects of his care must be adjusted. He should continue to have his serum bilirubin level monitored to ensure threshold levels are not exceeded; he must have fluids and nutrition to meet his needs; his parents must be informed of his condition and its management with encouragement of their continued participation in his care; his general health must be monitored to ensure that there is no deterioration.

If *any* of the characteristics of physiological jaundice are not met, the jaundice is deemed to be due to a pathological cause. The cause must be investigated and specifically treated, but the jaundice must also be treated to prevent the bilirubin levels rising to too high a level, where there is a danger of kernicterus (bilirubin encephalopathy, i.e. yellow staining of the basal ganglia by bilirubin).

Kernicterus can be fatal, but survivors are severely handicapped by athetoid cerebral palsy, classically with accompanying sensorineural deafness, paralysis of upgaze and dental enamel dysplasia. The level of unconjugated bilirubin at which kernicterus can occur in healthy term babies is not known, but appears to lie somewhere between 425 and 600 µmol/L.

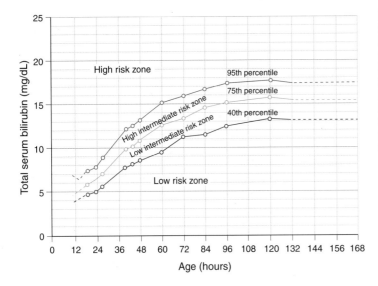

**Figure 19.2** Hour-specific bilirubin values from more than 13 000 healthy babies. Conversion of mg/dL to μmol/L requires multiplication by 17.1. (From Bhutani VK, Honson L, Sivieri MS, 1999. Predictive ability of a predischarge hour specific serum bilirubin for subsequent significant hyperbilirubinaemia in healthy term and near term newborns. Reproduced with permission from *Pediatrics*, vol. 103, pages 6–14, copyright 1999.)

A level above 425 μmol/L is reached by only 1 in 770 normal term babies.

The key to successful kernicterus prevention lies in detecting the very few healthy but usually ineffectively breast fed babies who are likely to develop a serum unconjugated bilirubin of more than 425 μmol/L, and in carefully monitoring serum bilirubin levels in preterm babies. Babies 'track' for serum bilirubin, so that a baby who is on the 50th centile at 48 hours (136 μmol/L) will not develop a dangerous level unless a new complication develops or he has an undiagnosed haemolytic disease (Figure 19.2). A baby with a similar level at 24 hours, however, is already tracking along the 95th centile and needs a repeat estimation. Such a baby is not suitable for early discharge unless the parents are willing to return to the hospital for repeat serum bilirubin measurements.

Midwives need to understand the assessment of jaundice as the early signs of bilirubin encephalopathy (lethargy, irritability, poor suck, shrill cry) can be ignored. Assessing the level of jaundice from clinical examination can be difficult, especially in Afro-Caribbean and Asian babies. Various transcutaneous bilirubinometers are under evaluation and may eventually assist in reducing the traffic of blood samples (and babies) to and from hospitals.

The treatment of jaundice involves the use of phototherapy and usually this requires readmission to hospital, although home phototherapy is used in some areas for specific babies. Phototherapy, used correctly, is a remarkably effective treatment and is capable of converting a fifth of the circulating unconjugated bilirubin to harmless photoisomers within a few hours. Very occasionally, the serum bilirubin will rise dramatically (usually with haemolytic disease) and an exchange transfusion is performed to remove and dilute the circulating bilirubin.

## Infection, skin care and hygiene

### Infection

Babies can acquire infections via the placenta, the amniotic fluid, the birth canal or from cross-infection via hands, equipment or droplet infections after birth. Because they are relatively immunodeficient, babies are particularly vulnerable to infection. The more preterm the baby, the more immunodeficient he is and the more infection he is exposed to; therefore, he is even more vulnerable than the term baby. Immunodeficiency can result in easy spread of the infection in the baby, and septicaemia and septic shock are serious potential risks.

The non-specific and specific defences mechanisms (innate and acquired immunity) are reduced in babies. Non-specific mechanisms include intact skin and mucous membranes, cilia, body secretions, phagocytic leucocytes and lymphocytes, and the process of inflammation, all of which are limited or easily overcome. Specific mechanisms, immunoglobulins (antibodies) and cellular immunity develop as the baby is exposed to pathogens. During the third trimester of pregnancy, immunoglobulin (Ig) G is transferred across the placenta to the fetus and offers specific immunity for several months after birth. IgA, the secretory immunoglobulin, is contained in breast milk, as are many other immune protective substances, and these offer further protection against GI tract infections in particular.

Prevention of infection is, therefore, vital and the midwife has responsibilities to prevent infection in the mother, the baby and in herself. Prevention of congenital infection in the baby is closely linked to prevention of infection in the mother. While these cannot be fully discussed in this chapter, the midwife is recommended to review literature on the sexually transmitted diseases, toxoplasmosis and rubella to determine the treatment and prevention strategies. Early onset Group B streptococcal infection is the most frequent cause of severe early-onset infection in newborn babies, with a 10 per cent mortality and a risk of deafness or cerebral palsy in survivors that may be as high as 40–50 per cent. Specific guidelines for the prevention and management of this infection should be consulted (Royal College of Obstetricians and Gynaecologists 2003).

Prevention of postnatal infection in the baby includes the most important factor (i.e. that of thorough and frequent washing of hand and arms with soap and water, or an alcohol rub). Other important strategies include the provision of a clean and safe environment at home and in the hospital, using aseptic and clean techniques for procedures, using individual equipment for each baby, discouraging visitors with infections, and the promotion of breast feeding.

Prevention of infection in the midwife depends on adherence to universal precautions. These should be a part of routine practice and not reserved for situations where there is a higher risk of contamination.

The midwife must be alert for signs of infection in the baby and help the mother to appreciate what these are. This is the principal reason for the daily midwifery examination of the baby. Babies may exhibit non-specific signs of infection, such as temperature instability, lethargy, poor feeding, rash, hypoglycaemia, bradycardia, apnoea and jaundice, with sudden cardiorespiratory collapse a sign of overwhelming sepsis. If an organ system is involved, there may be specific signs (e.g. in a respiratory infection, there may be increased signs of respiratory distress and increasing oxygen requirements).

If an infection is suspected, investigations must be undertaken and would include: a full physical examination; a complete blood cell count; blood, urine and faeces for culture; and possibly a lumbar puncture, chest X-ray and ultrasound scan.

Congenital infection can result in miscarriage, preterm birth, severe congenital abnormalities and low birth weight. The baby may show signs of hepatosplenomegaly, petechial rash, jaundice or seizures. A viral screen would be undertaken as well as the investigations above.

The specific management of a neonatal infection is the administration of antibiotics but other supportive care for the baby is also essential.

### Skin care and hygiene

As the baby's skin is more susceptible to damage and pathogens can enter via this route, it is appropriate to consider skin care and hygiene along with infection.

The skin is the largest organ in the body but the younger the gestation of the baby, the thinner the skin, and thus the greater the risk of damage. Ensuring the integrity of the skin is part of midwifery care and will include helping the mother to do the following:

- avoid friction against hard or rough surfaces;
- handle the baby gently;
- minimize the contact time between skin and irritants, such as urine or stool;
- use only cleansing products recommended for use on babies' skin and rinse them off with clean water;
- use only non-biological detergent and avoid fabric conditioners and starch;
- avoid the use of adhesives.

These principles also apply if the baby requires care in the NNU, although some aspects are more difficult to achieve. The secure placement of tubes and catheters usually requires adhesives, but there are products available to protect and preserve the skin's integrity (Lund et al. 1999).

Daily bathing of the baby is unnecessary; however, the mother should feel confident to bath her baby and may request that she has supervised practice of this skill by the midwife. The baby's face may require more regular cleaning and plain water is sufficient for this. The eyes do not require specific cleaning and, if there is a discharge, the cause should be investigated and treated if necessary. Cleansing the buttock area with each nappy change is recommended. Barrier creams can be used, although they can interfere with action of certain disposable nappies.

The umbilical cord clamp/tie should be removed when the stump is dry, usually by day 3 of life. The cord should be washed with plain water and kept dry to encourage the normal separation process to occur. The nappy should be tucked below the cord to avoid contamination with excreta. If the cord has not separated completely by day 7–10 of life, investigations as to the cause should be undertaken.

## Pain and neurological problems

### Pain

It is now accepted that babies feel pain, although there is still controversy concerning the experience of pain at different gestations. However, neonatal care should aim to prevent pain and to minimize the baby's experience of pain, if painful procedures have to be undertaken.

The signs of pain have behavioural, physiological and metabolic aspects:

- *behavioural signs* include irritability, crying, grimacing and withdrawal of limbs;
- *physiological signs* include tachycardia or bradycardia, apnoea or tachypnoea and hypertension;
- *metabolic signs* include hyperglycaemia, glycosuria and proteinuria.

It is recommended that a successful pain management strategy must include environmental aspects, such as reducing the noise and light, minimizing handling and providing soft clothing and bedding so that the baby feels comfortable and secure. The strategy should also plan for the necessity of undertaking painful procedures. In this case, the baby may feel consoled if he is swaddled or cuddled and given the opportunity to suck on a soother/dummy or breast feed before, during and after the procedure. Kangaroo care, where the baby is held securely against the parent's chest, either skin-to-skin or clothed, can also be consoling. Talking to the baby, rocking and massage may also help the baby recover from a painful experience.

For the actual procedure, the equipment must be that which has been recommended (e.g. automated devices must be used for heel stabs, not lancets). The operator must be fully prepared with all the equipment at hand; the technique used must follow best practice guidelines; the operator must be experienced in undertaking the technique or be supervised by someone who is; there must be a limit to unsuccessful attempts before a more experienced operator is used; and the baby must be given time to rest and recover between attempts in all but emergency situations.

For any surgical and some invasive procedures, adequate analgesia and anaesthesia must be administered, usually under the guidance of the anaesthetist. For other painful procedures, analgesia is essential. It is suggested that pharmacological treatment will be less than successful if the other aspects of pain management discussed above are not in place.

Babies may demonstrate neurological signs, similar to those associated with pain, when they have a neurological problem; therefore, it is important that differentiation is made to ensure appropriate management.

### Neurological problems

The neurological problems babies can suffer include haemorrhage owing to trauma at birth that may cause cephalhaematoma, subaponeurotic and subdural haemorrhages. Hypoxia can also result in haemorrhage into the subarachnoid space, the periventricular area, the ventricles and the cerebrum.

Having knowledge of the predisposing factors can help but the midwife should always be alert for neurological signs, such as: disruptions to tone, consciousness and cry; deviations from normal temperature, heart rate and respiratory function; poor feeding and vomiting; sudden fall in haemoglobin level; bulging anterior fontanelle and abnormal eye movements; sudden collapse; and seizure activity.

Usually, a cephalhaematoma can be diagnosed and managed by the midwife but, if the signs of neurological problems present, referral to a doctor is essential and further investigations will be undertaken including ultrasound scan, X-ray and full blood count. The involvement of a neurologist may be required. Management of neurological problems can be difficult but is aimed at reducing the risk of further damage, reducing the risk of complications and giving full supportive care to meet the baby's needs. Replacement blood transfusion may be required and anticonvulsants can control seizure activity.

The baby will require follow-up assessment by a neurologist and careful evaluation of growth and development is essential.

Neonatal abstinence syndrome (NAS) is increasingly apparent in babies causing them considerable disturbance. The age at which this occurs, and the extent to which the baby is affected depends on the substance or substances taken by the mother. The neurological signs exhibited by the baby can be varied, but a high-pitched persistent cry, inability to settle to sleep and poor sucking ability are the most common. The combination of even these signs can make caring for these babies very difficult and, if the mother's habit continues, there may be even more difficulties encouraging the parents to take appropriate responsibility for their baby's care.

The care of babies with NAS is structured around a quiet, subtly lit environment with little stimulation to try to encourage sleep. Rocking, swaddling and kangaroo care may also be helpful. Gastric feeding may have to supplement the baby's attempts to feed normally until his ability to coordinate sucking develops. Trying to keep the mother and baby together appears to be beneficial, so admission to the NNU is restricted to those babies with NAS who have other significant problems. For babies who suffer severe NAS, replacement drugs can be given and controlled weaning undertaken and/or sedation given until the baby's signs subside. If the mother is on a stable drug programme, breast feeding can be used, although this is controversial. The baby will maintain his dependence until he is weaned from the breast and, therefore, from the drug.

Involvement of social and drugs workers is important in the total care of the family.

## Sleep, rest and self-regulation

Sleep is vital for neonates and deep sleep is most beneficial for recovery and growth. A healthy term baby will sleep for most of the time in the first days of life, wakening only for feeds. He can cope with minor disruptions to this pattern, but can sleep through some procedures and even visits from relatives. The more preterm the baby, the more disruptions to sleep he will encounter and the less able he is to cope with these. In the NNU, strategies are in place to try to reduce these disruptions so that sleep opportunities are enhanced. Reducing noise, light and handling, providing soft fabric-covered 'nests' and facilitating parents to use kangaroo care are some of the strategies that have been shown to be helpful.

Term babies are neurologically better prepared to cope with the stresses of extrauterine life than are preterm babies, in that they have the ability to self-regulate. This means that they can comfort themselves when they experience stress, thus their negative

experience of stress is reduced. Self-consolation includes bracing limbs, hand to mouth and sucking, and crying.

As preterm babies have limited ability to self-regulate, they do not cope as well with stressors and can quickly demonstrate signs of negative stress, such as disruptions to vital signs, colour, tone, eye movements, cry; and frantic body movements; fixed positions; and gaze aversion. In the NNU, the strategies for encouraging sleep and reducing the experience of pain may also help reduce the stress babies can experience. In addition, specific flexed supported positioning can encourage midline orientation and hand to mouth consolation.

Preterm babies are at risk of neuromuscular developmental problems, as they have not benefited from the physiological flexion the uterus facilitates during the last weeks of pregnancy. The supported flexed positions that these babies are encouraged to adopt in the NNU can positively influence future development.

## Care of the dying baby and his family

Some babies die, and midwives must develop skills to care for the dying baby and his family. The care the baby requires is usually as for any baby until his condition deteriorates, and then the care focuses on ensuring symptomatic relief and comfort for the baby as he dies. This usually involves being held in a warm, subtly lit area preferably by his parents or by a member of staff known to the parents, if they cannot undertake this role themselves, possibly nutritive or non-nutritive sucking, and having any pain controlled by sufficient analgesia. The parents may want privacy for their final contact with their baby and this should be respected. Any other interventions are usually dependent on the condition affecting the baby. Parents may request to take their baby home or to a hospice to die, and suitable arrangements should be made for this.

The care the baby requires after death can be given by the parents, if they choose to, or by the midwife. Bathing, dressing and holding the baby after death can be an emotional experience for all concerned, but should be undertaken with dignity and respect. The parents should be given as much time as they wish to say goodbye to their baby, with mementos taken, if the parents request, such as photographs, footprints, etc.

The legal requirements are complex and vary slightly from country to country, and different religions and cultures expect certain rituals to be performed. It is, therefore, important that the midwife is aware of these possibilities, and has resources easily accessible to ensure the requirements and expectations are complied with. Discussion with the parents is essential to ensure their needs can be met.

## Social/emotional needs

Babies are social beings, and need and enjoy appropriate contact and interactions, especially with their parents. Such interaction should be encouraged from birth with opportunities given for parents to hold, watch, talk with, feed and examine their baby within the first hours of life. Thereafter, the parents are encouraged to be the main caregivers for their baby and the interaction opportunities this affords them are invaluable.

Even if the baby requires care in the NNU, parents should be able to see and touch their baby before transfer. The father usually accompanies the baby to the NNU. The mother will be encouraged to visit the baby as soon as she is able and as often as she wishes. The parents' involvement in the baby's care will depend on their wishes and how ill the baby is but, generally, involvement is encouraged from birth. However, there may be some adjustment to the usual interaction activities depending on the baby's gestation and condition.

## Educational needs of the parents

Parents have varying experience of caring for a baby. For those with no experience, there is a wealth of literature readily available in print or on the internet, and there are prenatal preparation for parenthood classes the parents can access to develop some understanding of what it means to care for a baby. However, it is not until the baby is actually born and his dependence on his parents for his every need becomes apparent that some parents realize what this new role will mean for them.

They are usually keen to learn as much as they can about caring for their baby, and will use the midwife and other resources for this purpose. Midwives should be able to offer evidence-based information and choices, thus helping parents develop/further develop decision-making skills in relation to many aspects of parenting that they can use after discharge from the midwife's care.

Specific discharge teaching pathways to guide appropriate interventions have been developed and can be used formally or informally by midwives, and especially by NNU staff, as the preterm or sick baby recovers and the parents are preparing for discharge.

The midwife must be alert to changes in policy about baby care so that the parents have up-to-date information from which to make their choices. For example, the prevention of sudden infant death guidance was updated to include the slogan 'feet to foot' (baby's feet to the bottom of the cot) to augment the 'back to sleep' message, thus midwives had to change their practice in hospital as well as the information they gave to parents. Controversies about immunization guidelines are ongoing and the midwife must update her understanding of the arguments so that she can help parents discuss the options available to them.

Staff in the NNU have longer contact with parents to help them develop their parenting skills, but the emotional turmoil these parents must work through is considerable and can negatively influence their learning. Therefore, teaching is an ongoing part of the care of parents that can be continued in the community by NNU staff once the baby is discharged.

## Conclusion

Neonatal care is a vast topic and the content of this chapter represents only an overview of some of the main aspects that should be understood by the midwife. The physical needs of the baby must be considered as well as his social/emotional needs. The parents' educational needs must also be taken into account in the overall plan of care. The midwife should work in partnership with parents in all aspects of care, supporting their efforts to parent their baby and undertaking care as required, if the parents are unable to do this. The midwife should be able to organize care of the healthy term baby and his family independently, and should participate in the care of the baby who requires special care in a NNU, along with the rest of the neonatal team.

## CASE HISTORY: HYPOGLYCAEMIA

John was born at term to a 35-year-old primigravida who went into spontaneous labour. The admission cardiotocograph was normal, but later showed reduced baseline variability and an emergency Caesarean section was carried out. John weighed 2.76 kg (third centile), and was in good condition with Apgar scores of $7^1$ and $9^5$. He was transferred to the postnatal ward. He fed hungrily at first, taking both breast and formula feeds. At the age of about 55 hours, John refused a feed and became floppy. His temperature had fallen to 35.5°C. He was placed in an incubator but took only 15 mL of formula and remained floppy. His blood glucose was low, and overnight he remained floppy, cyanosed and intermittently jittery; a 10 per cent dextrose infusion was placed and run at a rate equivalent to 6 mg/kg per minute. John then developed seizures and required increased amounts of dextrose to maintain his glucose levels. He had significant disability at follow-up, with visual impairment and developmental delay. Magnetic resonance imaging of his brain showed changes considered to be characteristic of those seen as a result of hypoglycaemic damage at term.

### What interventions might have been helpful at the age of 55 hours when his temperature and blood glucose levels were low?

Incubator care and additional heat conservation/generation measures to ensure his temperature was within normal limits in 1 hour, immediate nasogastric feeds of a measured volume of milk to meet his needs, with repeat feeds at least every 3 hours plus intravenous dextrose infusion and a limited bolus of dextrose, if the blood sugar level was very low.

## References

Baston H, Durward H. *Examination of the newborn. A practical guide.* London: Routledge, 2001.

British Association of Perinatal Medicine. *Guidelines for good practice in the management of neonatal respiratory distress syndrome.* London: BAPM, 1998. www.bapm.org/ (accessed November 2004).

British Association of Perinatal Medicine (BAPM) (2001) *Standards for hospitals providing neonatal intensive and high dependency care,* 2nd edition. London: BAPM December 2001. www.bapm.org/ (accessed November 2004).

Lang S. *Breastfeeding special care babies.* Edinburgh: Balliere Tindall, 2002.

Lund C, Kuller J, Lane A, et al. Neonatal skin care: the scientific basis for practice. *Neonatal Network* 1999; **18**:15–27.

Mifflin PC. *Saving very premature babies.* Edinburgh: Books for Midwives, 2003.

Rennie JM, Roberton NRC. *A manual of neonatal intensive care,* 4th edition. London: Arnold, 2002.

Resuscitation Council – UK. *Newborn life support: resuscitation guidelines.* 2005. www.resus.org.uk/pages/guide.htm (accessed June 2006).

Royal College of Obstetricians and Gynaecologists. *Prevention of early onset neonatal Group B streptococcal disease* (36). November 2003. www.rcog.org.uk/guidelines.asp?PageID= 106&GuidelineID=56 (accessed November 2004).

## Annotated bibliography

Boxwell G (ed.). *Neonatal intensive care nursing.* London: Routledge, 2000.

An excellent nursing text contributed to by neonatal nurses and experts from across the UK that gives detailed information about many of the conditions that affect babies, the investigations and the medical and nursing management.

Rennie JM (ed.). *Robertson's textbook of neonatology,* 4th edition. London: Churchill Livingstone, 2004.

An updated version of a very comprehensive and well-known textbook on all aspects of neonatology that is excellent for reference.

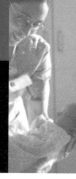

# Law and ethics relating to midwifery practice

## OVERVIEW

The nature of contemporary midwifery practice is characterized by increasing uncertainties about what is right and wrong. Midwives can, therefore, find themselves faced with dilemmas and consequently have to make decisions in situations where there may be an absence of any robust clinical evidence. The ongoing advances and developments in reproductive health and fetal medicine, where risks to the woman and fetus are considerable, raise further legal and ethical issues for the practising midwife. Not only may there be the potential for misjudgement or mismanagement by the attending doctors and midwives, but also the potential for a conflict of interest to develop between the various health care professionals involved, and the woman. Furthermore, over the last 20 years, there have been a number of government reforms that have resulted in changes in health care provision. The publishing of *The patient's charter* [Department of Health (DoH) 1991] and *Your guide to the NHS* (DoH 2001) have not only helped to increase the public's awareness of the choices available to them, but have also raised their expectations regarding involvement in making care decisions. This final chapter aims to address some of the pertinent legal and ethical issues relating to the practising midwife in the twenty-first century.

## Legal issues

### Responsibility, sphere of practice and delegation

The Nursing and Midwifery Order 2001 (SI 2002, No. 253) is the statutory legislation that currently governs the midwifery profession and endorsed the formation of the governing body: the Nursing and Midwifery Council (NMC). The Activities of a Midwife: Article 4 of the EU Second Midwifery Directive (80/155/EEC) are clearly defined in the *Midwives rules and standards* (NMC 2004a), and thus provides each midwife with the legal framework in which to practise as an accountable practitioner within the context of normal midwifery for which she has been duly trained

and has the appropriate expertise. Rule 6 (NMC 2004a) further clarifies the midwife's responsibility and sphere of practice in that she should refer to other appropriately qualified health professionals whenever any deviation occurs that is outside her current sphere of practice.

A midwife who does not practise according to these rules and standards could find herself before the NMC Professional Conduct Committee with a possible suspension from practice and/or removal from the professional register. It is also important to note that a midwife cannot delegate her midwifery responsibilities to anyone other than a practising midwife or registered medical practitioner. However, when supervising student midwives, the midwife remains professionally accountable for what the student does, including the consequences of their actions and omissions.

## Postregistration education and practice (PREP)

In order for all nurses, midwives and specialist community public health nurses to retain their name on the professional register, they have to fulfil the requirements of postregistration education and practice (NMC 2006), which are as follows:

- undertake a minimum of 35 hours study relevant to their practice every 3 years;
- maintain a personal professional profile of their learning activity;
- complete a notification of intention to practise form;
- have practised for 450 hours minimum over 3 years;
- undertake a return to practice programme, if they have been out of practice for 3 years or more.

From a legal perspective, it is each midwife's responsibility to ensure she remains professionally up to date with developments in practice, is clinically competent to fulfil her role and that her practice is evidence-based. Legally, it is no defence for the midwife to disregard developments in practice and continue to use out-of-date protocols. All employers are required to provide regular programmes of education and training, either within the workplace or alternative educational institutions, and support midwives in meeting their professional development needs. The role of the Supervisor of Midwives can also assist in this respect during the annual supervisory visit undertaken with each midwife. Furthermore, in order to reduce future litigation claims, in some universities and maternity units, there has been much development in the area of interprofessional learning and working, where midwives, doctors and other support staff, practise their management of maternity emergencies, such as shoulder dystocia, massive obstetric haemorrhage, eclampsia, etc. in simulated drills, this being a recommendation from the Confidential Enquiries into Maternal Deaths report (Lewis and Drife 2004).

## Record keeping

Records relating to the care of women and babies are a fundamental aspect of the midwifery and obstetric practice to aid communication between the midwife, the woman and others who are providing care and should be made contemporaneously (Rule 9; NMC 2004a, 2005). Good midwifery practice is based on careful assessment of the clinical situation, followed by instigation of an appropriate management plan: both of which the midwife should clearly document in the clinical records. Such records should be as clear, concise and accurate as possible, and reflect the advice given to the woman, the ensuing discussions and consequently the care/procedures that were either undertaken/declined. Every page in the woman's records should have her name clearly stated with each entry being dated, timed and signed (including the name printed legibly below) by the midwife. Abbreviations should be avoided unless universally recognized. All entries should be made in dark ink so that photocopying is facilitated should the records need to be scrutinized by experts, where the care and management provided is legally questioned.

All records relating the care of the woman and baby must be kept for 25 years as defined by the Congenital Disabilities (Civil Liabilities) Act 1976. This also includes work diaries, if clinical information is contained in them. The retention of other documents, such as duty rotas, may depend on local policy but, where national guidelines are available, these should be followed. Claims can arise up to 25–30 years after the baby's birth and, if the documentation is lost, it is difficult for the case to be successfully defended.

## Standards, guidelines and protocols

Although the fear of litigation appears to be a major factor of modern midwifery and obstetric practice, the development of risk management and clinical governance strategies have made an improvement to clinical practice with the establishment of common standards. Through the National Institute for Health and Clinical Excellence (NICE), there has been the introduction of national guidelines that standardize certain aspects of maternity care provision. It is important that all staff working in the maternity services are familiar with these guidelines, including all local protocols. Deviation from guidelines or protocols does not necessarily constitute a breach of duty of care to the woman. However, the reasons for deviating from any protocol should be clearly stated within the clinical records. It is important that these protocols are dated and regularly updated according to best possible evidence. Such documents should always be retained whenever they have been updated, in case they need to be used years later in defence of practice alongside the Bolam Standard.

## Consent

Within law, informed consent is taken to mean the reasonable person standard or the Bolam Standard. This means that a woman should be given as much information as any reasonable person could be expected to understand in order to make a decision about her care/treatment. This implies that the woman is deemed competent to make such a decision, that is, she is legally an adult (18 years or over) or is not mentally incapacitated in any way. In the case of minors, if they can demonstrate they understand the implications of the proposed care/treatment, they are considered Gillick competent to make their own decisions. As midwives are increasingly becoming involved with caring for pregnant teenagers, it is also advisable that the child's parents or other accompanying adults are kept informed of any clinical decisions that are made.

The purpose of any procedure/treatment, including any significant or potential complication, should also be discussed with the woman by the midwife or doctor. Ideally, the health professional who is going to perform the procedure should be the one to obtain the woman's consent, otherwise details of the discussion and decision made should be clearly documented in the woman's records for colleagues to see that consent had been duly obtained or refused.

Wherever possible, the woman should be given time to contemplate her decision to either consent or decline the proposed procedure/treatment, and should never be forced to comply under duress. Should a midwife undertake a procedure without first obtaining consent from a woman, that midwife would be liable for trespass to the person.

Although the law protects the rights of the woman, the fetus has no rights until it is born. Thus, a mentally competent pregnant woman cannot be legally forced to have a Caesarean section for a risk to the fetus. Should a woman refuse an intervention that may endanger the life of the fetus, while accepting the law, it is an uncomfortable moral and ethical dilemma for any midwife or obstetrician to have to sit back and let a fetus die. In such situations, cases may be referred to court for an emergency application to authorize the intervention to take place legally.

## Cardiotocography

While the majority of pregnancies may be considered to be of low risk, it is important that the midwife recognizes when a complication develops during labour that consequently warrants continuous electronic fetal monitoring. As most obstetric claims often revolve around the interpretation of intrapartum cardiotocography (CTG) tracings, midwives and obstetricians, therefore, have a professional responsibility for their continued personal development in this area according to the NICE guidelines (2001) concerning the use of electronic fetal monitoring.

When a trace is commenced, it is good practice to include the woman's identification details/label, and ensure that the date and time the recording takes place corresponds to what is actually printed on the CTG trace. The maternal pulse and any other incidents occurring during the tracing (e.g. the woman moving position/vomiting), which may affect the recording of the fetal heart, are also written on the trace. Upon completion, the trace should be securely attached in the woman's clinical records. If the recordings of either the fetal heart rate pattern or the tocography tracing are inadequate, every effort should be made to rectify this (e.g. by repositioning the woman or using a fetal scalp electrode). Reliance on intermittent auscultation, using a Pinard's stethoscope or sonicaid, is preferable to an inadequate CTG recording. Such details should be clearly written in the clinical records. The timing of any intervention, and whether the timing was appropriate, often becomes an important medicolegal issue. For example, if a decision is taken to perform an emergency Caesarean section, the conventional standard is that the baby should have been delivered within 30 minutes of the decision being taken. However, this 30-minute time interval is not evidence based and cannot always be attained.

## Claims in midwifery and obstetric practice

Some mistakes in clinical practice are obvious, such as the obstetrician leaving a swab inside the abdomen at Caesarean section. However, most medicolegal cases are much more contentious. The most significant claims arise from brain damage and cerebral palsy. These are based on the allegation that there was negligence on the part of the health professionals involved in the management, resulting in fetal asphyxia and consequently neurological damage to the baby.

As with all medicolegal cases, for the claimant to be successful, the following need to be established.

- There was a breach of duty of care to the woman. This means that the attending staff owed the woman a duty of care and that the standard of care afforded to her was below a standard that she could reasonably have expected.
- The injury sustained was caused by the substandard care.

However, in many cases where a child suffers brain damage and develops cerebral palsy, while it may be accepted that the care afforded was substandard, it is more difficult to prove causation (i.e. whether the substandard care actually resulted in the disability). The situation is complicated by the knowledge that only 10–15 per cent of infants born with significant brain damage acquire their disability as a result of the events of labour and birth. The problem that all health professionals working in the maternity services face is that parents who give birth to a child with a neuro-developmental handicap will seek to ascribe the damage to issues of management during the intrapartum period. When allegations are made, experts assess the case on behalf of both the claimant (either and/or both the woman and baby) and the defendant (usually the hospital Trust). Consideration of issues of causation is often far from straightforward and it is usual that many different medicolegal expert opinions are obtained, from neonatologists, paediatric neurologists and obstetricians, before finally reaching a conclusion.

## Ethical issues

Throughout history, there has always been the potential for moral dilemma and ethical debate concerning issues relating to fertility, pregnancy and childbirth. In recent years, as technology and expectations advance, and with recognition of the individual's right to exercise their own autonomy over their own health and body, issues are crystallized, and cast more sharply into public and professional arenas. However, it must not be forgotten that such discussions and decisions impact deeply and personally on the lives of those involved.

There are many excellent texts available that are devoted to general ethics and also specifically to applied ethics in midwifery and health care (Rambold 1992, Jones 2000, etc.; please see additional reading section

at the end of this chapter). Therefore, this section will be confined to brief clarification of some of the theories and principles, and exploration of fictitious cases, where these points can be applied.

It must be stressed that there can be no single 'right' answer to any ethical debate. Each individual parent and professional is entitled to their own moral views. However, each professional is charged with the responsibility to reflect and consider her/his own moral code; to recognize the position of influence and power that they have as a professional; and to refrain from allowing their own moral views to colour or affect, in any way, the care of those who entrust their health and well-being to them.

## Terminology

Ethics and morals are frequently used and interchanged synonymously with each other. While this is only of real concern to the purists, there are differences between them. For general accuracy, ethics relates to the wider picture, the larger impact, and morality relates to the individual.

The Code of Professional Conduct: standards for conduct, performance and ethics (NMC 2004b) is seen as an ethical *and* a professional code for registered nurses, midwives and health visitors; and as a professional body, midwives also have a separate code of ethics, the *International code of ethics for midwives* (International Confederation of Midwives 1993). These and other documents identify the expected behaviour and practice of all the individuals registered and working in these professions. Ethical working and business practices also include promoting individual's rights, fair trade and treatment, respect towards and no abuse of individuals, such as institutional racism or bullying, etc.

Morality relates more closely to the individual and their own personal code of thoughts and behaviour. The moral codes of like individuals are reflective of the ethical code that they professionally ascribe to, but their individual morality is generally more specific. Moral codes are shaped in early life, being influenced by family, school and social life, and by life events, both personally experienced, and from those of friends, in books or the media.

Individual morality is the blueprint from which each person makes life choices. On a day-to-day basis, this may be from telling children not to lie, then promoting the use of deception to gain a child's compliance (i.e. be good for Father Christmas to visit with presents) to valuing honesty yet knowingly taking excess change from mistaken cash transactions. In relation to major life events, the individual's moral code relates to personal views about abortion and euthanasia, for example.

It is from the individual's own moral code that initial assessments of the rightness or wrongness of other's behaviour and actions are made. However, as professional midwives, we must exercise caution and restraint. For, just as others seldom have the right to interfere in how we run our lives, so we have to consider what right we have to dictate to or judge those we serve.

## Philosophical ethical theory

Detailed understanding of philosophical ethical theory is not essential to good midwifery practice. However, basic knowledge in this area assists in the recognition and appreciation of possible motivations for the actions or/and omissions of others, and the impact of these on the whole or wider picture. This section gives a brief overview, so please refer to other ethics-related texts for greater insight.

If one imagines a philosophical continuum: at one end are the outcome-based theories, such as utilitarianism, consequentialism and teleology, and at the opposite end sits the duty-based theory of deontology. Other theories lie between.

Outcome-based theories, such as *utilitarianism*, maintain that moral and ethical judgements of right and wrong are based entirely on the *effect produced* by the action or inaction. An action is considered right or wrong according to its consequences. For example, a war may be considered just and right if it results in the overthrow of a tyrannical regime and the freedom of an oppressed people. But equally, the same war may be wrong and unjust if one tyrant is replaced by another, and the people continue to live a life of oppression, starvation, etc., and with loss of considerable numbers of lives. In midwifery, maintaining a correct and effective ratio of appropriately qualified staff to women, within the confines of a reducing financial and resource budget, against a backdrop of raising expectations of outcome, is an ethical as well as a managerial issue.

*Deontology*, while recognizing that consequences can have serious implications, cannot and does not consider them. The theory relates to the *duties* each individual has, and how they discharge those duties to others, and not on the consequences of them. The rightness of an action or inaction is determined on the features, and the intrinsic qualities of that action or inaction (for some, this also includes the motivation behind the action or inaction). Therefore, some things are right and obligatory as they uphold a duty; such as supporting autonomous decisions, as this supports the duty to respect others as an end in themselves, and not the means to another's end. Other things are wrong and indefensible, as they would breach a duty; such as lying to or deceiving an individual about the prognosis of a condition, as this robs them of acting autonomously with the remainder of their life, and fails to respect them as an autonomous moral subject. In the purest considerations of the theory, it is for the individuals themselves to determine which duty they feel is their absolute and inviolate (or categorical imperative) one, and the order of how the remaining are then ranked.

Along the length of the continuum, other theories sit between utilitarianism and deontology. These include: *particularism*, a flexible approach combining common sense and morality; *situationalism*, where each situation is considered on its own merits and influencing characteristics; and *response ethics*, which considers the influencing factors in a given situation in actual practice that require an 'immediate' response. Each of these theories combines elements of the two major theories and applies them to fit the given position; however, whilst they appear flexible, some argue that they do not seem to have clear consistency or focus. Another theory is that of ethical egoism.

*Ethical egoism* maintains that each person ought to act to serve her/his own self-interests. However, this self-interest may often relate to another and to promoting what is best for them (i.e. a parent to their child/children) or an activist to their cause. The ethical egoist acts in a manner to maximize the long-term aim or well-being for that which is important to them; and what is right and just is the action or inaction that achieves this. Such reasoning does not exclude actions that may be considered either morally good or bad – stealing, being honest, helping others, etc. But these actions are acceptable or not acceptable, to the ethical egoist, only because they produce the required outcome for them or their specific cause, not because they are laudable or good or bad things in themselves: if you help others, they will help you; if you do not steal from them, then they will not steal from you, and so on.

It must be recognized that the descriptions of the various theories here are extremely brief and provide an overview only. Further reading of these is strongly recommended.

## Ethical principles

The generally accepted four cardinal principles in bioethical discussion are autonomy, non-maleficence, beneficence and justice. However, the principles of confidentiality, truth telling, informed choice and consent also require great consideration, as they are very pertinent in any health care arena. These and other principles pertaining to ethical professional midwifery practice and the record keeping of the same, can be found in many texts, and additional reading is recommended to supplement the information given here.

*Autonomy* relates to the person's ability to make or to exercise self-determining choices. Frequently included in this concept is the notion of 'respect for persons', that is, treating or respecting persons as dignified, moral subjects worthy of respect in their own right. It is generally accepted that, provided an autonomous person's actions do not impinge on the autonomous actions of others, that person should have the freedom to perform whatever action he or she wishes, regardless of any specific possible consequences to themselves. Autonomy, however, is not simply doing because one can. It also includes individuals taking responsibility for their own self-determined choices. It could be argued that many people exercise self-determination, but fewer operate with total autonomy.

In terms of appropriate ethical care, autonomy relates to evidence of the care and entries in records that clearly and intrinsically show respect for the individual client. Evidence that information is given, care is relevant and responsive to the individual's needs, and informed consent is always obtained prior to procedures further identifies a respect for the personhood and autonomy of the individual client.

*Non-maleficence* is the moral obligation each person in society owes to the others, of not deliberately inflicting evil or harm upon them. It does not require the 'giver' to do anything, rather it requires each of us *not* to harm. Harm, however, is not just an obvious

injury, but can also be seen as a failure to act when one has or had a reasonable duty to do so. Thus, it is not only incorrectly, unjustifiably or carelessly acting that can result in injury or harm, but also failing to act and/or excessive interventions.

Within the arena of ethical professional care, clear evidence of breaching the principle of non-maleficence must be accompanied with justifications and counter actions as necessary. Painful treatment or surgery to remove or reduce suffering, or save a life, are examples of a possible justification for breaching the principle of non-maleficence, as is a vaccination that produces a localized painful reaction but provides the individual with immunity to a specific disease.

The principle of *beneficence* is frequently closely linked to the principle of non-maleficence, and is often seen as a justification for it being breached. Relating to actively promoting or doing good, beneficence as a principle is often seen as fundamental to the health care professional's interactions with clients. When health care professionals act in the benefit of others, it is believed that a positive contribution is made, which promotes the client's health and well-being. Extreme care must be exercised, however, to ensure that, in acting to promote the client's good, health care professionals do not act paternalistically in what they consider to be in the best interests of the individual without discussing this with them, and thus robbing the person of self-determined autonomous and informed choice. Evidence of appropriate beneficent care and treatment should be apparent in all health care interactions.

The principle of *justice* is the most nebulous of the four, and is still the subject of disagreements amongst scholars. For the basis of this application, it relates to two linked concepts: justice as fairness, and justice as equal distribution of benefits and burdens. Much debate still continues about the relative justice of health care provision and access (e.g., specific screening tests and water birth), and equal provision and access to equitable care across the country.

In terms of demonstrating appropriate care, each should ensure that, as health care professionals, we are seen to act justly towards all clients, and that each person has what is due or owed to them. Scrutiny of records should be able to confirm that this principle is upheld and, where there is doubt, explanation must be given. Situations such as disproportionately long waits for care or treatment, for example, should be explained.

Elements of ethical professional practice require each midwife to demonstrate respect for their clients in relation to these principles, and to honour their obligations relating to the principles of *confidentiality*, *truth-telling* and promoting *informed choice* in order to obtain valid *consent*.

Understanding the importance of protecting *confidential* information is not a new concept in health care arenas. Legal and professional guidance is available, and all health care professionals should be well aware of how to protect confidential information and avoid possible confidentiality breaches. Protecting confidentiality is part of the unique relationship any health care professional has with her/his client, and is intrinsic to the relationship of fidelity. Clients invariably share, and entrust private and personal information, thoughts and feelings with their carers, and this is especially true of women and their midwives. The midwife must completely respect the spirit in which the information is entrusted to her, and breach that trust only after careful thought and consideration, and in accordance with professional guidelines available to her.

All too often, professionals do breach confidentiality in what may be classed as 'soft settings' and extra vigilance is required to ensure this possibility does not continue to occur. Where telephones are fitted with silence or discrete settings, these must be used when leaving a caller waiting for any reason and for any length of time. Staff should not discuss their day, clients or stresses together while in public corridors, lifts and rest areas. Staff must remember that curtains, open windows and doors, and some walls are not sound proofed, and personal discussions always seem more interesting when overheard.

Each of us must be vigilant to protect the confidential information others entrust to us. What is remarkable enough to be interesting and to be discussed, is frequently also that which is unique enough to be traceable back to the source. This is upsetting for those who feel that their trust as well as private information has been betrayed, and it could also give rise to professional misconduct proceedings.

*Truth-telling* is probably the one principle to which everyone would say that they totally subscribe; however, in practice, it is the one most likely to be subjugated. Humans value truthfulness, but find the truth hard to handle. Frequently people say that they want to be told the truth, but actually want to hear only the part of it with which they feel comfortable. Thus, truth-telling can be a moral minefield.

In the first instance, the professional must be in complete possession and knowledge of all the facts, and must have a deep understanding of how these impact on the situation. Second, communication of what is known is also fraught with potential problems. The manner and order in which the facts are imparted influences how they are perceived. In addition, all persons do and have to alter how and what they say depending on the recipients, the time frame and urgency, and other elements of the situation. The midwife must use all her skills in communication, and her knowledge of midwifery and human nature so that she may appropriately inform her clients of the facts material to them in order to promote and protect client autonomy.

Professionals should accept, however, that they do not know everything, and may not be able to be exact about outcomes, effects, degrees of influence, etc., and, in these cases, honesty is paramount. White lies, prevarications and omissions all have the potential to erode client autonomy, as well as professional/client relationships, and careful consideration and justification must always be applied if any of these are to be used. The maxim must be 'How would I feel if this were done to me?'

The principles of non-maleficence and beneficence are frequently used to justify breaching the principle of truth-telling, in that it is said to be in the client's best interests not to know x, or to be told only part of y. This may well be justified in some situations, but it is for each practitioner to consider carefully the validity of any principle trade-off, and how this rests with their own moral code and professional practice. Failure to inform fully, to omit or to deceive all have a direct impact on *informed choice and valid consenting*.

In order to exercise informed choice and to give or withhold a valid consent, the individual must know and understand that which has material importance to them. To choose without knowledge is to be robbed of autonomy, but to have knowledge is also to have to accept the potential of unwanted outcomes. Midwives must be aware, however, that some women are not used to making such far-reaching choices, and may never have had to exercise their autonomy in this way before, or ever had to consider life and death outcomes for someone important to them.

Much is published on the legal and professional considerations of consent, and the Department of Health has also produced information and guidance on informed consent, including a 12-point good practice and legal guide for practitioners (www.dh.gov.uk). Failure to gain informed consent prior to any treatment or care may leave the practitioner liable both legally and professionally, as previously considered in this chapter. However, apart from the legal and professional considerations of consent, there is also an ethical dimension to it. Several definitions of 'ethical' consent exist and most refer to the following elements as requirements intrinsic to the concept of an ethically acceptable informed consent.

The process is voluntary and uncoerced. There is sufficient information at a level the individual can comprehend, with adequate time for deliberation and any further clarification as necessary. Good accounts of the proposed action/s are given, with all possible side effect and perceived benefits, plus any other possible and practicable alternative, and what is likely to happen if no action is taken. The professional may consider including a recommendation for the client, which is balanced, informative and justified (although great care must be exercised if this line of action is considered). Finally, there is a recognition that the individual is at liberty, with no fear of criticism, to accept or reject the proposed course of action/s that may affect her/him.

It could be argued that there may be urgent situations where there is not sufficient time for the above process to occur. This may be true. However, pregnancy and labour are usually long enough for midwives to be able to discuss with and inform women fully of a great many things, so that final clarification and informed consent gaining may still be possible within a tight time frame.

## Moral and ethical application to fictitious cases

Consider the following cases and discuss them with colleagues. Try to apply the theories and principles in a balanced way, with justifications for your thought processes.

There is no single right answer for any of these dilemmas but the midwife must be able to balance and justify her actions or inactions for each, applying the triangular approach of ethical, professional and legal duties and responsibilities in order to serve all these masters, and stay true to her own moral code and the trust women place in her as a midwife.

## DISCUSSION CASES – DOES THE FETUS HAVE ANY RIGHTS?

The legal status of the fetus is clear. Ethically, the situation is not so straightforward. Some individuals may feel that the right to life of the fetus supersedes that of the mother's right to choose. Consider the following two scenarios, then compare your reasoning for both.

Woman A is expecting her second child. Her first child, a boy, was born at term with good Apgar scores, a good birth weight, was breast-fed and is now 2 years old. She has smoked 20 or more cigarettes a day for the past 4 years. She is now 34 weeks pregnant; there is severe intrauterine growth restriction and the predicted birth weight of the baby at term of below the fifth centile. The mother is well, there is no clear cause for the growth restriction, but her smoking is considered to be a serious influencing factor. Should Woman A be 'persuaded' to stop smoking and, if so, how? What are the justifications for this, any other or no action?

Woman B is in labour at term with her first baby. Her pregnancy and labour to this point have both progressed smoothly and with no identified problems. The fetal head is almost crowning, but now acute and severe fetal distress is apparent with cord entanglement the suspected cause. It is believed that the use of an episiotomy would effect an immediate and safe delivery of the fetus, resulting in no lasting harm to either the mother or her baby. Woman B refuses an episiotomy. There is no indication that she is not autonomous or informed. Severe fetal compromise or death is imminent. Consider if the midwife should perform an episiotomy in the presence of an informed refusal? Justify your response.

Consider any differences found between the two cases and explore the possible reasons for them.

What are your thoughts on the sanctity of the life of the fetus? Consider if this is affected if there is a serious reduction in the quality of the life of the baby and intact long-term survival is not possible. Should the mother's right to choose what is best for herself and her baby, as she sees it, be supported by the midwife when the midwife feels the woman's actions are wrong? What are the midwife's responsibilities to protect the woman's autonomy and to be her advocate?

## DISCUSSION CASES – MATERNAL RIGHT TO CHOOSE?

There is much written on the value of choice for woman in childbirth, the potential for good and positive outcomes for low-risk women choosing a home confinement and the potential for the medicalization of childbirth for low-risk women delivering in hospitals.

Consider the following scenarios and then compare your reasoning for each.

Woman C lives in a rural area and is expecting her seventh baby. This is a planned pregnancy, as were all her previous ones. All previous labours and deliveries have been uneventful. The first four were planned for and born in hospital. The last two were planned for hospital confinements but were both unattended home births. In each, Woman C did not realize how advanced the labour had been, she called for appropriate assistance when she did realize, but delivered just as the services arrived. She requests a home confinement for this birth. Her community midwife has never undertaken a home confinement and the GP practice has withdrawn support for them. Her GP considers home confinement to be potentially very dangerous, and explains his views and reasoning to Woman C when she tries to pursue one.

Consider this scenario. What could happen and why? Use ethical, professional and legal reasoning and justifications in your considerations.

Woman D is expecting her seventh child. This is a planned pregnancy, as were all her previous ones. All previous labours and deliveries have been uneventful, none were born in hospital. The first four were planned and attended home births. The last two were also planned home confinements, but were unattended births as Woman D did not realize how advanced her labour was and called for appropriate assistance when she did realize, but delivered just as the services arrived. She requests a home confinement for this birth. The community midwife has never undertaken a home confinement and the GP practice has withdrawn support for them. Woman D is a traveller and is not registered with a GP, but when she went to register was told by a GP that he considers home confinement to be potentially very dangerous, and especially so in her case and refused to take on her care.

Consider this scenario. What could happen and why? Use ethical, professional and legal reasoning and justifications in your considerations.

Consider any differences found between the two cases and explore the possible reasons for them.

Consider also the cost of home confinement in terms of midwifery, paramedic, medical and aligned professional support. What would happen if 50 per cent of women booking today requested a home confinement? Are the choices currently offered ethically based?

## References

Department of Health. *Your guide to the NHS*. London: HMSO, 2001.

Department of Health. *The patient's charter*. London: HMSO, 1991.

Department of Health. *12 Key points on consent: the law in England*. London, HMSO, 2001. *www.dh.gov.uk*

European Union. *Second midwifery directive (80/155/EEC)*. Brussels: European Union, 1980.

International Confederation of Midwives. *International code of ethics for midwives*. London: ICM, 1993.

Jones SR. *Ethics in midwifery*, 2nd edition. Edinburgh: Mosby, 2000.

Lewis G, Drife J (eds). *Confidential Enquiry into Maternal and Child Health; why mothers die 2000–2002*. Sixth report of the confidential enquiry into maternal deaths in the United Kingdom. London: RCOG Press, 2004.

National Institute for Health and Clinical Excellence. *The use of electronic fetal monitoring: the use and interpretation of cardiotocography in intrapartum fetal surveillance*, London: NICE, 2001.

Nursing and Midwifery Council. *Code of Professional Conduct: standards for conduct, performance and ethics*, London: NMC, 2004b.

Nursing and Midwifery Council. *Midwives' rules and standards*, London: NMC, 2004a.

Nursing and Midwifery Council. *Guidelines for records and record keeping*, London: NMC, 2005.

Nursing and Midwifery Council. *The PREP Handbook*, London: NMC, 2006.

*Nursing and Midwifery Order 2001* (SI 2002 No 253).

Rambold G. *Ethics in nursing and midwifery practice*. London: Southbank, 1992.

## Key additional reading

Bartter K (ed.). *Ethical issues in advanced nurse practice.* London: Elsevier Science, 2002.

Dimond B. *Legal aspects of midwifery,* 3rd edition. Edinburgh: Books for Midwives, 2006.

Frith L, Draper H. *Ethics and midwifery: issues in contemporary practice,* 2nd edition. Edinburgh: Books for Midwives, 2004.

Jones SR, Jenkins R. *The law and the midwife,* 2nd edition. Oxford: Blackwell Publishing, 2004.

Raynor MD, Marshall JE, Sullivan A. *Decision making in midwifery practice.* Edinburgh: Churchill Livingstone, 2006.

Singleton J, McLaren S. *Ethical foundations of health care.* London: Mosby, 1995.

Thompson I, Melia K, Boyd K. *Nursing ethics.* Edingburgh: Churchill Livingstone, 2000.

# Levels of evidence

Professional midwifery practice is in a state of constant change. Today, more than ever, clients demand a high standard of professional care and practice from midwives, and all health care professionals. As practitioners we have an obligation to ensure that our practice is based on sound knowledge and understanding, and on good research evidence where this exists.

In all areas of health care practice, the applicable and relevant research evidence base available is not without gaps. It is also not a static process. New research is becoming available all the time. Each midwife must continue to keep up to date with changes, and read and be critical of what is written. Thus, lifelong learning is not simply a catchy phrase to use at reviews or interviews, but must be a way of life.

Practice can not be supported by custom, tradition or best guess work; but must be well considered, evidence based and able to be justified and defended. But how are health care professionals to determine the significance of the evidence used to support one practice over another? Indeed, all research – even excellent pieces – should not be automatically transferred directly into the practice setting, but must be examined closely for its applicability to that setting. There is a confusing array of terminology used in this area, and the following boxes offer some guidance though this.

The first box shows some common phrases from the clinical field and gives accompanying clarifications of these.

## Common phrases from the clinical field

### Clinical guidelines
These give guidance on the accepted practice in clinical situations. All practitioners must be well versed with the ones in force where they work. The guidelines should be clear, unambiguous, reliable, clinically applicable, effective and flexible enough to be able to respond to the individual needs of women. They should also be frequently revised and evidence based and, if possible, this should be research evidence. These may also be known as protocols or procedures. The National Institute for Clinical Excellence (NICE) guidelines are one example of guidelines produced by a respected body that should be used to support local clinical guidelines.

### Evidence-based practice
This is the conscious, conscientious, explicit and judicious use of current best evidence by the practitioner, for all care and intervention decisions and practices.

### Best research evidence
This is significant and clinically relevant research. It may originate from a midwifery, paediatric, medical, pharmacological or other aligned professional source, but is especially appropriate if it is professional or client-centred clinical research. It is peer reviewed and published in a respected professional journal, showing sufficient detail on the process and initial findings for the reader to draw their own, as well as the published considerations on the findings and results.

### Clinical expert
This is an individual who has usually undertaken additional study to Masters' level, but remains in clinical practice. This individual demonstrates excellent clinical skills and judgement; has significant past practice experiences and practice intuition; is able to make a rapid identification of each individual client's health status, present condition and expected health outcomes; has excellent working knowledge of the impact of any physical, psychological and pharmacological input; is

able, with excellent communication skills, to interact with and involve other appropriate professionals and the client in clinical discussions and decisions; is able to synthesize up-to-date research and best-practice guidelines, and to assimilate these into the current situation; and is confident in their own professional judgement.

The second box gives an adapted classification of the standard evidence tables used by the Scottish Intercollegiate Guidelines Network (SIGN) as shown in *Obstetrics by ten teachers* (Baker 2004). Further information on SIGN can be found in the book edited by Craig and Smyth (2002) entitled *The evidence-based practice manual for nurses*.

### Classification of evidence levels

Ia Evidence obtained from meta-analysis of randomized controlled trails

Ib Evidence obtained from at least one randomized controlled trail

II Evidence obtained from at least one well-designed controlled study without randomization, or from at least one other type of well-designed quasi-experimental study

III Evidence obtained from well-designed, non-experimental, descriptive studies, such as comparative studies, correlation studies and case studies

IV Evidence obtained from expert committee reports or opinions and/or clinical experience of respected authorities.

This classification of evidence levels is valuable as a grading method of the reliability of evidence, which can then be applied to research studies used to support given practices or changes of practice. In itself, this is a good basis. The midwife must, however, also consider how this evidence might be applied. The third box identifies further criteria that the midwife might use to help in these considerations.

### Further criteria

- Is the study large enough, or focus specific enough to be applicable to my practice area?
- Is the quality of the study good enough for me to use the results?
- Are the research participants or the subject matter data reflective of my clients or my practice?
- Can the evidence be applied to and in my practice context?
- Reflective and critical practice is the key to evidence-based professional health care

These tables identify levels of evidence and measures of reliability, but they can only be used as guides. All midwives must have knowledge and understanding of the research process, and be able to use this knowledge to analyse research studies critically as well as other evidence used to advocate one practice over another.

## References

Baker PN (ed.). *Obstetrics by ten teachers*. London: Hodder Arnold, 2006.

Craig, J, Smyth R. (2002) *The evidence-based practice manual for nurses*. Edinburgh: Churchill Livingstone, 2002.

# Index